Computers and Medicine

Helmuth F. Orthner, Series Editor

Springer
New York
Berlin
Heidelberg
Barcelona
Budapest
Hong Kong
London
Milan
Paris
Santa Clara
Singapore
Tokyo

Computers and Medicine

Charles P. Friedman
Jeremy C. Wyatt

Evaluation Methods in Medical Informatics

Foreword by Edward H. Shortliffe

With 40 Illustrations

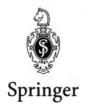

Springer

Charles P. Friedman, Ph.D.
Formerly Assistant Dean for Medical
   Education and Informatics, University of
   North Carolina
Professor and Director
Center for Biomedical Informatics
University of Pittsburgh
8074 Forbes Tower
Pittsburgh, PA 15213, USA

Jeremy C. Wyatt, M.B., B.S., D.M., M.R.C.P.
Consultant, Medical Informatics
Imperial Cancer Research Fund
P.O. Box 123
Lincoln's Inn Fields
London WC2A 3PX, UK

Contributors:
Bonnie Kaplan, Ph.D.
Associate Professor, Computer Science/
   Information Systems
Director, Medical Information Systems Program
School of Business
Quinnipiac College
Hamden, CT 06518, USA

Allen C. Smith, III, Ph.D.
Assistant Professor and Associate Director
Office of Educational Development
CB 7530–322 MacNider Building
University of North Carolina School of
   Medicine
Chapel Hill, NC 27599, USA

Series Editor:
Helmuth F. Orthner, Ph.D.
Professor of Medical Informatics
University of Utah Health Sciences Center
Salt Lake City, UT 84132, USA

Library of Congress Cataloging-in-Publication Data
Evaluation methods in medical informatics/Charles P. Friedman,
   Jeremy C. Wyatt, with contributions by Bonnie Kaplan, Allen C. Smith III
       p. cm.—(Computers and medicine)
     Includes bibliographical references and index.
     ISBN 0-387-94228-9 (hardcover: alk. paper)
     1. Medical informatics—Research—Methodology. 2. Medicine—Data
processing—Evaluation. I. Friedman, Charles P. II. Wyatt, J.
(Jeremy) III. Series: Computers and medicine (New York, N.Y.)
     [DNLM: 1. Medical informatics. 2. Technology, Medical.
3. Decision Support Techniques. W 26.55.A7 E92 1996]
R858.E985 1996
610'.285—dc20
                                    96-18411

Printed on acid-free paper.

Production coordinated by Carlson Co. and managed by Natalie Johnson; manufacturing supervised
by Jeffrey Taub.
Typeset by Carlson Co., Yellow Springs, OH, from the authors' electronic files.
Printed and bound by Braun-Brumfield, Inc., Ann Arbor, MI.
Printed in the United States of America.

9 8 7 6 5 4 3 2 1

ISBN 0-387-94228-9 Springer-Verlag New York Berlin Heidelberg   SPIN 10424646

To Pat and Sylvia

Foreword

As director of a training program in medical informatics, I have found that one of the most frequent inquiries from graduate students is, "Although I am happy with my research focus and the work I have done, how can I design and carry out a practical evaluation that proves the value of my contribution?" Informatics is a multifaceted, interdisciplinary field with research that ranges from theoretical developments to projects that are highly applied and intended for near-term use in clinical settings. The implications of "proving" a research claim accordingly vary greatly depending on the details of an individual student's goals and thesis statement. Furthermore, the dissertation work leading up to an evaluation plan is often so time-consuming and arduous that attempting the "perfect" evaluation is frequently seen as impractical or as diverting students from central programming or implementation issues that are their primary areas of interest. They often ask what compromises are possible so they can provide persuasive data in support of their claims without adding another two to three years to their graduate student life.

Our students clearly needed help in dealing more effectively with such dilemmas, and it was therefore fortuitous when, in the autumn of 1991, we welcomed two superb visiting professors to our laboratories. We had known both Chuck Friedman and Jeremy Wyatt from earlier visits and professional encounters, but it was coincidence that offered them sabbatical breaks in our laboratory during the same academic year. Knowing that each had strong interests and skills in the areas of evaluation and clinical trial design, I hoped they would enjoy getting to know one another and would find that their scholarly pursuits were both complementary and synergistic. To help stir the pot, we even assigned them to a shared office that we try to set aside for visitors, and within a few weeks they were putting their heads together as they learned about the evaluation issues that were rampant in our laboratory.

The contributions by Drs. Friedman and Wyatt during that year were marvelous, and they continue to have ripple effects today. They served as local consultants as we devised evaluation plans for existing projects, new proposals, and student research. By the spring they had identified the topics and themes that needed to be understood better by those in our laboratory, and they offered a well-received seminar on evaluation methods for medical information systems. It was out of the class notes formulated for that course that the present volume evolved.

Its availability will allow us to rejuvenate and refine the laboratory's knowledge and skills in the area of evaluating medical information systems, so we have eagerly anticipated its publication.

This book fills an important niche that is not effectively covered by other medical informatics textbooks or by the standard volumes on evaluation and clinical trial design. I know of no other writers who have the requisite knowledge of statistics coupled with intensive study of medical informatics and an involvement with creation of applied systems as well. Drs. Friedman and Wyatt are scholars and educators, but they are also practical in their understanding of the world of clinical medicine and the realities of system implementation and validation in settings that defy formal controlled trials. Thus the book is not only of value to students of medical informatics but will be a key reference for all individuals involved in the implementation and evaluation of basic and applied systems in medical informatics.

EDWARD H. SHORTLIFFE, M.D., PH.D
Section of Medical Informatics
Stanford University School of Medicine

Series Preface

This monograph series intends to provide medical information scientists, health care administrators, physicians, nurses, other health care providers, and computer science professionals with successful examples and experiences of computer applications in health care settings. Through these computer applications, we attempt to show what is effective and efficient, and hope to provide guidance on the acquisition or design of medical information systems so that costly mistakes can be avoided.

The health care provider organizations such as hospitals and clinics are experiencing large demands for clinical information because of a transition from a "fee-for-service" to a "capitation-based" health care economy. This transition changes the way health care services are being paid for. Previously, nearly all heath care services were paid for by insurance companies after the services were performed. Today, many procedures need to be pre-approved, and many charges for clinical services must be justified to the insurance plans. Ultimately, in a totally capitated system, the more patient care services are provided per patient, the less profitable the health care provider organization will be. Clearly, the financial risks have shifted from the insurance carriers to the health care provider organizations. In order for hospitals and clinics to assess these financial risks, management needs to know what services are to be provided and how to reduce them without impacting the quality of care. The balancing act of reducing costs but maintaining health care quality and patient satisfaction requires accurate information of the clinical services. The only way this information can be collected cost-effectively is through the automation of the health care process itself. Unfortunately, current health information systems are not comprehensive enough, and their level of integration is low and primitive at best. There are too many "islands" even within single health care provider organizations.

With the rapid advance of digital communications technologies and the acceptance of standard interfaces, these "islands" can be bridged to satisfy most information needs of health care professionals and management. In addition, the migration of health information systems to client/server computer architectures allows us to re-engineer the user interface to become more functional, pleasant, and also responsive. Eventually, we hope, the clinical workstation will become the tool that health care providers use interactively without intermediary data entry support.

Computer-based information systems provide more timely and legible information than traditional paper-based systems. In addition, medical information systems can monitor the process of health care and improve quality of patient care by providing decision support for diagnosis or therapy, clinical reminders for follow-up care, warnings about adverse drug interactions, alerts to questionable treatment or deviations from clinical protocols, and more. The complexity of the health care workplace requires a rich set of requirements for health information systems. Further, the systems must respond quickly to user interactions and queries in order to facilitate and not impede the work of health care professionals. Because of this and the requirement for a high level of security, these systems can be classified as very complex and, from a developer's perspective, also as "risky" systems.

Information technology is advancing at an accelerated pace. Instead of waiting for three years for a new generation of computer hardware, we are now confronted with new computing hardware every 18 months. The forthcoming changes in the telecommunications industry will be revolutionary. Within the next five years, and certainly before the end of this century, new digital communications technologies, such as the Integrated Services Digital Network (ISDN), Asynchronous Data Subscriber Loop (ADSL) technologies, and very high speed local area networks using efficient cell switching protocols (e.g., ATM), will not only change the architecture of our information systems, but also the way we work and manage health care institutions.

The software industry constantly tries to provide tools and productive development environments for the design, implementation, and maintenance of information systems. Still, the development of information systems in medicine is an art, and the tools we use are often self-made and crude. One area that needs desperate attention is the interaction of health care providers with the computer. While the user interface needs improvement and the emerging graphical user-interfaces form the basis for such improvements, the most important criterion is to provide relevant and accurate information without drowning the physician in too much (irrelevant) data.

To develop an effective clinical system requires an understanding of what is to be done and how to do it, as well as an understanding on how to integrate information systems into an operational health care environment. Such knowledge is rarely found in any one individual; all systems described in this monograph series are the work of teams. The size of these teams is usually small, and the composition is heterogeneous, i.e., health professionals, computer and communications scientists and engineers, statisticians, epidemiologists, and so on. The team members are usually dedicated to working together over long periods of time, sometimes spanning decades.

Clinical information systems are dynamic systems, their functionality constantly changing because of external pressures and administrative changes in health care institutions. Good clinical information systems will and should change the operational mode of patient care which, in turn, should affect the functional requirements of the information systems. This interplay requires that medical information systems be based on architectures that allow them to be adapted rapidly and with minimal expense. It also requires a willingness by management of the health care institution to adjust its operational procedures, and, most of all, to provide end-user education in the use of information technology. While medical information systems should be functionally integrated, these systems should also be modular so that incremental upgrades, additions, and deletions of modules can be done in order to match the pattern of capital resources and investments available to an institution.

We are building medical information systems just as automobiles were built early in this century, i.e., in an ad-hoc manner that disregarded even existent standards. Although technical standards addressing computer and communications technologies are necessary, they are insufficient. We still need to develop conventions and agreements, and perhaps a few regulations that address the principal use of medical information in computer and communications systems. Standardization allows the mass production of low cost parts which can be used to build more complex structures. What exactly are these parts in medical information systems? We need to identify them, classify them, describe them, publish their specifications, and, most importantly, use them in real health care settings. We must be sure that these parts are useful and cost effective even before we standardize them.

Clinical research, health service research, and medical education will benefit greatly when controlled vocabularies are used more widely in the practice of medicine. For practical reasons, the medical profession has developed numerous classifications, nomenclatures, dictionary codes, and thesauri (e.g., ICD, CPT, DSM-III, SNOMED, COSTAR dictionary codes, BAIK thesaurus terms, and MESH terms). The collection of these terms represents a considerable amount of clinical activities, a large portion of the health care business, and access to our recorded knowledge. These terms and codes form the glue that links the practice of medicine with the business of medicine. They also link the practice of medicine with the literature of medicine, with further links to medical research and education. Since information systems are more efficient in retrieving information when controlled vocabularies are used in large databases, the attempt to unify and build bridges between these coding systems is a great example of unifying the field of medicine and health care by providing and using medical informatics tools. The Unified Medical Language System (UMLS) project of the National Library of Medicine, NIH, in Bethesda, Maryland, is an example of such an effort.

The purpose of this series is to capture the experience of medical informatics teams that have successfully implemented and operated medical information systems. We hope the individual books in this series will contribute to the evolution of medical informatics as a recognized professional discipline. We are at the threshold where there is not just the need but already the momentum and interest in the health care and computer science communities to identify and recognize the new discipline called Medical Informatics.

I would like to thank the editors of Springer-Verlag New York for the opportunity to edit this series. Also, many thanks to the present and past departmental chairmen who allowed me to spend time on this activity: William S. Yamamoto, M.D., and Thomas E. Piemme, M.D., of the Department of Computer Medicine at

George Washington University Medical Center in Washington, D.C., and Homer R. Warner, M.D., Ph.D., and Reed M. Gardner, Ph.D., of the Department of Medical Informatics at the University of Utah Health Sciences Center in Salt Lake City, Utah. Last, but not least, I am thanking all authors and editors of this monograph series for contributing to the practice and theory of Medical Informatics.

HELMUTH F. ORTHNER, PH.D.
Salt Lake City, Utah, USA

Preface:
Counting the Steps on Box Hill

In February 1995, during a visit by the American coauthor of this volume to the home of the Wyatt family in the United Kingdom, one afternoon's activity involved a walk on Box Hill in Surrey. In addition to the coauthors of this volume, Jeremy's wife Sylvia and the two Wyatt children were present. We walked down a steep hill. As we began ascending the hill, the group decided to count the number of earthen steps cut into the path to make climbing easier. When we arrived at the top, each of us had generated a different number.

There ensued a lively discussion of the reasons the numbers differed. Clearly, one or more of us may have lost attention and simply miscounted, but there emerged on analysis three more subtle reasons for the discrepancies.

- First, not all of the steps on our return trip went upward. Do the downward steps count at all toward the total; and if so, do they add or subtract from the count? *We realized that we had not agreed to all of the rules for counting because we did not know in advance all of the issues that needed to be taken into account.*

- Second, the path was so eroded by recent heavy rain that it was not always easy to distinguish a step from an irregularity. What counts as a step? In a few instances along the way, we had discussions about whether a particular irregularity was a step, and apparently we had disagreed. *It is not clear if there is any verifiably right answer to this question unless there existed plans for the construction of the steps. Even then, should a step now eroded almost beyond recognition still count as a step?*

- Third and finally, one of the children, having decided in advance that there were 108 steps, simply stopped counting once she had reached this number. She wanted there to be no more steps and made it so in her own mind. *Beliefs, no matter how they develop, are real for the belief holders and must be taken seriously.*

Even an apparently simple counting task had led to disagreements about the results. Each of us thought himself or herself perfectly correct, and we realized there was no way to resolve our differences without one person exerting power over the others by dictating the rules or arbitrating the results of our disagreements.

It struck us that this pleasant walk in the country had raised several key themes that confront anyone designing, conducting, or interpreting an evaluation. These issues of anticipation, communication, measurement, and belief were distinguishing issues that should receive major emphasis in a work focused on evaluation in contrast to one covering methods of empirical research more generally. As such, these issues represent a point of departure for this book and direct much of its organization and content. We trust that anyone who has performed a rigorous data-driven evaluation can see the pertinence of the Box Hill counting dilemma. We hope that anyone reading this volume will in the end possess both a framework for thinking about these issues and a methodology for addressing them.

More specifically, we have attempted to address in this book the major questions relating to evaluation in informatics.

1. Why should information resources be studied? Why is it a challenging process? (Chapter 1)
2. What are all the options for conducting such studies? How do I decide what to study? (Chapters 2 and 3)
3. How do I design, carry out, and interpret a study using a particular set of techniques?
   a. For objectivist or quantitative studies (Chapters 4 through 7).
   b. For subjectivist or qualitative studies (Chapters 8 and 9).
4. How do I conduct studies in the context of health care organizations? (Chapter 10)
5. How do I communicate study designs and study results? (Chapter 11)

We set out to create a volume useful to several audiences: those training for careers in informatics who as part of their curricula must learn to perform evaluation studies; those actively conducting evaluation studies who might derive from these pages ways to improve their methods; and those responsible for information systems in medical centers who wish to understand how well their services are working, how to improve them, and who must decide whether to purchase or use the products of medical informatics for specific purposes. This book can alert such individuals to questions they might ask, the answers they might expect, and how to understand them. This book is intended to be germane to all health professions and professionals, even though we, like many in our field, used the word "medical" in the title. We have deliberately given emphasis to both quantitative (what we call "objectivist") methods and qualitative ("subjectivist") methods, as both are vital to evaluation in informatics. A reader may not choose to become proficient in or to conduct studies using both approaches, but we see an appreciation of both as essential.

The organizing principle for this volume is a textbook for a graduate level course, although we hope and intend that the work will also prove useful as a general reference. The subject matter of this volume has been the basis of a graduate course offered at the University of North Carolina since 1993. Someone reading the book straight through should experience a linear development of the subject, as it touches on most of the important concepts and develops several key methodological skill areas. To this end, "self-test" exercises with answers and "food for thought" questions have been added to many chapters.

In our view, evaluation is different from an exercise in applied statistics. This work is therefore intended to complement, not replace, basic statistics courses offered at most institutions. (We assume the reader to have only a basic knowledge of statistics.) The reader will find in this book material derived from varying methodological traditions including psychometrics, statistics and research design, ethnography, clinical epidemiology, decision analysis, organizational behavior, and health services research, as well as the literature of informatics itself. We have found it necessary to borrow terminology, in addition to methods, from all of these fields, and we have deliberately chosen one specific term to represent a concept that is represented differently in these traditions. As a result, some readers may find the book using an unfamiliar term to describe what, for them, is a familiar idea.

Several chapters also develop in some detail examples taken either from the informatics literature or from as yet unpublished studies. The example studies were chosen because they illustrate key issues and because they are works with which we are highly familiar, either because we have contributed directly to them or because they have been the work of our close colleagues. This proximity gave us access to the raw data and other materials from these studies, which allowed us to generate pedagogic examples differing in emphasis from the published literature about them. Information resources forming the basis of these examples include the Hypercritic system developed at Erasmus University in The Netherlands, the TraumAID system developed at the Medical College of Pennsylvania and the University of Pennsylvania, and the T-HELPER system developed at Stanford University.

We consciously did *not* write this book specifically for software developers or engineers who are primarily interested in formal methods of verification. In the classic distinction between validation and verification, this book is more directed at validation. Nor did we write this book for professional methodologists who might expect to read about contemporary advances in the methodological areas from which much of this book's content derives. Nonetheless, we hope that individuals from a broad range of professional backgrounds, who are interested in applying well-established evaluation techniques specifically to problems in medical informatics, will find the book useful.

In conclusion, we would like to acknowledge the many colleagues and collaborators whose contributions made this work possible. They include contributing chapter authors Allen Smith and Bonnie Kaplan; Ted Shortliffe and the members of the Section on Medical Informatics at Stanford for their support and ideas during our sabbatical leaves there in 1991–1992, where the ideas for this book took shape; Fred Wolf and Dave Swanson, who offered useful comments on several chapters; and colleagues Johan van der Lei, Mark Musen, John Clarke, and Bonnie Webber for the specific examples that derive from their own research.

Chuck specifically thanks his students at UNC and Duke for challenging him repeatedly both in and out of class. He particularly wishes to thank Randy Cork,

Joe Mirrow, and Keith Cogdill for their contributions to and their vetting of many chapters. Chuck also thanks Stuart Bondurant, Dean of the UNC School of Medicine from 1979 to 1994, for his unfailing support, which made possible both this volume and the medical informatics program at UNC. Three MIT physicists Chuck has been very fortunate to know and work with—the late Nathaniel Frank, the late Jerrold Zacharias, and Edwin Taylor—taught him the importance of meeting the needs of students who are the future of any field. Finally, Chuck wishes to thank his family—Pat, Ned, and Andy—for their support and forbearance during his many hours of sequestration in the study.

Jeremy acknowledges the many useful insights gained from coworkers during collaborative evaluation projects, especially from Doug Altman (ICRF Centre for Statistics in Medicine, Oxford) and David Spiegelhalter (MRC Biostatistics Unit, Cambridge). The UK Medical Research Council funded the traveling fellowship that enabled Jeremy to spend a year at Stanford in 1991–1992. Finally, Jeremy thanks his family, Sylvia, David, and Jessica and his parents for their patience and support during the long gestation period of this book.

C.P.F. AND J.C.W.
Chapel Hill, North Carolina, USA
London, UK

Contents

1

Challenges of Evaluation in Medical Informatics

This chapter develops in a general and intuitive way many issues that are explored in more detail in later chapters of this book. It gives a first definition of evaluation, describes why evaluation is needed, and notes some of the problems of evaluation in medical informatics that distinguish it from evaluation in other areas. In addition, it lists some of the many clinical information systems and resources, questions that can be asked about them, and the various perspectives of those concerned.

First Definitions

Most people understand the term "evaluation" to mean measuring or describing something, usually to answer questions or help make decisions. Whether we are choosing a holiday destination or a word processor, we evaluate the options and how well they fit key objectives or personal preferences. The form of the evaluation differs widely, according to what is being evaluated and how important the decision is. So, in the case of holiday destinations, we may ask our friend which Hawaiian island she prefers and then browse the World Wide Web, whereas for a word processor we may focus on more technical details, such as the time to open and spell-check a 3000-word document or its compatibility with our printer. Thus the term "evaluation" describes a wide range of data collection activities designed to answer questions ranging from the casual "What does my friend think of Maui?" to the more focused "Is word processor A quicker than word processor B on my computer?"

In medical informatics we study the collection, processing, and dissemination of health care information; and we build "information resources"—usually consisting of computer hardware or software—to facilitate these activities. Such information resources include systems to collect, store, and retrieve data about specific patients (e.g., clinical workstations and databases) and systems to assemble, store, and reason using medical knowledge (e.g., medical knowledge acquisition tools, knowledge bases, decision-support systems, and multimedia educational systems). Thus there is a wide range of medical information resources to evaluate.

1

To further complicate the picture, each information resource has many aspects that can be evaluated. The technically minded might focus on inherent characteristics, asking such questions as: "How many columns of data are there per database table?" or "How many probability calculations per second can this tool sustain?" Clinicians, however, might ask more pragmatic questions, such as: "Is the information in this system completely up to date?" or "How long must we wait till the decision-support system produces its recommendations?" Those with a broader perspective might wish to understand the impact of these resources on users or patients, asking questions such as: "How well does this database support clinical audit?" or "What effects will this decision-support system have on working relationships and responsibilities?" Thus evaluation methods in medical informatics must address a wide range of questions, ranging from technical characteristics of specific systems to their effects on people and organizations.

In this book we do not exhaustively describe how each evaluation method can be used to answer each kind of question. Instead, we describe the range of techniques available and focus on those that seem most useful in medical informatics. We introduce in detail methods, techniques, study designs, and analyses that apply across a wide range of evaluation problems. In the language of software engineering, our focus is much more on software validation (checking that the "right" information resource was built, which involves determining that the specification was right and the resource is performing to specification) than software verification (checking whether the resource was built to specification). As we introduce methods for validating clinical software in detail, we distinguish the study of software functions from the study of its impact or effects on users and the wider world. Although software verification is important, we merely summarize some of the relevant principles in Chapter 3 and refer the reader to general computer science and software engineering texts.

Reasons for Performing Evaluations

Like any complex, time-consuming activity, evaluation can serve multiple purposes. There are five major reasons we evaluate clinical information resources.[1]

1. *Promotional:* To encourage the use of information systems in medicine, we must be able to reassure physicians that the systems are safe and benefit both patients and institutions through improved cost-effectiveness.

2. *Scholarly:* If we believe that medical informatics exists as a discipline, ongoing examination of the structure, function, and impact of medical information resources must be a primary method for uncovering its principles.[2] In addition, some developers examine their information resources from different perspectives out of simple curiosity to see if they are able to perform functions that were not in the original specifications.

3. *Pragmatic:* Without evaluating their systems, developers can never know which techniques or methods are more effective, or why certain approaches

failed. Equally, other developers are not able to learn from previous mistakes and may reinvent a square wheel.

4. *Ethical:* Before using an information resource, health care providers must ensure that it is safe and be able to justify it in preference to other information resources and the many other health care innovations that compete for the same budget.

5. *Medicolegal:* To reduce the risk of liability, developers of an information resource should obtain accurate information to allow them to assure users that it is safe and effective. Users need evaluation results to enable them to exercise their professional judgment before using systems, thus helping the law to regard the user as a "learned intermediary." An information resource that treats the users merely as automatons without allowing them to exercise their skills and judgment risks being judged by the strict laws of product liability instead of the more lenient principles applied to provision of professional services.[3]

Every evaluation study is motivated by one or more of these factors. Awareness of the major reason for conducting an evaluation often helps frame the major questions to be addressed and avoids any disappointment that may result if the focus of the study is misdirected.

Who Is Involved in Evaluation and Why?

We have already mentioned the range of perspectives in medical informatics, from the technical to the organizational. Figure 1.1 shows some of the actors involved in paying for (solid arrows) and regulating (shaded arrows) the health care process. Any of these actors may be affected by a medical information resource, and each may have a unique view of what constitutes benefit. More specifically, in a typical clinical information resource project the key "stakeholders" are the developer, the user, the patients whose management may be affected, and the person responsible for purchasing and maintaining the system. Each of these individuals or groups may have different questions to ask about the same information resource (Fig. 1.2). Thus, whenever we design evaluation studies, it is important to consider the perspectives of all stakeholders in the information resource. Any one study can satisfy only some of them. A major challenge is to distinguish those persons who must be satisfied from those whose satisfaction is optional.

What Makes Evaluation So Difficult?

Evaluation, as defined earlier, is a general investigative activity applicable to many fields. Many evaluation studies have been performed, and much has been written about evaluation methods. Why, then, write a book specifically about evaluation in medical informatics?

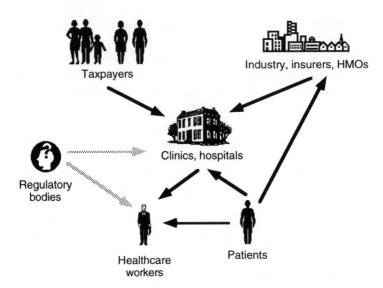

FIGURE 1.1. Actors involved in health care delivery and regulation.

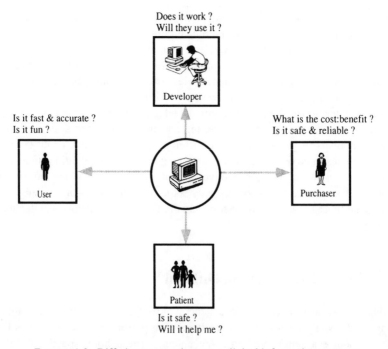

FIGURE 1.2. Differing perspectives on a clinical information resource.

The evaluation of clinical information resources lies at the intersection of three areas, each notorious for its complexity (Fig. 1.3): medicine and health care delivery, computer-based information systems, and the general methodology of evaluation itself. Because of the complexity of each area, any work that combines them necessarily poses serious challenges. These challenges are discussed in the sections that follow.

Problems Deriving from Medicine and Health Care Delivery

The goal of this section is to introduce nonclinicians to some of the complexities of medicine and both nonclinicians and clinicians to some of the implications of this complexity for evaluating clinical information resources.

Donabedian informed us that any health care innovation may influence three aspects of the health care system.[4]

1. *Structure* of the health care system, including the space it occupies, equipment available, financial resources required, and the number, skills, and interrelationships of staff
2. *Processes* that take place during health care activity, such as the number and appropriateness of diagnoses, investigations, and therapies administered
3. *Outcomes* of health care for both individual patients and the community, such as quality of life, complications of procedures, and length of survival

Thus when evaluating the impact of an information resource on a health care system, its effects can be seen on any of these three aspects. Complexity arises because an information resource may lead to an improvement in one area (patient

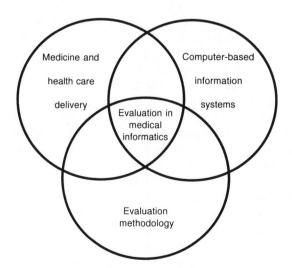

FIGURE 1.3. Complexity of evaluation in medical informatics.

outcomes, for example) accompanied by deterioration in another (the costs of running the service perhaps).

It is well known that the roles of nursing and clinical personnel are well defined and hierarchical in comparison to those in many other professions. It means that information resources designed for a specific group of professionals, such as a residents' information system designed for one hospital,[5] may hold little benefit for others. It often comes as a surprise to those developing information systems that, despite the obvious hierarchy, junior physicians cannot be obliged by their senior counterparts to use a specific information resource, as is the case in the banking or airline industries where these practices have become "part of the job." Thus compliance may be a limiting factor when testing the effects of information resources on health care workers.

Because health care is a safety-critical area, and possibly because there may be more skeptics than in other professions, more rigorous proof of safety and effectiveness is required when evaluating information resources here than in areas such as retail or manufacturing. Clinicians are rightly skeptical of innovative technology but may be unrealistic in their demand for proof of efficacy if the innovation threatens their current practices. Because we are usually skeptical of new practices and accept existing ones, the standard required for proving the effectiveness of computerized information resources may be inflated beyond that required for existing methods for handling clinical information, such as the paper medical record.

Complex regulations apply to those developing or marketing clinical therapies or investigational technology. It is not yet clear whether these regulations apply to all computer-based information resources or only to those that manage patients directly, without a human intermediary.[6] If the former, developers must comply with a comprehensive schedule of testing and monitoring procedures, which may form an obligatory core of evaluation methods in the future.

Medicine is well known to be a complex domain, with students spending a minimum of 7 years to gain qualifications. A single internal medicine textbook contains approximately 600,000 facts[7]; practicing experts have as many as 2 million to 5 million facts at their fingertips.[8] Medical knowledge itself[7] and methods of health care delivery change rapidly, so the goalposts for a medical information resource may move during the course of an evaluation study.

Patients often suffer from multiple diseases, which may evolve over time at differing rates, and may undergo a number of interventions over the course of the study period, confounding the effects of changes in information management. There is variation in the interpretation of patient data among medical centers. What may be regarded as an abnormal result or an advanced stage of disease in one setting may pass without comment in another because it is within their laboratory's normal limits or is an endemic condition in their population. Thus simply because an information resource is safe and effective when used in one center on patients with a given diagnosis, one is not entitled to prejudge the results of evaluating it in another center or in patients with a different disease profile.

The causal links between introducing an information resource and achieving improvements in patient outcome are long and complex compared to direct patient care interventions such as drugs (Fig. 1.4). In addition, the functioning of an information resource and its impact may depend critically on input from health care workers or patients (Fig. 1.4, shaded arrows). It is thus unrealistic to look for quantifiable changes in patient outcome following the introduction of many information resources until one has documented changes in the structure or processes of health care delivery. For example, MacDonald et al. showed during the 1980s that the Regenstreif system with its alerts and reminders affected clinical decisions and actions.[9] Almost 10 years later clear evidence of a reduction in the length of stay was obtained,[10] but we still lack direct evidence that the system leads to improved patient outcomes. In Chapter 3 we discuss circumstances in which it may be sufficient to evaluate the effects of an information resource on a clinical process, such as the proportion of patients with heart attacks given the clot-dissolving drug streptokinase, and avoid the need to launch a study large enough to document changes in patient outcome.

In some cases changes in clinical processes are difficult to interpret because the resulting improved information management or decision-taking merely clears one logjam and reveals another, which in turn impedes patient care. An example of this situation occurred during the evaluation of the ACORN chest pain decision-aid, designed to facilitate more rapid and accurate diagnosis of patients with acute

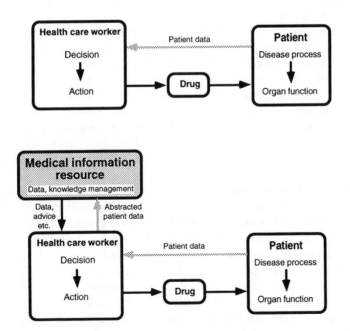

FIGURE 1.4. Mode of action of a drug compared to a medical information resource.

ischemic heart disease in the emergency room.[11] Although ACORN allowed emergency room staff to rapidly identify patients requiring admission to the cardiac care unit (CCU), it uncovered an additional problem: the lack of beds in the CCU and delays in transferring other patients out of them.[12]

The processes of medical decision-making are complex and have been extensively studied.[13, 14] Clinicians make many kinds of decisions—including diagnosis, monitoring, choice of therapy, and prognosis—using incomplete and fuzzy data, some of which are appreciated intuitively and not recorded in the clinical notes. If an information resource generates more effective management of both patient data and medical knowledge, it may intervene in the process of medical decision-making in a number of ways, so it may be difficult to decide which component of the resource is responsible for the observed changes.

Data about individual patients are typically collected at several locations and over periods of time ranging from an hour to decades. Unfortunately, clinical notes usually contain only a subset of what was observed and seldom contain the reasons actions were taken.[15] Because reimbursement agencies often have access to clinical notes, the notes may even contain data intended to mislead chart reviewers or conceal important facts from the casual reader.[16, 17] Thus evaluating an electronic medical record system by examining the accuracy of its contents may not give a true picture.

There is a general lack of "gold standards" in medicine. For example, diagnoses are rarely known with 100% certainty, partly because it is unethical to do all possible tests in every patient (or even to follow up patients without good cause) and partly because of the complexity of the human body. When attempting to establish a diagnosis or the cause of death, even if it is possible to perform a postmortem examination correlating the observed changes with the patients' symptoms or findings before death may prove impossible. Determining the "correct" management for a patient is even worse, as there is wide variation in so-called consensus opinions,[18] which is reflected in wide variations in clinical practice even in neighboring areas. An example is the use of endotracheal intubation in patients with severe head injuries, which varied from 15% to 85% among teaching hospitals, even within California (B. Jennett, personal communication). Also, getting busy physicians to give their opinions about the correct management of patients for comparison with a decision support system's advice may take as much as a full year.[19]

Doctors practice under strict legal and ethical obligations to give their patients the best care available, to do them no harm, to keep them informed about the risks of all procedures and therapies, and to maintain confidentiality. These obligations may well impinge on the design of evaluation studies. For example, because health care workers have imperfect memories and patients take holidays and participate in the unpredictable activities of real life, it is impossible to impose a strict discipline for data recording, and study data are often incomplete. Before a randomized controlled trial can be undertaken, health care workers and patients are entitled to a full explanation of the possible benefits and disadvantages of being allocated to the control and intervention groups prior to giving their consent.

Problems Deriving from the Complexity of Computer-Based Information Resources

From a computer science perspective, the goal of evaluating a computer-based information resource is to predict its function and impact from knowledge of its structure. However, although software engineering and formal methods for specifying, coding, and evaluating computer programs have become more sophisticated, even systems of modest complexity challenge these techniques. To rigorously verify a program (obtain proof that it performs all and only those functions specified) requires testing resources that increase exponentially according to the program's size. This is an "NP-hard" problem. Put simply, to test a program rigorously requires application of every combination of possible input data in all possible orders. This entails at least N factorial experiments, where N is the number of input data items.

A broad range of computer-based information resources has been applied to medicine (Table 1.1), each with different target users, input data, and goals. Computer-based information resources are a novel technology in medicine and require new methods to assess their impact. New problems arise, such as the need for decision-aids to be shown to be valuable before users believe their advice. This is known as the "evaluation paradox" and is discussed in later chapters. Many applications do not have their maximum impact until they are fully integrated with hospital information systems and become part of routine clinical practice.[20]

In some projects, the goals of the new information resource are not precisely defined. Developers may be attracted by technology and produce applications without first demonstrating the existence of a clinical problem that the application is designed to meet.[12] An example was a conference entitled "Medicine Meets Virtual Reality: *Discovering Applications* for 3D Multimedia" [our italics]. The lack of a clear need for the information resource makes some medical informatics projects difficult to evaluate.

Some computer-based systems are able to adapt to their users or to data already acquired, or they may be deliberately tailored to a given institution. Hence it may be difficult to compare the results of one evaluation with a study of the same information resource conducted at a different time or in another location. Also the notoriously rapid evolution of computer hardware and software means that the time course of an evaluation study may be greater than the lifetime of the information resource itself.

Medical information resources often contain several distinct components, including interface, database, reasoning, and maintenance programs as well as patient data, static medical knowledge, and dynamic inferences about the patient, the user, and the current activity of the user. Such information resources may perform a wide range of functions for users. It means that if evaluators are to answer questions such as: "What part of the information resource is responsible for the observed effect?" or "Why did the information resource fail?" they must be familiar with each component of the information resource, their functions, and their potential interactions.[11]

TABLE 1.1. Range of computer-based information resources in medicine

Clinical data systems	Clinical knowledge systems
Clinical databases	Computerized textbooks (e.g., *Scientific American Medicine* on CD-ROM)
Communications systems (e.g., picture archiving and communication systems)	Teaching systems (e.g., interactive mult-media anatomy tutor)
On-line signal processing (e.g., 24-hour ECG analysis system)	Patient simulation programs (e.g., inter-active acid-base metabolism simulator)
Alert generation (e.g., ICU monitor, drug interaction system)	Passive knowledge bases (e.g., MEDLINE bibliographic system)
Laboratory data interpretation	Patient-specific advice generators (e.g., MYCIN antibiotic therapy advisor)
Medical image interpretation	Medical robotics

Problems of the Evaluation Process Itself

Evaluation studies, as envisioned in this book, do not focus solely on the structure and function of information resources; they also address their impact on care providers who are customarily its users and on patient outcomes. To understand users' actions, investigators must confront the gulf between peoples' private opinions, public statements, and actual behavior. What is more, there is clear evidence that the mere act of studying performance changes it, a phenomenon usually known as the Hawthorne effect.[21] Finally, humans vary widely in their responses to stimuli, from minute to minute and from one to another, making the results of measurements subject to random and systematic errors. Thus evaluation studies of medical information resources require analytical tools from the behavioral and social sciences, statistics, and other fields.

Evaluation studies require test material (e.g., clinical cases) and information resource users (e.g., physicians or nurses). These are often in shorter supply than the study design requires: The availability of patients is usually overestimated, sometimes manyfold. In addition, it may be unclear what kind of cases or users to recruit to a study. Often study designers are faced with a trade-off between selecting cases or users with high fidelity to real life and those who can help achieve adequate experimental control. Finally, one of the more important determinants of the results of an evaluation study is the manner in which case data are abstracted and presented to users. For example, one would expect differing results in a study of an information resource's accuracy depending on whether the test data were abstracted by the developers or by the intended users.

There are many reasons for performing evaluations, ranging from assessing a student's work to making national health policy decisions or understanding a specific technical advance. There are inevitably many actors in evaluation studies (see above), including information resource developers, users, and patients, all of whom may have different perspectives on which questions to ask and how to interpret the answers. Table 1.2 lists some sample questions that may arise about the resource itself and its impact on users, patients, and the health care system.

TABLE 1.2. Possible questions that may arise during evaluation of a medical information resource

Questions about the resource	Questions about the impact of the resource
Is there a clinical need for it?	Do people use it?
Does it work?	Do people like it?
Is it reliable?	Does it improve users' efficiency?
Is it accurate?	Does it influence the collection of data?
Is it fast enough?	Does it influence users' decisions?
Is data entry reliable?	For how long do the observed effects last?
Are people likely to use it?	Does it influence users' knowledge or skills?
Which parts cause the effects?	Does it help patients?
How can it be maintained?	Does it change consumption of resources?
How can it be improved?	What might ensue from widespread use?

The multiplicity of possible questions creates challenges for the designers of evaluation studies. Any one study inevitably fails to address some questions and may fail to answer adequately some questions that are explicitly addressed.

Addressing the Challenges of Evaluation

No one could pretend that evaluation is easy. This entire book describes ways that have been developed to solve the many problems discussed in this chapter. First, evaluators should recognize that a wide range of evaluation approaches are available and should adopt a specific "evaluation mindset," as described in Chapter 2. This mindset includes awareness that every study is to some extent a compromise. To help overcome the many potential difficulties, evaluators require knowledge and skills drawn from a range of disciplines including medicine, computer science, statistics, measurement theory, psychology, sociology, and anthropology. To avoid committing excessive evaluation resources at too early a stage, the intensity of evaluation activity should be titrated to the stage of development of the information resource: It is clearly inappropriate to subject a prototype from a 3-month student project to a multicenter randomized trial.[22] It does not imply that evaluation can be deferred to the end of a project. Evaluation plans should be appropriately integrated with system design and development from the outset.

If the developers are able to enunciate clearly the aims of an information resource, defining the questions to be answered by an evaluation study becomes easier. As we see in later chapters, evaluators should always watch for adverse or unexpected effects. Life is also easier for evaluators if they can build on the work of their predecessors. For example, if there is a commonly applied measure of patient outcome or quality of care, they should use it in their study rather than developing a new measure, which would have to undergo a thorough, time-consuming process of validation. One valuable role evaluators may play is to dampen the often unbridled enthusiasm of developers for their own systems, focusing their attention on a small number of specific benefits it is reasonable to expect.

As illustrated above, there are many potential problems when evaluating clinical information resources, but it is possible; and many useful evaluations have already been performed. For example, Johnston et al.[23] reviewed the results of 28 randomized controlled trials of decision support systems and concluded that most showed clear evidence of an impact on clinical processes, and a smaller number changed patient outcomes. Designing experiments to detect changes in patient outcome due to the introduction of an information resource is possible using control patients or control providers, as discussed in a later chapter. We do not wish to deter evaluators, merely to open their eyes to the complexity of this area.

Place of Evaluation Within Informatics

Medical informatics is a complex, derivative field. Informatics draws its methods from many disciplines and from many specific lines of creative work within these disciplines.[24] Some of the fields undergirding informatics are what may be called basic. They include, among others, computer science, information science, cognitive science, decision science, statistics, and linguistics. Other fields supporting informatics are more applied in their orientation, including software and computer engineering, clinical epidemiology, and evaluation itself. One of the strengths of informatics has been the degree to which individuals from these different disciplinary backgrounds but with complementary interests have learned not only to coexist but to collaborate productively.

This diverse intellectual heritage for informatics can, however, make it difficult to define creative or original work in the field.[25] The "tower" model, shown in Figure 1.5, asserts that creative work in informatics occurs at four levels that build on one another. Projects at every level of the tower can be found on the agenda of professional meetings in informatics and published in journals within the field. The topmost layer of the tower embraces empirical studies of information resources (systems) that have been developed using abstract models and perhaps also installed in settings of ongoing health care or education. Because informatics is so intimately concerned with the improvement of health care, the value or worth of resources produced by the field is a matter of significant ongoing interest.[26] Studies occupy the topmost layer because they rely on the existence of models, systems, and settings where the work of interest is under way. There must be *something* to study. As we see later, studies of information resources usually do not await the ultimate installation or deployment of these resources. Conceptual models may be studied empirically, and information resources themselves can be studied through successive stages of development.

Studies occupying the topmost level of the tower model are the focus of this book. Empirical studies include measurement and observations of the performance of information resources and the behavior of people who in some way use these resources, with emphasis on the interaction between the resources and the people and the consequences of these interactions. Included under empirical studies are activities that have traditionally been called "evaluation." We chose to

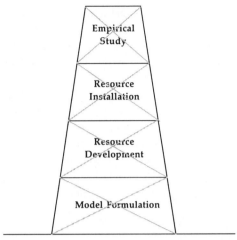

FIGURE 1.5. Tower model. (Adapted from the *Journal of the American Medical Informatics Association,* with permission.)

include the term "evaluation" instead of "empirical methods" in the title of this book because the former term is most commonly used in the field. The importance of evaluation and, more generally, empirical methods is becoming recognized by those concerned with information technology. In addition to papers reporting specific studies using the methods of evaluation, books on the topic, apart from this one, have begun to appear.[27-29]

Finally, if abstract principles of medical informatics exist,[2, 30] then evaluating the structure, function, and impact of medical information resources should be one of our primary methods for uncovering these principles. Without evaluation, medical informatics becomes an impressionistic, anecdotal, multidisciplinary subject, with little professional identity or chance of making progress toward greater scientific understanding and more effective clinical systems. Thus overcoming the problems described in this chapter to evaluate a wide range of resources in various clinical settings has intrinsic merit and can contribute to the development of medical informatics as a field. Evaluation is not merely a possible, but a necessary, component of medical informatics activity.[30]

Food for Thought

1. Choosing any alternative area of biomedicine as a point of comparison (e.g., drug trials), list as many factors as you can that make studies in medical informatics more difficult to conduct successfully than in your chosen area. Given these difficulties, is it worthwhile to conduct empirical studies in medical informatics, or should we use intuition or the marketplace as the primary indicator of the value of an information resource?

2. Many writers on evaluation of clinical information resources believe that the evaluations that should be done should be closely linked to the stage of development of the resource under study. Do you believe this position is reasonable? What other logic or criteria may be used to help decide what studies should be performed in any given situation?

3. Suppose you were running a philanthropic organization that supported medical informatics. When investing the scarce resources of your organization, you might have to choose between funding system/resource development and empirical studies of resources already developed. Faced with this decision, what weight would you give to each? How would you justify your decision?

4. To what extent is it possible to ascertain the effectiveness of a medical informatics resource? What are the most important criteria of effectiveness?

References

1. Wyatt J, Spiegelhalter D: Evaluating medical expert systems: what to test, and how? Med Inf (Lond) 1990;15:205–217.
2. Heathfield H, Wyatt J: The road to professionalism in medical informatics: a proposal for debate. Methods Inf Med 1995;34:426–433.
3. Brahams D, Wyatt J: Decision-aids and the law. Lancet 1989;2:632–634.
4. Donabedian A: Evaluating the quality of medical care. Millbank Mem Q 1966; 44:166–206.
5. Young D: An aid to reducing unnecessary investigations. BMJ 1980;281:1610–1611.
6. Brannigan V: Software quality regulation under the Safe Medical Devices Act, 1990: hospitals are now the canaries in the software mine. In: Clayton P (ed) Proceedings of the 15th Symposium on Computer Applications in Medical Care. New York: McGraw-Hill, 1991:238–242.
7. Wyatt J: Use and sources of medical knowledge. Lancet 1991;338:1368–1373.
8. Pauker S, Gorry G, Kassirer J, Schwartz W: Towards the simulation of clinical cognition: taking a present illness by computer. Am J Med 1976;60:981–996.
9. McDonald CJ, Hui SL, Smith DM, et al: Reminders to physicians from an introspective computer medical record: a two-year randomized trial. Ann Intern Med 1984; 100:130–138.
10. Tierney WM, Miller ME, Overhage JM, McDonald CJ: Physician order writing on microcomputer workstations. JAMA 1993;269:379–383.
11. Wyatt J: Lessons learned from the field trial of ACORN, an expert system to advise on chest pain. In: Barber B, Cao D, Qin D (eds) Proceedings of the Sixth World Conference on Medical Informatics, Singapore. Amsterdam: North Holland, 1989:111–115.
12. Heathfield HA, Wyatt J: Philosophies for the design and development of clinical decision-support systems. Methods Inf Med 1993;32:1–8.
13. Elstein A, Shulman L, Sprafka S: Medical Problem Solving: An Analysis of Clinical Reasoning. Cambridge, MA: Harvard University Press, 1978.
14. Evans D, Patel V (eds): Cognitive Science in Medicine. London: MIT Press, 1989.
15. Van der Lei J, Musen M, van der Does E, in't Veld A, van Bemmel J: Comparison of computer-aided and human review of general practitioners' management of hypertension. Lancet 1991;338:1504–1508.

16. Musen M: The strained quality of medical data. Methods Inf Med 1989;28:123–125.
17. Wyatt JC: Clinical data systems. Part I. Data and medical records. Lancet 1994; 344:1543–47.
18. Leitch D: Who should have their cholesterol measured ? What experts in the UK suggest. BMJ 1989;298:1615–1616.
19. Gaschnig J, Klahr P, Pople H, Shortliffe E, Terry A: Evaluation of expert systems: issues and case studies. In: Hayes-Roth F, Waterman DA, Lenat D (eds) Building Expert Systems, Reading, MA: Addison-Wesley, 1983.
20. Wyatt J, Spiegelhalter D: Field trials of medical decision-aids: potential problems and solutions. In: Clayton P (ed) Proceedings of the 15th Symposium on Computer Applications in Medical Care, Washington. New York: McGraw-Hill, 1991:3–7.
21. Roethligsburger F, Dickson W: Management and the Worker. Cambridge, MA: Harvard University Press, 1939.
22. Stead W, Haynes RB, Fuller S, et al: Designing medical informatics research and library projects to increase what is learned. J Am Med Inf Assoc 1994;1:28–34.
23. Johnston ME, Langton KB, Haynes RB, Matthieu D: A critical appraisal of research on the effects of computer-based decision support systems on clinician performance and patient outcomes. Ann Intern Med 1994;120:135–142.
24. Greenes RA, Shortliffe EH: Medical informatics: an emerging academic discipline and institutional priority. JAMA 1990;263:1114–1120.
25. Friedman CP: Where's the science in medical informatics? J Am Med Inf Assoc 1995;2:65–67.
26. Clayton P: Assessing our accomplishments. Symp Comput Applications Med Care 1991;15:viii–x.
27. Anderson JG, Aydin CE, Jay SE (eds): Evaluating Health Care Information Systems. Thousand Oaks, CA: Sage, 1994.
28. Cohen P: Empirical Methods for Artificial Intelligence. Cambridge, MA: MIT Press, 1995.
29. Jain R: The Art of Computer Systems Performance Analysis. New York: Wiley, 1991.
30. Wyatt JC: Medical informatics: artifacts or science? Meth Inf Med 1996;35:3.

2

Evaluation as a Field

The previous chapter should have succeeded in convincing the reader that evaluation in medical informatics, for all its potential benefits, is difficult in the real world. The informatics community can take some comfort in the fact that it is not alone. Evaluation is difficult in any field of endeavor. Fortunately, many good minds—representing an array of philosophical orientations, methodological perspectives, and domains of application—have explored ways to address these difficulties. Many of the resulting approaches to evaluation have met with substantial success. The resulting range of solutions, the field of evaluation itself, is the focus of this chapter.

If this chapter is successful, the reader will begin to sense some common ground across all evaluation work while simultaneously appreciating the range of tools available. This appreciation is the initial step in recognizing that evaluation, though difficult, is possible.

Evaluation Revisited

For decades, behavioral and social scientists have grappled with the knotty problem of evaluation. As it applies to medical informatics, we can begin to express this problem as the need to answer a basic set of questions. To the inexperienced, these questions might appear deceptively simple.

- An information resource is developed. Is the resource performing as intended? How can it be improved?
- Subsequently, the resource is introduced into a functioning clinical or educational environment. Again, is it performing as intended, and how can it be improved? Does it make any difference in terms of clinical or educational practice? Are the differences it makes beneficial? Are the observed effects those envisioned by the developers or different effects?

Note that we can append "why or why not?" to each of these questions. In actuality, there are many more potentially interesting questions than have been listed here.

Out of this multitude of possible questions comes the first challenge for anyone planning an evaluation: to select the best or most appropriate set of questions to explore a particular situation. This challenge was introduced in Chapter 1 and is reintroduced here. The issue of what can and should be studied is the primary focus of Chapter 3. The questions to study in any particular situation are not inscribed in stone and would probably not be miraculously handed down if one climbed a tall mountain in a thunderstorm. Many more questions can be stated than can be explored; and it is often the case that the most interesting questions reveal their identity only after a study is begun. Further complicating the situation, evaluations are inextricably political. There are legitimate differences of opinion over the relative importance of particular questions. Before any data are collected, those conducting an evaluation may find themselves in the role of referee between competing views and interests as to what should be on the table.

Even when the questions can be stated in advance, with consensus that they are the "right" questions, they can be difficult to answer persuasively. Some would be easy to answer if we possessed a unique kind of time machine which might be called an "evaluation machine." As shown in Figure 2.1, the evaluation machine would enable us to see how our clinical environment would appear if our resource had never been introduced. By comparing real history with the fabrication created by the evaluation machine, we could potentially draw accurate conclusions about the effects of the resource. Even if we had an evaluation machine, however, it could not solve all our problems. It could not tell us why these effects occurred or how to make the resource better. To obtain this information we would have to communicate directly with many of the actors in our real history to understand how they used the resource and their views of the experience. There is usually more to evaluation than demonstrations of causes and effects.

In part because we do not possess an evaluation machine but also because we need ways to answer additional, important questions for which the machine would be of little help, there can be no single solution to the problem of evaluation. There is, instead, an interdisciplinary field of evaluation with an extensive methodological literature.[1-3] This literature details many diverse approaches to evaluation, all of which are currently in use. We introduce these approaches later in the chapter. These approaches differ in the kinds of questions that are seen as primary, how specific questions get onto the agenda, and the data collection methods ultimately used to answer the questions. In informatics it is important that such a range of methods is available because the questions of interest can vary dramatically: from the focused and outcome-oriented (Does implementation of this system affect morbidity and/or mortality?) to the practical, and market-oriented questions, such as those frequently stated by Barnett.[*]

1. Is the system used by real people for real use with real patients?
2. Is the system being paid for with real money?

---

[*] These questions were given to the authors in a personal communication on December 8, 1995. A slightly different version of these questions is found in Blum[4] on page 286.

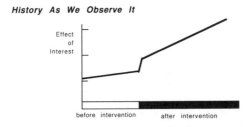

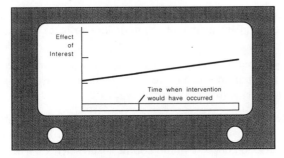

FIGURE 2.1. Hypothetical "evaluation machine."

3. Has someone else taken the system, modified it, and claimed they developed it?

Evaluation is challenging in large part because there are so many options and there is almost never an obvious best way to proceed. The following points bear repeating.

1. In any evaluation setting, there are many potential questions to address. What is asked shapes (but does not totally determine) what is answered.
2. There may be little consensus on what constitutes the best set of questions.
3. There are many ways to address these questions, each with advantages and disadvantages.
4. There is no such thing as a perfect study.

Individuals conducting evaluations are in a continuous process of compromise and accommodation. The challenge of evaluation, at its root, is to collect and communicate useful information while acting in this spirit of compromise and accommodation.

Deeper Definitions of Evaluation

Not surprisingly, there is no single accepted definition of evaluation. A useful goal for the reader may be to evolve a personal definition that makes sense, can be concisely articulated, and can be publicly defended without obvious embarrassment. We advise the reader not to settle firmly on a definition now. It is likely to change, many times, based on later chapters of this book and other experiences. To begin development of a personal definition, we offer three discrete definitions from the evaluation literature and some analyses of their similarities and differences. All three of these definitions have been modified to apply specifically to medical informatics.

Definition 1 (adapted from Rossi and Freeman[1]): Evaluation is the systematic application of social research procedures to judge and improve the way information resources are designed and implemented.

Definition 2 (adapted from Guba and Lincoln[3]): Evaluation is the process of describing the implementation of an information resource and judging its merit and worth.

Definition 3 (adapted from House[2]): Evaluation leads to the settled opinion that something about an information resource is the case, usually but not always leading to a decision to act in a certain way.

The first definition of evaluation is probably the most mainstream. It ties evaluation to the empirical methods of the social sciences. How restrictive this is depends, of course, on one's definition of the social sciences. The authors of this definition would certainly believe that it includes experimental and quasi-experimental methods that result in quantitative data. Judging from the contents of their book, the authors probably do not see the more qualitative, observational methods derived from ethnography and social anthropology as highly useful in evaluation studies.* Their definition further implies that evaluations are carried out in a planned, orderly manner, and that the information collected can engender two types of results: improvement of the resource and some determination of its value.

The second definition is somewhat broader. It identifies descriptive questions (How is the resource being used?) as an important component of evaluation while implying the need for a complete evaluation to result in some type of judgment. This definition is not as restrictive in terms of the methods used to collect information. This openness is intentional, as these authors embrace the full gamut of methodologies, from the experimental to the anthropological.

The third definition is the least restrictive and emphasizes evaluation as a process leading to deeper understanding and consensus. Under this definition an evaluation could be successful even if no judgment or action resulted, so long as the study resulted in a clearer or better shared idea by some significant group of individuals regarding the state of affairs surrounding an information resource.

When shaping a personal definition, the reader should keep in mind something implied by the above definitions as a group but not explicitly stated: that evaluation is an empirical process. Data of varying shapes and sizes are always collected. It is also important to view evaluation as a service activity. Evaluation is

---

* The authors state (p. 265) that "assessing impact in ways that are scientifically plausible and that yield relatively precise estimates of net effects requires data that are quantifiable and systematically and uniformly collected."

tied to and shaped by the resource under study. Evaluation is useful to the degree that it sheds light on issues such as the need for, functioning, and utility of the information resource under study.

The Evaluation Mindset: Distinction Between Evaluation and Research

The previous sections probably make evaluation look like a difficult thing to do. If scholars of the field disagree in fundamental ways about what evaluation is and how it should be done, how can relative novices proceed at all, much less with confidence? To address this dilemma we introduce a mindset for evaluation, a general orientation that anyone conducting an evaluation might constructively bring to the undertaking. As we introduce several important characteristics of this mindset, some of the differences between evaluation and research should also come into clearer focus.

1. *Tailor the study to the problem.* Every evaluation is made to order. Evaluation differs profoundly from mainstream views of research in that an evaluation derives importance from the needs of "clients" (those with the "need to know") rather than the unanswered questions of an academic discipline. If an evaluation contributes new knowledge of general importance to an academic discipline, that is a serendipitous by-product.
2. *Collect data useful for making decisions.* As discussed previously, there is no theoretical limit to the questions that can be asked and, consequently, to the data that can be collected in an evaluation study. What is done is determined by the decisions that need ultimately to be made and the information seen as useful to inform these decisions.
3. *Look for intended* and *unintended effects.* Whenever a new information resource is introduced into an environment, there can be many consequences. Only some of them relate to the stated purpose of the resource. During a complete evaluation it is important to look for and document effects that were anticipated as well as those that were not and to continue the study long enough to allow these effects to manifest. The literature of innovation is replete with examples of unintended consequences. During the 1940s rural farmers in Georgia were trained and encouraged to preserve their vegetables in jars in large quantities to ensure they would have a balanced diet throughout the winter. The campaign was so successful that the number of jars on display in the farmers' homes became a source of prestige. Once the jars became a prestige factor, however, the farmers were disinclined to consume them, so the original purpose of the training was subverted.[5] On a topic closer to home, the QWERTY keyboard became a universal standard even though it was actually designed to *slow* typing out of concern for jamming a mechanical device that has long since vanished.[4]
4. *Study the resource while it is under development and after it is installed.* In

general, the decisions evaluation can facilitate are of two types. *Formative* decisions are made as a result of studies undertaken while a resource is under development and these affect the resource before it can probably go on line. *Summative* decisions are made after a resource is installed in its envisioned environment and deal explicitly with how effectively the resource performs in that environment. Often it takes many years for an installed resource to stabilize within an environment. Before conducting the most useful summative studies, it may be necessary for this amount of time to pass.

5. *Study the resource in the laboratory and in the field.* Completely different questions arise when an information resource is still in the laboratory and when it is in the field. In vitro studies, conducted in the developer's laboratory, and in vivo studies, conducted in an ongoing clinical or educational environment, are both important aspects of evaluation.

6. *Go beyond the developer's point of view.* The developers of an information resource usually are empathic only up to a point and are often not predisposed to be detached and objective about *their* system's performance. Those conducting the evaluation often see it as part of their job to get close to the end-user and to portray the resource as the user sees it.[6]

7. *Take the environment into account.* Anyone who conducts an evaluation study must be, in part, an ecologist. The function of an information resource must be viewed as an interaction between the resource, a set of "users" of the resource, and the social/organizational/cultural "context," which does much to determine how work is carried out in that environment. Whether a new resource functions effectively is determined as much by its goodness-of-fit with its environment as by its compliance with the resource designers' operational specifications as measured in the laboratory.

8. *Let the key issues emerge over time.* Evaluation studies are dynamic. The design for an evaluation, as it might be stated in a project proposal, is typically just a starting point. Rarely are the important questions known with total precision or confidence at the outset of a study. In the real world, evaluation designs must be allowed to evolve as the important issues come into focus.

9. *Be methodologically catholic and eclectic.* It is best to derive data collection methods from the questions to be explored, rather than bringing some predetermined methods or instruments to a study. Some questions are better addressed with qualitative data collected through open-ended interviews and observation. Others are better addressed with quantitative data collected via structured questionnaires, patient chart audits, and logs of user behavior. For evaluation, quantitative data are not clearly superior to qualitative data. Most comprehensive studies use data of both types. Accordingly, those who conduct evaluations must know rigorous methods for collection and analysis of both.

This evaluator's mindset is different from that of a traditional researcher. The primary difference is in the binding of the evaluator to a "client," who may be one or two individuals, a large group, or several groups who share a "need to know" but may be interested in many different things. What these clients want to know— not what the evaluator wants to know—largely determines the evaluation's agenda. By contrast, the researcher's allegiance is usually to a focused question or problem. In research a question with no immediate impact on what is done in the world can still be important. Within the evaluation mindset, this is not the case. Although many important scientific discoveries have been accidental, researchers as a rule do not actively seek out unanticipated effects. Evaluators often do. Whereas researchers usually value focus and seek to exclude from a study as many extraneous variables as possible, evaluators seek to be comprehensive. A complete evaluation of a resource focuses on developmental as well as in-use issues. Research laboratory studies often carry more credibility because they are conducted under controlled circumstances and can illuminate cause and effect relatively unambiguously. During evaluation, field studies often carry more credibility because they illustrate more directly the utility of the resource. Researchers can afford to, and often must, lock themselves into a single data collection paradigm. Even within a single study, evaluations often employ many paradigms.

Anatomy of Evaluation Studies

Despite the fact that there are no a priori questions and a plethora of approaches, there are some structural elements that all evaluation studies have in common (Fig. 2.2). As stated above, evaluations are guided by someone's or some group's need to know. No matter who that someone is—the development team, funding agency, or other individuals and groups—the evaluation must begin with a process of negotiation to identify the questions that will be a starting point for the study. The outcomes of these negotiations are an understanding of how the evaluation is to be conducted, usually stated in a written contract or agreement as well as an initial expression of the questions the evaluation seeks to answer. The next element of the study is investigation, the collection of data to address these questions and, depending on the approach selected, possibly other questions that arise during the study. The mechanisms are numerous, ranging from the performance of the resource on a series of benchmark tasks to observation of users working with the resource.

The next element is a mechanism for reporting the information back to the

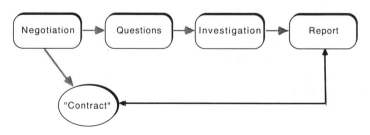

FIGURE 2.2. Anatomy of an evaluation study.

individuals with the need to know. The format of the report must be in line with the stipulations of the contract; the content of the report follows from the questions asked and the data collected. The report is most often a written document but does not have to be. The purposes of some evaluations are well served by oral reports or live demonstrations. We emphasize that it is the evaluator's obligation to establish a process through which the results of his or her study are communicated, thus creating the potential for the study's findings to be put to constructive use. No investigator can guarantee a constructive outcome for a study, but there is much that can be done to increase the likelihood of a salutary result. Also note that a salutary result of a study is not necessarily one that casts the resource under study in a positive light. A salutary result is one where the "stakeholders" learn something important from the study findings.

The diagram of Figure 2.2 may seem unnecessarily complicated to students or researchers who are building their own information resource and wish to evaluate it in a preliminary way. To these individuals we offer a word of caution. Even when they appear simple and straightforward at the outset, evaluations have a way of becoming complex. Much of this book deals with these complexities and how they can be anticipated and managed.

Philosophical Bases of Evaluation

Several authors have developed classifications (or "typologies") of evaluation methods or approaches. Among the best was that developed in 1980 by Ernest House.[2] A major advantage of House's typology is that each approach is elegantly linked to an underlying philosophical model, as detailed in his book. This classification divides current practice into eight discrete approaches, four of which may be viewed as "objectivist" and four "subjectivist." This distinction is important. Note that these approaches are *not* entitled "objective" and "subjective," as those words carry strong and fundamentally misleading connotations: of scientific precision in the former case and of imprecise intellectual voyeurism in the latter.

The objectivist approaches derive from a logical-positivist philosophical orientation—the same orientation that underlies the classical experimental sciences. The major premises underlying the objectivist approaches are as follows.

- In general, attributes of interest are properties of the resource under study. More specifically, this position suggests that the merit and worth of an information resource—the attributes of most interest during the evaluation—can in principle be measured, with all observations yielding the same result. Any discrepancies would be attributed to measurement error. It is also assumed that an investigator can measure these attributes without affecting how the resource under study functions or is used.
- Rational persons can and should agree on what attributes of a resource are important to measure and what results of these measurements would be identified as a most desirable, correct, or positive outcome. In medical informatics,

this premise is tantamount to stating that a gold standard of resource performance can always be identified, and that all rational individuals can be brought to consensus on what this gold standard is.

- Because numerical measurement allows precise statistical analysis of performance over time or performance in comparison with some alternative, numerical measurement is prima facie superior to a verbal description. Qualitative data may be useful in preliminary studies to identify hypotheses for subsequent, precise analysis using quantitative methods.
- Through these kinds of comparisons, it is possible to prove beyond reasonable doubt that a resource is superior to what it replaced or to some competing resource.

Chapters 4–7 of this book address objectivist methods in detail.

Contrast the above with a set of assumptions that derive from an "intuitionist-pluralist" world view that gives rise to a set of subjectivist approaches to evaluation.

- What is observed about a resource depends in fundamental ways on the observer. Different observers of the same phenomenon might legitimately come to different conclusions. Both can be "objective" in their appraisals even if they do not agree. It is not necessary that one is right and the other wrong.
- Merit and worth must be explored in context. The value of a resource emerges through study of the resource as it functions in a particular patient care or educational environment.
- Individuals and groups can legitimately hold different perspectives on what constitutes a gold standard or the most desirable outcome of introducing a resource into an environment. There is no reason to expect them to agree, and it may be counterproductive to try to lead them to consensus. An important aspect of an evaluation would be to document the ways in which they disagree.
- Verbal description can be highly illuminating. Qualitative data are valuable in and of themselves and can lead to conclusions as convincing as those drawn from quantitative data. The value of qualitative data therefore goes far beyond that of identifying issues for later "precise" exploration using quantitative methods.
- Evaluation should be viewed as an exercise in argument, rather than demonstration, because any study, as House[2] pointed out (p. 72), appears equivocal when subjected to serious scrutiny.

The approaches to evaluation that derive from this subjectivist philosophical perspective may seem strange, imprecise, and "unscientific" when considered the first time. This stems in large part from widespread acceptance of the objectivist world view in biomedicine. The importance and utility of subjectivist approaches to evaluation are, however, emerging. Within medical informatics there is growing support for such approaches.[6–8] As stated earlier, the evaluation mindset includes methodological eclecticism. It is important for those trained in classical experimental methods at least to understand, and possibly even embrace, the subjectivist world view if they are going to conduct fully informative evaluation studies. Chapters 8 and 9 of this book address subjectivist approaches in detail.

Multiple Approaches to Evaluation

House[2] classified evaluation into eight approaches, which should be considered archetypes. Although most evaluation studies conducted in the real world can be unambiguously tied to one or a superposition of these approaches, some studies exhibit properties of several approaches and are not cleanly classified. The label "approach" has been deliberately chosen, so it is not confused with "methods." Methods refer specifically to the procedures for collecting and analyzing data, whereas an approach is a broader term connoting the general strategy directing the design and execution of a study. Following this exposition of eight approaches is an exercise for the reader to classify each of a set of evaluation studies in medical informatics into one of these categories.

Objectivist Approaches

The first four approaches derive from the objectivist position.

Comparison-Based Approach

The comparison-based approach employs experiments and quasi-experiments. The information resource under study is compared to a control condition, a placebo, or a contrasting resource. The comparison is based on a relatively small number of "outcome variables" that are assessed in all groups. This approach thus seeks to simulate the "evaluation machine" using randomization, controls, and statistical inference to argue that the information resource was the cause of any differences observed. Examples of comparison-based studies include the work of McDonald et al. on physician reminders[9] and the studies from Stanford on rule-based systems.[10, 11] The 28 controlled trials of medical decision support systems, reviewed by Johnston et al.,[12] fall under the comparison-based approach. The Turing test[13] can be seen as a specific model for a comparison-based evaluation.

Objectives-Based Approach

The objectives-based approach seeks to determine if a resource meets its designers' objectives. Ideally, such objectives are stated in great detail, so there is little ambiguity when developing procedures to measure their degree of attainment. These studies are comparative only in the sense that the observed performance of the resource is viewed in relation to stated objectives. The concern is whether the resource is performing up to expectations, not if the resource is outperforming what it replaced. The objectives that are the benchmarks for these studies are typically stated at an early stage of resource development. Although clearly suited to laboratory testing of a new resource, this approach can also be applied to testing an installed resource. Consider the example of a resource to provide advice to emergency room physicians.[14] The designers might set as an objective that the system's advice be available within 10 minutes of the time the patient is first seen. An evaluation study that measures the time for this advice to be delivered and compares it to this objective would be objectives-based.

Decision Facilitation Approach

With the decision facilitation approach, evaluation seeks to resolve issues important to developers and administrators, so these individuals can make decisions about the future of the resource. The questions posed are those that the decision-makers state, although those conducting the evaluation may help the decision-makers frame these questions so they are more amenable to empirical study. The data collection methods follow from the questions posed. These studies tend to be "formative" in focus. The results of studies conducted at the early stages of resource development are used to chart the course of further development, which in turn generates new questions for further study. A systematic study of alternative formats for computer-generated advisories, conducted while the resource to generate the advisories is still under development, provides a good example of this approach.[15]

Goal-Free Approach

With the three approaches described above, the evaluation is guided by a set of goals for the information resource or specific questions the developers either state or play a profound role in shaping. Therefore any study is polarized by these manifest goals and much more sensitive to anticipated rather than unanticipated effects. With the "goal-free" approach, those conducting the evaluation are purposefully blinded to the intended effects of an information resource and pursue whatever evidence they can gather to enable them to identify all the effects of the resource, regardless of whether intended or not.[16] This approach is rarely applied in practice but is useful to individuals designing evaluations to remind them of the multiplicity of effects an information resource can engender.

Subjectivist Approaches

There are four subjectivist approaches to evaluation.

Quasi-legal Approach

The quasi-legal approach establishes a mock trial or other formal adversary proceeding to judge a resource. Proponents and opponents of the resource offer testimony and may be examined and cross-examined in a manner resembling standard courtroom procedure. A jury witness to the proceeding can then, on the basis of this testimony, make a decision about the merit of the resource. As in a debate, the issue can be decided by the persuasive power of rhetoric as well as the persuasive power of that which is portrayed as fact. There are few examples of this technique formally applied to medical informatics, but the technique has been applied to facilitate difficult decisions in other medical areas.[17]

Art Criticism Approach

The art criticism approach relies on formal methods of criticism and the principle of "connoisseurship."[18] Under this approach, an experienced and respected critic, who may or may not be trained in the domain of the resource but has a great deal of experience with resources of this generic type, works with the resource over a period of time. She or he then writes a review highlighting the benefits and short-comings of the resource. Clearly, the art criticism approach cannot be definitive if the critic is not expert in the subject matter domain of a medical informatics resource, as the critic is then unable to judge the clinical or scientific accuracy of the resource's knowledge base or the advice it provides. Nonetheless, the thoughtful and articulate comments of an experienced reviewer can help others appreciate important features of a resource. Because society does not routinely expect critics to agree, the lack of interobserver agreement does not invalidate this approach. Although they tend to be more informal and tend to reflect less direct experience with the resource than would be the case in a complete "art criticism" study, software reviews that routinely appear in technical journals and magazines are examples of this approach in common practice.

Professional Review Approach

The professional review approach is the well-known "site visit" approach to evaluation. It employs panels of experienced peers who spend several days in the environment where the resource is installed. Site visits are often guided by a set of guidelines specific to the type of project under study but sufficiently generic to accord the reviewers a great deal of control over the conduct of any particular visit. They are generally free to speak with whomever they wish and to ask of these individuals whatever they consider it is important to know. They may request documents for review. Over the course of a site visit, unanticipated issues may emerge. Site visit teams frequently have interim meetings to identify these emergent questions and generate ways to explore them. As a field matures, it becomes possible to articulate guidelines that could be the focus of site visits, supporting application of the professional review approach. In medical informatics, the evolving evaluation criteria for computer-based patient records[19] are one example of such guidelines.

Responsive/Illuminative Approach

 The responsive/illuminative approach seeks to represent the viewpoints of those who are users of the resource or an otherwise significant part of the clinical environment where the resource operates.[20] The goal is understanding, or "illumination," rather than judgment. The methods used derive largely from ethnography. The investigators immerse themselves in the environment where the resource is operational. The designs of these studies are not rigidly predetermined. They develop dynamically as the investigators' experience accumulates. The study team begins with a minimal set of orienting questions; the deeper questions that receive thoroughgoing study evolve over time. Many examples of studies using this approach can be found in the literature of medical informatics.[21-23]

Self-Test 2.1

The answers to these exercises appear at the end of this chapter.

1. Associate each of the following hypothetical studies with a particular approach to evaluation:
   a. A comparison of different user interfaces for a computer-based medical record system, conducted while the system is under development.
   b. A site visit by the U.S. National Library of Medicine's Biomedical Library Review Committee to the submitters of a competing renewal of a research grant.
   c. Inviting a noted consultant on user interface design to spend a day on campus to offer suggestions regarding the prototype of a new system.
   d. Conducting patient chart reviews before and after introduction of an information resource without telling the reviewer anything about the nature of the information resource or even that the intervention was an information resource.
   e. Videotaping attending rounds on a service where a knowledge resource has been implemented and periodically interviewing members of the ward team.
   f. Determining if a new version of a resource executes a standard set of performance tests at the speed the designers projected.
   g. Randomizing patients so their medical records are maintained, either by a new computer system or standard procedures, and then seeking to determine if the new system affects clinical protocol recruitment and compliance.
   h. Staging a mock debate at a research group retreat.

Why Are There So Many Approaches?

From the above examples, it should be clear that it is possible to employ almost all of these approaches to evaluation in medical informatics. Why, though, are there so many approaches to evaluation? The intuitive appeal—at least to those schooled in experimental science—of the comparison-based approach seems unassailable. Why do it any other way if we can demonstrate the value of a medical information resource, or lack thereof, definitively with a controlled study?

The goal-free approach signals one shortcoming of comparison-based studies that employ classical experimental methods. Although these studies can appear definitive when proposed, they inevitably rely on intuitive, arbitrary, or political choice of questions to explore or outcomes to measure. What *is* measured is often what *can be* measured with the kind of quantitative precision the philosophical position underlying this approach demands. It is often the case that the variables that are most readily obtainable and most accurately assessed (e.g., length of hospital stay), and which therefore are employed as outcome measures in studies, are difficult to relate directly to the effects of a medical information resource because there are numerous intervening factors. Studies may have null results, not because there are no effects but because these effects are not manifested in the general or global outcome measures pursued. In other circumstances, outcomes cannot be unambiguously assigned a positive value. For example, if use of a computer-based tutorial program is found to raise students' national licensure examination scores, which are readily obtained and highly reliable, it usually does not settle the argument about the value of this resource. It merely kindles a new argument about the validity of the examination used as an outcome measure. In the most general case, a resource can produce several effects: some positive and some negative. Unless the reasons for these mixed effects can somehow be further explored, the total impact of a resource cannot be understood or may be seriously misestimated.

Consider, for example, a resource developed to identify "therapeutic misadventures"—problems with drug therapy of hospitalized patients—before these problems can become medical emergencies.[24] Such a resource would employ a knowledge base encoding rules of proper therapeutic practice and would be connected to a hospital information system containing the clinical data about inpatients. When the resource detected a difference between the rules of proper practice and the data about a specific patient, it would issue an advisory to the clinicians responsible for the care of that patient. If comparison-based study of this system's effectiveness employed only global outcome measures, such as length of stay or morbidity and mortality, and the study yielded null results, it would not be clear what to conclude. It may be that the resource is having no beneficial effect, but it may also be that a problem with the implementation of the system—which, if detected, can be rectified—is accounting for the null results. The failure of ward clerks to place the advisories in a visible place in a timely fashion could account for an apparent dysfunction of the resource. In this case, a study using the decision facilitation approach or the responsive/illuminative approach might reveal the problem with the resource and, from the perspective of the evaluator's mindset, be a much more valuable study.

Other reasons many evaluation approaches exist and should be employed stem from specific features of the information resources that are studied and from the challenges, as discussed in Chapter 1, of studying these resources. First, medical information resources are frequently revised; the system may change in significant ways, for legitimate reasons, before there is time to complete a comparison-based study. Second, subjectivist approaches are well suited to developing an understanding of how the resource works within a particular environment. The success or failure may be attributable more to match or mismatch with the environment than intrinsic properties of the resource itself. Without such understanding it is difficult to know how exportable a particular resource is and what factors are important to explore as the resource is considered for adoption by a site other than the place of its development. Third, there is need to understand how users employ medical information resources, which requires an exercise in description, not judgment or comparison. If the true benefits of information and knowledge resources emerge from interaction of person and machine, approaches to evaluation that can take the idiosyncratic nature of human cognition into account must figure into a complete set of investigative activities. Finally, subjectivist approaches also offer a unique contribution in their ability to help us understand *why* something happened in addition to *that* something happened. The results of a comparison-based study may be definitive in demonstrating that a resource had a specific impact on patient care, but these results may tell us little about what aspect of the resource made the difference or about the chain of events through which this effect was achieved.

This section spoke primarily in defense of the subjectivist methods, but only because their validity is not commonly accepted in the biomedical settings of which medical informatics is a part. The section should be interpreted, above all, as another plea for catholicism, for open-mindedness, suggesting that a mode of study from which something important can be learned is a mode of study worth pursuing. For evaluation, we cannot give any particular method of study higher status than the problem under study.

Roles in Evaluation Studies

Another important way to see the complexity of evaluation is via the multiple roles that are played in the conduct of a study. A review of these roles is useful to help understand the process of evaluation and to help those who are planning studies to anticipate everything that needs to be done. At the earliest stage of planning a study, and particularly when the evaluation contract is being negotiated, attention to these roles and their interworkings helps ensure that the contract will be complete and will serve well in guiding the conduct of the study.

The roles and how they interrelate are illustrated in Figure 2.3. It is important to note from the outset of this discussion that the same individual may play multiple roles, and some roles are shared by multiple individuals. The smaller the scale of the study, the greater is the overlap in roles.

The first set of roles relates to the individuals who conduct the study. These individuals include the director of the evaluation who is the person professionally responsible for the study, and any staff members who might work for the director. As soon as more than one person is involved in the conduct of a study, interper-

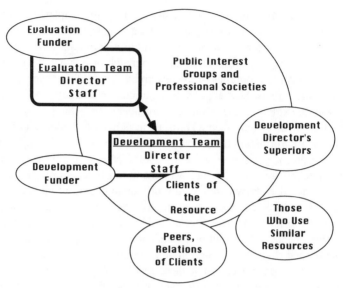

FIGURE 2.3. Roles in an evaluation study.

sonal dynamics among members of this group become an important factor contributing to the success or failure of the study.

There is a separate set of roles related directly to the development of the resource under study. Those who fulfill these roles include the director of the resource's development team, his or her staff, and the clients of the resource. There are two potential client groups: those who use the resource (e.g., health care professionals) and those whose interests the resource directly serves (e.g., patients).

The third set of roles includes individuals or groups (or both) who, although they are not developing the resource or are direct participants in the evaluation study, nonetheless may have a profound interest in the study's outcome. In the jargon of evaluation, these individuals are generally known as "stakeholders." These individuals or groups include those who fund the development of the resource, funders of the evaluation (who may be different from the funders of the resource), supervisors of the director of development of the resource, those who use similar resources in other settings, peers and relations of the clients, and a variety of public and political groups with interest in the resource or the results of studying its effects.

At the first stage of planning a study, it is an excellent idea to make a list of these roles and indicate which individuals or groups occupy each one. Sometimes it requires a few educated guesses, but the exercise should still be undertaken at the outset.

Self-Test 2.2

Below is a description of the evaluation plan for the T-HELPER project at Stanford University.[25, 26] This description is intentionally incomplete for purposes of constructing a practice exercise. After reading the description, answer each of the following questions. [Answers to questions 1 and 2 are found at the end of this chapter.]

1. Indicate who, in this study, played each of the roles discussed above and depicted in Figure 2.3.
2. The project evaluation focuses on two questions relating to protocol enrollment and user attitudes. If you were designing an evaluation to address these questions, what approach(es) would you consider using?
3. What other evaluation questions, not addressed in the study, might have been of interest for this project?

Case Study: T-HELPER: Computer Support for Protocol-Directed Therapy

This project developed computer-based techniques for clinical data and knowledge management in the area of acquired immunodeficiency syndrome (AIDS) therapy and to implement those methods in a system that can be used for patient care and that can be evaluated in clinical settings. Clinicians used the new system, called THERAPY-HELPER (or simply T-HELPER) to review and maintain the records of patients receiving protocol-directed therapy for human immunodeficiency virus (HIV) disease. The entire effort was supported by a 5-year grant to Stanford University from the Agency for Health Care Policy and Research.

The project was conducted in four stages:

1. T-HELPER I was developed to facilitate a data-management environment for patients with HIV infection. T-HELPER I provided a graphical medical record that allowed health care workers to review past data and to enter new information while perusing textual information regarding those protocols under which the patient is being treated or for which the patient might be eligible.
2. T-HELPER II, an enhanced version of T-HELPER I, incorporated active decision-support capabilities to encourage enrollment in and compliance with protocol-based therapy.
3. T-HELPER I and T-HELPER II were installed at two large county-operated AIDS clinics in northern California: the Immunocompromised Host Clinic at ABC Medical Center and the XYZ AIDS program.
4. A rigorous evaluation of the T-HELPER systems was undertaken. The studies explored the effect of each version of the system on (1) the rate of patient enrollment in clinical trial protocols, and (2) physician satisfaction with the T-HELPER system. The study design allowed assessment of the incremental value of the decision-support functions provided in T-HELPER II.

1. *Development group:* The project was divided into three general areas of effort: (1) system development (supervised by Dr. M); (2) system installation and user training (supervised by Dr. F); and (3) system evaluation (supervised by Dr. C). The project was

under the overall supervision of Dr. M. Several research staff members and graduate students were employed over the 5 years on various aspects of the project.

2. *Trial/evaluation sites:* ABC Medical Center is a 722-bed facility and a teaching hospital of the Stanford University School of Medicine. At the outset of the project, six HIV-related protocols from the California Cooperative Treatment Group (CCTG) were operative at this center. In addition, a number of privately sponsored protocols were in progress. Twenty-eight percent of HIV-infected residents in its home county seek care at ABC, a group that is estimated to be 22% Hispanic, 8% African-American, 9% female, and 14% intravenous (IV) drug users. At the project outset, the XYZ AIDS clinic provided care to an estimated 377 HIV-infected patients annually. The patient population was approximately 33% African-American, 16% Hispanic, 24% women, and 36% IV drug users.

3. *System installation:* Full utilization of the T-HELPER system required three main logistical requirements: (1) building local area networks in the two clinics, (2) interfacing with the registration systems at each clinic, and (3) arranging for laboratory data connections. The local area network is necessary to allow health care providers to use the system in multiple locations throughout the clinic. A fully wired clinic allowed for workstations in each examination room, in each provider workroom, and in the nursing and registration work areas. Registration data connections were necessary to simplify the entry of demographic data into T-HELPER and provide data about which patients are active in the clinic at a particular time. Laboratory data were required to provide input to the decision-support modules and to give additional clinical information to providers that would help attract users to the workstation to complete their paperwork. Each installation site expressed concerns for patient data confidentiality. This concern meant that the network installations had to be stand-alone and would not have any connectivity to other networked environments. Furthermore, because of differences in networking technology, it was not practical to directly link the T-HELPER local area network with the existing computer systems at each site. Instead, special-purpose point-to-point links were made to the registration and laboratory systems at ABC and XYZ.

4. *System evaluation:* The primary goal of the evaluation was to determine if the T-HELPER II system increased the rate of accrual of eligible and potentially eligible patients to protocols. In addition, the evaluation group examined physicians' knowledge and acceptance of the computer as an adjunct to patient care and in collaborative research. It then correlated these attitudes with use of and compliance with the T-HELPER systems.

Why It May Not Work Out as the Books Suggest

If we did possess an evaluation machine, life would be easier but not perfect. We would design and implement our information resources, let the machine tell us what would have happened had the resource not been implemented, and then compare the two scenarios. The difference would, of course, be a measure of the "effect" of the resource, but there may be many other factors, not detectable by the machine, that are important to investigate. We have seen throughout this chapter how the unavailability of the evaluation machine and other factors have led many creative individuals to devise a wide assortment of evaluation approaches. The richness and diversity of these approaches make it safe to say that an informative study can probably be designed to address any question of substantive interest in informatics.

Obviously, not every question can be formally investigated, and not every question should be. Still, sometimes questions that should be investigated are not, and sometimes otherwise well designed studies run amok. What goes wrong and what can be done about it?

There are two main reasons why deserving studies are not carried out. In both cases we see that attention to the roles in an evaluation (Fig. 2.3) and the importance of advance negotiation of an evaluation contract can both signal problems and help the study designers navigate through them.

- *Sometimes we'd rather not know* or *fear of the clear:* Some, perhaps many, resource developers believe they have more to lose than to gain from a thoroughgoing study of their resource. This possibility is more likely in the case of a resource perceived to be functioning successfully or one that generates a great deal of interest because of some novel technology it employs. There are three logical counterarguments to this viewpoint: (1) the perception of the resource's success may not be substantiated by the data; (2) the study, if it supports these perceptions, can show how and perhaps why the resource is successful; and (3) a study would generate information leading to improvement of even the most successful resource. With reference to Figure 2.3, stakeholders outside the development team can bring pressure on the resource developers to initiate a study, but studies carried out under these circumstances tend to progress with great difficulty. Trust typically does not exist between the evaluation team and the development team. However difficult it may be to accomplish, the evaluation contract must be specific, or it will usually not be possible to complete the study.
- *Differences in values:* Performance of an evaluation often requires the resource developers to engage in tasks they would not normally undertake; at a minimum it requires some modifications in the project's implementation timeline. If the development group does not value the information they obtain from a study, they may, for example, be unwilling to await the results of a study before designing some aspect of the resource that could be shaped by these results, or they may be reluctant to freeze the production version of a system long enough for a study to be completed. Underlying differences in values may also be revealed as a form of perfectionism. The resource developers or other stakeholders may argue that less-than-perfect information is of no utility because it cannot be trusted. ("Indeed, if all evaluations are equivocal when subjected to serious scrutiny, why bother?") Because everyone on earth makes important decisions based on imperfect information every day, such a statement is usually not meant to be taken literally but as a reflection of a belief that a study is not justified by the results that will be generated. Some differences in belief can be reconciled, others cannot.

The potential for these clashes of values to occur underscores the importance of the negotiations leading to an evaluation contract. If these negotiations come to a halt over a specific issue, it may be indicative of a gap in values that cannot be spanned, making the study impossible in the end. On the other hand, the evaluators must respect the values of the developers and design studies that have minimal detrimental impact on the developmental activities and timeline. We underscore that it is the responsibility of the evaluation team and study director to identify these potential value differences and to initiate a collaborative effort to address them by way of generating an evaluation contract. The evaluation team should not expect the system developers to initiate such efforts and under no circumstances should they defer resolution of such issues in the interest of getting a study started. When the development and evaluation teams overlap, the problem is no less sticky and requires no less attention. In this case, individuals and groups may find themselves internally conflicted unless they undertake conversations among themselves, alternating between the developers' and the evaluators' positions, about how to resolve value differences imposed by the conduct of an study in the context of resource development.

When evaluation works well, as it often does, the development and evaluation teams perceive each other as part of a common enterprise, with shared goals and interests. Communication is honest and frequent. Because no evaluation contract can anticipate every problem that may arise during the conduct of a study, problems are resolved through open discussion, using the evaluation contract as a basis. Most problems are resolved through compromise.

Conclusion

Evaluation, like medical informatics itself, is a derivative field. What is done—the specific questions asked and the data collected to illuminate these questions—derives from what interested individuals want to know. In Chapter 3 we present a catalog of evaluation questions pertinent to medical informatics in order to give enhanced shape and substance to our often-repeated claim about the large numbers of questions that exist. We also present a typology of the "kinds" of studies people in informatics tend to undertake. These catalogs and typologies are too general to offer more than a first level of guidance to designers of a study. The real issues emerge from knowledge of the resource in question and the environment, if any, into which the resource is being placed.

Food for Thought

To deepen your understanding of the concepts presented in this and the previous chapter, you may wish to consider the following questions:

1. Are there any a priori evaluation questions in medical informatics or questions that must be a part of every evaluation?
2. In your opinion, what is the difference between research and evaluation in medical informatics?
3. Do you believe that independent, unbiased observers of the same behavior or outcome should agree on the *quality* of that outcome?

4. Many of the evaluation approaches assert that a single unbiased observer is a legitimate source of information during an evaluation, even if that observer's data or judgments are unsubstantiated by others. What are some examples in our society where we vest important decisions in a single experienced and presumed impartial individual?

5. Do you agree with the statement that all evaluations appear equivocal when subjected to serious scrutiny?

Answers to Self-Tests

Self-Test 2.1

Question 1
   a. Decision-facilitation
   b. Professional review
   c. Art criticism
   d. Goal free
   e. Responsive/illuminative
   f. Objectives-based
   g. Comparison-based
   h. Quasi-legal

Self-Test 2.2

1. *Evaluation funder:* Agency for Health Care Policy and Research. *Evaluation team:* Director was Dr. C with unnamed staff. *Development funder:* Agency for Health Care Policy and Research. *Development team:* Director was Dr. M. (subdivided into two groups under Dr. M and Dr. F). *Clients:* The care providers at ABC and XYZ as well as the patients with HIV who use these facilities. *Development director's superiors:* Unnamed individuals at Stanford University who direct the center or department in which the project was based. *Peers, relations of clients:* Friends and relatives of HIV patients, and care providers, at the two clinics. *Those who use similar resources:* The community of care providers who work with HIV patients who are on clinical protocols. *Public interest groups and professional societies:* The full gamut of patient support and advocacy groups as well as professional societies relating to AIDS/HIV.

2. The first evaluation question, as stated, seems based suited to a comparison-based approach. The second question could be addressed by the comparison-based approach as well but would also be well served by a subjectivist, responsive/illuminative approach. Note that because this study was federally sponsored, the professional review approach may also have been used, as it is

not unusual for a project of this duration and extent to be site-visited at some point.

References

1. Rossi PH, Freeman HE: Evaluation: A Systematic Approach. Newbury Park, CA: Sage, 1989.
2. House ER: Evaluating with Validity. Beverly Hills: Sage, 1980.
3. Guba EG, Lincoln YS: Effective Evaluation. San Francisco: Jossey-Bass, 1981.
4. Blum BI: Clinical Information Systems. New York: Springer-Verlag, 1986.
5. Rogers EM, Shoemaker FF: Communication of Innovations. New York: Free Press, 1971.
6. Forsythe DE, Buchanan BG: Broadening our approach to evaluating medical information systems. Symp Comput Applications Med Care 1992;16:8–12.
7. Anderson JG, Aydin CE, Jay SJ (eds): Computers in Health Care: Research and Evaluation. Newbury Park, CA: Sage, 1995.
8. Rothschild MA, Swett HA, Fisher PR, Weltin GG, Miller PL: Exploration of subjective vs. objective issues in the validation of computer-based critiquing advice. Comput Method Programs Biomed 1990;31:11–18.
9. McDonald CJ, Hui SL, Smith DM, et al: Reminders to physicians from an introspective computer medical record: a two-year randomized trial. Ann Intern Med 1984;100:130–138.
10. Yu VL, Fagan LM, Wraith SM, et al: Antimicrobial selection by computer: a blinded evaluation by infectious disease experts. JAMA 1979;242:1279–1282.
11. Hickam D, Shortliffe EH, Bischoff M, et al: The treatment advice of a computer-based cancer chemotherapy protocol advisor. Ann Intern Med 1985;103:928–936.
12. Johnston ME, Langton KB, Haynes RB, Matthieu D: A critical appraisal of research on the effects of computer-based decision support systems on clinician performance and patient outcomes. Ann Intern Med 1994;120:135–142.
13. Turing AM: Computing machinery and intelligence. Mind Q Rev Psychol Philos 1950;59:433–460.
14. Wyatt J: Lessons learned from the field trial of ACORN, an expert system to advise on chest pain. In: Barber B, Cao D, Qin D (eds) Proceedings of the Sixth World Conference on Medical Informatics, Singapore. Amsterdam: North Holland, 1989:111–115.
15. De Bliek R, Friedman CP, Speedie SM, Blaschke TF, France CL: Practitioner preferences and receptivity for patient-specific advice from therapeutic monitoring system. Symp Comput Applications Med Care 1988;12:225–228.
16. Scriven M: Goal free evaluation. In: House ER (ed) School Evaluation. Berkeley, CA: McCutchan, 1973.
17. Smith R: Using a mock trial to make a difficult clinical decision. BMJ 1992;305:284–287.
18. Eisner EW: The Enlightened Eye: Qualitative Inquiry and the Enhancement of Educational Practice. New York: Macmillan, 1991.
19. CPR Systems Evaluation Work Group: Draft CPR Project Evaluation Criteria, 1994 (available from the Computer-based Patient Record Institute, 919 N. Michigan Avenue, Chicago, IL 60611).
20. Hamilton D, MacDonald B, King C, Jenkins D, Parlett M (eds): Beyond the Numbers Game. Berkeley, CA: McCutchan, 1977.

21. Kaplan B, Duchon D: Combining qualitative and quantitative methods in information systems research: a case study. MIS Quarterly 1988;4 :571–586.
22. Fafchamps D, Young CY, Tang PC: Modelling work practices: input to the design of a physician's workstation. Symp Comput Applications Med Care 1991;15:788–792.
23. Forsythe D: Using ethnography to build a working system: rethinking basic design assumptions. Symp Comput Applications Med Care 1992;16:505–509.
24. Speedie SM, Skarupa S, Oderda L, et al: MENTOR: continuously monitoring drug therapy with an expert system. MEDINFO 1986:237–239.
25. Musen MA, Carlson RW, Fagan LM, Deresinski SC, Shortliffe EH: T-HELPER: automated support for community-based clinical research. Symp Comput Applications Med Care 1992;16:719–723.
26. Musen MA: Computer Support for Protocol-Directed Therapy. Final Report of AHCPR Grant HS06330, August 1995.

3

Studying Clinical Information Resources

In Chapter 1 we introduced the challenge of conducting evaluations in medical informatics and discussed specific sources of complexity that give rise to these challenges. In Chapter 2 we introduced the range of approaches that can be used to conduct evaluations in medical informatics and across many areas of human endeavor. Chapter 2 also stressed that the evaluator can address many of these challenges by viewing each evaluation as anchored by specific purposes. Each study is conducted for some identifiable client group, often to inform specific decisions that must be made by members of that group. The work of the evaluator is made possible by focusing on the specific purposes the particular study is designed to address, often framing them as a set of questions and choosing the approach or approaches best suited to those purposes. A study is successful if it provides credible information to help members of an identified audience make decisions.

In this chapter the focus returns to informatics per se as we explore the specific purposes of evaluation studies of clinical information resources. The emphasis changes from *how* to study to *what* to study. Whereas in Chapter 2 we provided a tour of the various evaluation approaches, in this chapter we provide a tour of evaluation purposes ranging from validation of the resource design process to exploration of the impact of the resource on clinical outcomes after it is deployed in a health care setting. We also introduce the characteristics of clinical information resources that can be studied. Although the title of this chapter implies that we do, and the chapter largely does, address clinical resources, much of what follows applies to resources supporting education, administration, and biomedical research as well.

At this point the reader may be concerned that this book, at least Chapters 1–3, is merely a catalog or listing of everything that can be done, with no clear guidance about to how to choose what to study (and with what methods) in any particular situation. This concern is legitimate. To address the concern in part, this chapter closes with some general strategies employed by experienced evaluators to match studies to situations, but in the end the decision of what to study and how is exquisitely sensitive to each study's special circumstances. As we stated earlier, every evaluation must be custom-designed. Our "cataloguing" approach, by alerting the reader to all of the options broken down into logical groupings, can simplify the evaluation design process by allowing the novice evaluator to choose options from a list rather than having to invent them. This strategy also helps ensure that important possibilities are not overlooked. Even experienced investigators wrestle with the problem of deciding what to study and how. There is, unfortunately, no formula.

Full Range of What Can Be Studied

When evaluating a medical information resource, there are five major aspects of interest: the clinical need the resource is intended to address, the process used to develop the resource; the resource's intrinsic structure; the functions it carries out; and its impact on users, patients, and other aspects of the clinical environment. In a theoretically "complete" evaluation, separate studies of a particular resource might address each aspect. In the real world, however, it is difficult to be so comprehensive. Over the course of its development and deployment a resource may be studied many times, with the studies in their totality touching on many or most of these aspects; but few resources are completely studied, and many inevitably are studied in a partial way.

The evaluation focus changes as one studies the various aspects.

1. *Need for the resource:* Evaluators study the clinical status quo absent the resource: the nature of problems the resource is intended to address and how frequently these problems arise.
2. *Development process:* Evaluators study the skills of the development team and the methodologies they employed to understand if the design is likely to be sound.
3. *Resource's intrinsic structure:* The focus of the evaluation includes specifications, flow charts, program code, and other representations of the resource that can be inspected without actually running it.
4. *Resource's functions:* The focus is how the resource performs when it is used.
5. *Resource's impact:* The focus switches from the resource itself to its impact on users, patients, and health care organizations.

Several key factors characterize an evaluation study.

- *Focus of study:* As discussed above, the focus can be the status quo before introducing the information resource, the design process adopted, the resource's structure or function, the resource users' simulated decisions or real decisions, the clinical actions, and patient outcomes once the resource is made available in their place of work.
- *Study setting:* Studies of the design process, the resource's structure, and the resource's functions are best conducted outside the active clinical environment, in a "laboratory" setting. Studies to elucidate the need for a resource and studies of its impact on users would usually take place in real clinical settings. The same is true for studies of the impact of a resource on patients and health

care organizations, which can take place only in a true clinical setting where the resource is available for use at the time and where patient management decisions are made.

- *Clinical data employed:* For many studies the resource is actually "run." It requires clinical data, which can be simulated (not based on real patients), abstracted from real patients' records, or patient data. Clearly, the kind of data employed in a study has serious implications for the study results and the conclusions that can be drawn from them.

- *User of the resource:* Most information resources interact with one or more "users." In any particular study, the users of the resource can be members of the development team, the evaluation team, or other individuals not representative of those who will interact with the resource after it is deployed. Alternatively, the users in a study could be representative of the end-users for whose use the resource is ultimately designed. Again, the selection of resource users can affect study results profoundly.

- *Decisions affected by use of the resource:* Many information resources, by providing information or advice to clinicians, seek to influence the decisions made by these clinicians. As a study moves from the laboratory to the clinical setting, the information provided by the resource potentially has greater implications for the decisions being made. Depending on a study's design and purposes, perhaps no actual decisions are affected, perhaps only simulated decisions are affected (clinicians are asked what they "would" do, but no action is taken), or perhaps real decisions involving the care of patients are affected.

Taking these factors into account, Table 3.1 lists eight broad types of studies of clinical information resources that can be conducted, the focus of each type, the setting in which it occurs, the kind of clinical data employed as "input" to the resource, who uses the resource during the study, and the kinds of clinical decisions affected by the resource during the study. For example, a "laboratory user impact" study would be conducted outside the active clinical environment using simulated or abstracted clinical data. Although it would involve individuals representative of the "end-user" population, the primary results of the study would derive from simulated clinical decisions, so the clinical care of patients would not be affected by a study of this type. The reader may wish, similarly, to read across each row of the table to obtain an understanding of the contrasts among these study types. Self-Test 3.1 provides an opportunity to explore these contrasts.

Note that the study "types" given in Table 3.1 relate to the purposes, foci, settings, and logistics of evaluation studies. The evaluation approaches introduced in Chapter 2 address a complementary issue: What methods are to be used to identify specific questions and collect data as part of the conduct of these studies. Although it is perhaps extreme to state that every evaluation approach can apply to every type of study, there is certainly potential to use both objectivist and subjectivist approaches throughout Table 3.1. At the two extremes, for example, and as we shall see later, "need validation" studies and "clinical impact" studies provide opportunities to apply both subjectivist and objectivist approaches. The following sections of this chapter expand on the study types given in Table 3.1.

TABLE 3.1. Generic types of evaluation studies of clinical information resources

Type of study	Focus of study	Study setting	Kind of patient data	User of resource	Clinical decisions affected by use of the resource
Need validation	Status quo	Field	Real data	None	None
Design validation	Resource design process	Laboratory	None	None	None
Structure validation	Resource structure	Laboratory	None	None	None
Laboratory function	Resource function	Laboratory	Simulated or abstracted data	Developer, evaluator, or clinician	None
Field function	Resource function	Field	Real data	Developer, evaluator, or clinician	None
Laboratory user impact	Simulated decisions	Laboratory	Simulated or abstracted data	Clinician	Clinicians' simulated decisions
Field user impact	Simulated decisions	Field	Real data	Clinician	Clinicians' simulated decisions
Clinical impact	Patient care and outcomes	Field	Real data	Clinician	Clinicians' real decisions

Self-Test 3.1

For each of the following hypothetical evaluation scenarios, list which of the eight types of studies listed above in Table 3.1 they include. Some scenarios may include more than one type of study.

1. An order communication system is implemented in a small hospital. Changes in laboratory workload are assessed.
2. A study team performs a thorough analysis of the information required by psychiatrists to whom patients are referred by a community social worker.
3. A medical informatics expert is asked for her opinion about a PhD project. She requests copies of the student's code and documentation for review.
4. A new intensive care unit system is implemented alongside manual paper charting for a month. At the end of this time, the quality of the computerized data and data recorded on the paper charts is compared. A panel of intensivists is asked to identify, independently, episodes of hypotension from each data set.
5. A medical informatics professor is invited to join the steering group for a clinical workstation project in a local hospital. The only documentation available to critique at the first meeting is a statement of the project goal, description of the planned development method, and the advertisements and job descriptions for team members.
6. Developers invite clinicians to test a prototype of a computer-aided learning system as part of a user-centered design workshop
7. A program is devised that generates a predicted 24-hour blood glucose profile using seven clinical parameters. Another program uses this profile and other

patient data to advise on insulin dosages. Diabetologists are asked to prescribe insulin for the patient given the 24-hour profile alone and again after seeing the computer-generated advice. They are also asked their opinion of the advice.

8. A program to generate drug interaction alerts is installed in a geriatric clinic that already has a computer-based medical record system. Rates of clinically significant drug interactions are compared before and after installation of the alerting program.

Studying and Defining the Need for an Information Resource

The success of any clinical information resource depends on how well it fulfills a clinical need, assuming there is one.[1] Usually, before developers start to design an information resource, someone (often a representative of the potential user community) has identified an information management problem amenable to a computer-based solution. Sometimes, particularly with the newer information technology, the project is initiated by the developers without a clinical need; a suitable demonstration site is then located. Usually, the project deteriorates from this point as the developer tries to persuade the increasingly mystified clinicians of the potential of their breakthrough, but no one is sure of the need for the resource. Thus, defining the need for an information resource before it is developed is an important precursor to a development project.

Let us say, for the sake of argument, that a clinician notices that the postoperative infection rate on a certain ward is high, and that junior doctors seem to be failing to prescribe the prophylactic antibiotics that are known to be effective. The clinician may merely note the problem or try to define and study the need more precisely. In increasing order of complexity, he or she may discuss the problem with colleagues, conduct a wider survey to explore the extent of the perceived problem, or conduct a systematic evaluation of current clinical practices to document the problem objectively. The latter would include carefully defining what constitutes a postoperative infection (e.g., does it include chest infections as well as wound infections?) and then conducting an audit of postoperative infections and the drugs prescribed before and after surgery.

Defining the problem is insufficient, however, to justify a specific solution, such as an antibiotic reminder system. The system users and the developers of an information resource need to choose the appropriate kind of information to provide (advice to prescribe an appropriate antibiotic stocked on the ward), the appropriate time it is to be delivered (6 hours before to 2 hours after surgery), and the appropriate mode of delivery (advice on-screen to the resident or intern, or a printed reminder affixed to the front of the case record). Unless this requirements definition is carefully and thoroughly considered, important factors such as who the users are, their existing skills, the logistics of data entry and retrieval, and even if the problem is potentially soluable by providing information alone may be forgotten.

One of the problems of attempting to evaluate and define the need for an information resource before commencing development work is the impossibility of specifying in advance or on paper what functions users will need.[2] The problem is due to the fact that users typically cannot articulate which information they use to perform day-to-day tasks (the "paradox of expertise") and are unable to imagine how computer-based techniques might improve its quality or availability. When conventional systems analysis is conducted, users are typically unable to understand the written requirements documentation to visualize what is being proposed: They have neither the time nor the experience to imagine what the functioning software will look and feel like. An apparently functional prototype is required to help them formulate their requirements using a tangible product.[3, 4] It is for this reason that much software development now follows a "prototype and test" method, with emphasis on building prototypes of the resource, testing them with users, and revising them to rectify any identified deficiencies.[5] The reader is referred to the sections on capturing and defining user requirements through techniques such as rapid prototyping and user-centered design workshops in standard software engineering texts[4, 6] for further details.

To summarize, evaluating the need for an information resource means checking a wide variety of issues, including the following.

1. If there is a clinical problem; its characteristics and extent
2. What information is relevant to solving the problem
3. To whom the information must be delivered, when, and using what medium
4. Where the information can be obtained and in what format it must be presented
5. If the potential information resource users recognize the existence of the problem and what incentives they might need to use the information resource

Studying the Design and Development Process: Toward "Design Validation"

When information resources are designed for use in safety-critical areas such as medicine, it is tempting to try to prove from first principles that a certain structure for data and programs will lead to the desired functions and no others.[7] Despite progress in software engineering and "formal methods" for resource development, it is usually impossible to predict resource function from structure, as even resources of modest complexity challenge most current techniques. In addition, the effort required to prove that a piece of software does what it is meant to do and nothing else increases exponentially with the complexity of the tasks the program is designed to execute. This is an "NP-hard" problem. In the extreme case, to explore fully the behavior of an information resource requires an experiment involving approximately $(n*m)!$ observations, where n is the number of input data items and m is the mean number of values each can take, as every item of data must be presented in every permutation of value and order.

Because it is so difficult to prove that a piece of software performs as specified, the next best thing may be to assess a medical information resource by reviewing the design process that led to its construction. The assumption underlying evaluation of the design process is that if an information resource was designed correctly it is likely to contain the appropriate components arranged in a suitable architecture and thus to function correctly. Clearly, with our current incomplete knowledge of how to design software for a given purpose, this assumption is generous; even so, it often justifies a review of the design process. Suitable questions to ask as part of this review include the following.

- Was a design methodology, formal or informal, defined? Was it appropriate to the problem? Was the methodology followed by the resource designers?
- Did resource designers conduct a "walk through," or "inspection," of the resource design by software engineers not connected with the project and by user representatives to uncover any design errors?
- Did resource developers follow structured methods for data and task modeling such as an entity relation[8] or object-oriented modelling?
- Who took part in resource design and development? Were their skills appropriate; and, in particular, were representative resource users consulted?
- Were appropriate design and development tools used?

Studies to address these questions are not emphasized in this book, as the methods to conduct them involve a set of generic, technical, well-known procedures within the discipline of software engineering. They are, moreover, conducted in the same way for medical information resources as they are in any other domain of application. Readers are referred to standard works on software engineering for a discussion of these issues and how they might be addressed.

Studying the Structure of an Information Resource

The rationale for studying structure is as follows: If the resource contains appropriately designed components linked together in a suitable architecture, it is likely to function correctly. This assumption is again generous but somewhat more plausible than assuming that following the right design process can lead to a perfect resource. At a basic level, unless an information resource contains the right components, it is unlikely to work well. Checking how components interact is necessary to reassure oneself that it is likely to function as planned but is no substitute for evaluating the functions themselves.

The key components of an information resource are the hardware (including input and output devices); the interface between the user, the "information processor," and the internal data or knowledge structures; and the information processor itself, consisting of a variety of algorithms and inference methods (Fig. 3.1). Many resources also include auxiliary functions, such as installation and configuration tools, components to aid new users and developers, and tools to ensure that data are archived safely in case of hard disk failure.

Determining the exact boundaries of the resource is part of the study of a resource's structure. Whether the "resource" includes physical objects in the clini-

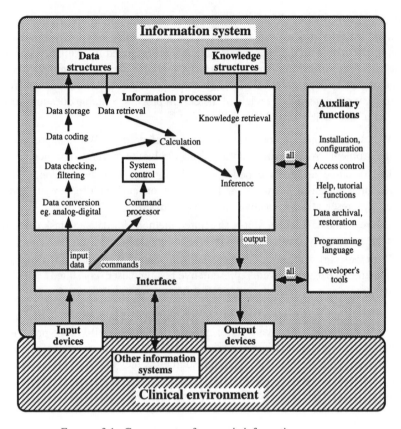

FIGURE 3.1. Components of a generic information resource.

cal environment (e.g., data collection forms), the interactions among users at the terminal or their telephone conversations with distant sites is determined by informed but fundamentally arbitrary decisions that are part of the design of every evaluation study. Once the boundaries around the resource have been drawn, however, it is essential that they not be changed over the course of a study. For example, it would be erroneous to claim that a computer decision-aid is responsible for improving diagnostic accuracy if some of the improvement is due to paper forms that are used to collect and organize patient data prior to keyboard entry[9] and the paper forms were defined earlier to be a component external to the resource.

There are certain components of the information resource that can be called "black boxes" because their structure is inherently difficult to comprehend or inspect.[10] Examples of such black boxes include neural networks, computer resources that adapt themselves dynamically to users or data, and programs which transgress the assumptions made by the originator of the algorithms they use. In such cases the structure of that component of the information resource is impenetrable, and only its functions[11] can be adequately observed or measured. In the case of neural networks or other data-derived classification resources, examining the data used to train the resource may possibly serve as a surrogate for evaluating its structure.[10]

The following sections address each key structural subcomponents of an information resource, as depicted in Figure 3.1, and how they may be studied.

Studying Input and Output Devices

Input devices include keyboard, pointing devices, a scanner for images or optical character recognition, microphone for speech input resources, and others. Output devices include the video display unit, printers, floppy disk drive, and other devices for data export. An example may help to illustrate some of the issues that can arise when studying such devices. In one project, a decision-aid installed on a small computer was mounted on a trolley so it could be wheeled to the patient's bedside. It was proposed to upgrade the resource by incorporating a mouse-driven graphic user interface, but the users pointed out that a mouse would not be an appropriate input device as it would fall off the trolley as it was moved, and it required free maneuvering space, which would require that the trolley be larger. A trackball was the solution. In the same project, users expressed doubt at the use of a computer with a low-contrast LCD display. However, after trying it, the users preferred this display to alternatives, as its narrow viewing angle meant that patients were unable to read the resource's advice.[1] In another project, clinicians failed to use a clinical database resource to help manage patients; careful observation and inquiry revealed that it was because of the noise and low quality generated by an impact printer. A laser printer solved both problems, and made the entire resource acceptable.

Studying the Structure of the Interface

From a structural perspective, a user interface can be described as the set of atomic elements (keyboard buttons, icons or buttons on the video screen, or sounds that can be played), the screens on which these elements are arranged, and the dialogue model that describes the relations between user events and the resource's responses (e.g., single or multiple screens, branching dialogue adaptive to the user's needs). Obviously, confining the evaluation to the structural components and their relations, ignoring the functionality of the interface, means constraining the study considerably, but in some cases lack of evaluation facilities may force investigators to this view. Suitable questions to ask about the structure of a user interface are what elements are used, how they are organized and presented, and what dialogue model has been implemented.

Studying the Structure of the Information Processor, Algorithms, and Inference Methods

The information processor consists of software components that collect data, process it, and generate output. Thus investigators can design studies to explore structural issues.

1. Structure and content of the information processor, cataloguing the functions specially implemented and use of documented libraries or public domain tools.
2. Algorithms or stored procedures used in databases to check data validity, transform data, and maintain consistency.
3. Inference mechanisms used in knowledge-based systems to propagate uncertainty, reason about time, and so on.
4. How the text of diagnostic help or routine output such as explanations is assembled.
5. How the various tasks carried out by the information processor are scheduled, and the opportunities for user control via the interface. Merely knowing that a program is event-driven at one extreme or follows a batch processing paradigm at the other can help evaluators understand a great deal about its likely functions and effects on users.

Studying Data Structures

Key attributes of data structures that can be studied include the database schema; the number and kind of entities or objects modeled; the level of detail, size, and number of possible elements; and the relations or messages that may connect the elements. Advocates of entity–relationship modeling have several criteria they routinely apply to determine if a database has been well modeled, such as the degree of normalization and parsimony of the model.[6] Some computer-aided software engineering environments (CASE tools) allow the user to carry out simple checks of consistency and completeness on the database schema. Such criteria are not yet as well developed for other data models (e.g., object-oriented databases). One area that should not be neglected is ensuring that the model represents a shared view and enjoys validity beyond the circle of users and systems analysts who developed it. This point can be assessed by asking outsiders to develop their own model from the same starting point and comparing the two models or by asking the outsiders to comment on the model already existing and make suggestions for improvement.

Evaluating Knowledge Bases

The advice or output generated by some information resources, such as decision-support systems, is based largely on the knowledge they contain and how this knowledge is represented. Thus the source and quality of the knowledge is a key issue. Attributes of medical knowledge-bases that can be evaluated include the following.

1. Source of the knowledge (e.g., from another resource, an expert, empirical data from rigorous studies such as randomized trials). It is disappointing that few information resources, conventional[12] or computer-based,[13] have been based on high-quality knowledge derived from clinical trials.
2. Accuracy and consistency of the knowledge.

3. Coverage of the knowledge across different kinds of decision tasks and across medical specialties. Some might argue that separate representation of decision-making methods is also necessary to ensure that the resource can generate adequate explanations.

4. Depth of the knowledge: its level of detail, whether causal knowledge or knowledge about anatomy or physiology is included, or simply associational "compiled" knowledge; if there is knowledge about how other knowledge can be used ("meta-knowledge"). For some resources, it is important that there is sufficient depth to support reasoning about time, uncertainty, and causality, as well as about anatomical and other relations.

5. If there are technical problems when representing the knowledge, such as redundancy or circularity.

The task of inspecting the contents of a knowledge base can be aided by computer-based tools. For example, in the case of rule-based resources, there are tools to detect circularity, dead-end rules whose antecedents are never met, and rules whose conclusions are never used.[14, 15] However, such tools function at the rule or syntactic level and so may distract attention from the more important "knowledge-level," or semantic, issues discussed above; they also often ignore important interactions between rules.[16]

Dynamic validation is another method for inspecting the knowledge base by applying synthetic test cases and examining the outputs for consistency. In the case of knowledge-based resources, the knowledge base itself may be used to generate the test cases,[17] or experts may "exercise" the knowledge base to uncover errors or omissions.[18] The latter is an example of studying the structure of a knowledge base by examining its function; it lies in the gray area between evaluations of structure and function. As mentioned earlier in the context of "black box" resources, for resources derived by machine learning, the only way to judge the quality of the knowledge may be to inspect the training data.[10]

Studying Resource Architecture and Links to Other Information Resources

Clearly, it is possible to build an information resource that contains appropriately designed components but still malfunctions because the necessary links between functional modules are absent or communicate irrelevant information. Thus it may be necessary to inspect diagrams of the resource architecture and documents describing the interfaces between important components.[6] Doubt should be cast if the architecture fails to allow significant data items to pass from one component to another, does not provide interfaces that transform data into required formats, if the transformations are inconsistent, or if data are routed indirectly through potential system bottlenecks when a simpler route is possible.

Because we are still unable to predict the output generated by interacting software components, it is important to evaluate the functions of the information resource as a whole (considered in the next two sections).

Necessity of Studying Resource Function and Impact

For some scientific disciplines, understanding the structure of a device allows one to predict how it will behave, and engineers can even design new objects with known characteristics directly from functional requirements. Examples of such devices are road bridges and conventional airliners: The principles of civil and aeronautical engineering are sufficiently well understood that, given a complex set of performance specifications such as traffic capacity or cost per passenger mile, a new bridge or a new airplane can be designed; field testing is expected to reveal relatively minor anomalies, which can be rapidly remedied. However, when the object concerned is a computer-based resource, not a bridge, the story is different. Software designers and engineers have incomplete theories linking the structure to the function of all but the most trivial computer-based resource.[19] Because of the lack of a theory connecting structure and function, there is no way to know that any revisions will bring about the desired effect until the next version of the resource is tested.

In sum, the only practical way of determining if a code does what it is intended to do is to test it. This informal participatory design, testing, and debugging activity is linked critically to the process of developing successful software. It is also not specific to medical resources. More formal evaluation studies, which are the foci of this book, can be undertaken before, during, and after the initial development of an information resource. Evaluation studies can guide further development, indicate if the resource is likely to be safe for use in a real patient-care setting, or elucidate if it has the potential to improve the users' decisions.

Other writings elaborate on the points offered here. Spiegelhalter[20] and Gaschnig et al.[21] discussed these phases of evaluation in more detail, drawing analogies from the evaluation of new drugs or the conventional software life cycle, respectively. Wasson et al.[22] discussed the evaluation of clinical prediction rules together with some useful methodological standards that apply equally to information resources. Lundsgaarde,[23] Miller,[24] Nykanen,[25] and Wyatt and Spiegelhalter[26] described, with differing emphases, the evaluation of clinical information resources, often focusing on decision support resources, which pose some of the most extreme challenges.

Studying Resource Function in Laboratory or Field Settings

Appendix A gives a sample of some of the many functions that can be examined for a range of information resource components, such as databases or user interfaces, and complete information resources. If one is adopting objectivist methods, it is often necessary to invent specific measures to "operationalize" the variables being addressed and to validate these new measures using established methods. When using subjectivist methods, the functions of interest provide an initial focus for the investigative process.

Settings for Functional Tests

Functional tests may take place in laboratory or field settings. For example, the most common approach to studying decision support resources is to collect case data for patients who are not currently receiving care and for the evaluator or clinician to enter it into the resource and then record and analyze the resource's output. Measures of the subjective experiences of the user may also be made at the same time but are considered later under the topic of the resource impact on users. When studying resources such as patient monitors or reminder resources, functional testing may take place in a field setting with the resource linked to live patient data, but the output would not be shown to clinicians who are managing these patients so as to avoid an unvalidated resource potentially changing their decisions (Table 3.1).

What Can Be Studied

As shown in Figure 3.1, information resources are built from many components, each with many functions that can be tested. Some of these general functions are listed in Table 3.2. A sample of the more specific functions that are most relevant to certain components or to intact clinical information resources of different kinds are listed in Appendix A.

Before disseminating any medical information resource that stores and communicates data or knowledge and is designed to influence clinical decisions, it is important to check that it is safe when used as intended. In the case of new drugs, it is a statutory duty of developers to perform extensive in vitro testing and in vivo testing in animals, before any human receives a dose. For information resources, equivalent safety tests might include measuring how fast the information resource functions compared to current procedures and estimating how often it corrupts or retrieves erroneous data or furnishes incorrect advice. It may be necessary to repeat these measurements following any substantial modifications to the information resource, as correction of errors may itself generate more errors or uncover previously unrecognized ones.

Examining an information resource for safe operation is particularly important when evaluating those that attempt to directly influence the decisions made by clinicians. Ensuring that such a resource is safe requires measurement of how often it gives poor advice using data representative of patients in whose management it is intended to assist and comparing the advice given with the decisions made by current decision-makers and expert judges.

Studying Resource Impact

Deciding which of the possible impact variables to include in a study and developing ways to measure them can be the most challenging aspect of an evaluation study design. (It receives the attention of two full chapers of this book.) Evaluators usually wish to limit the number of impact measures employed in a study

TABLE 3.2. General functions of components of information resources that may be evaluated

Input devices and interfaces
Number and types of data items; time taken; ease of correcting errors
Number and types of commands; time taken; number of functions available
Ability to integrate with other information resources at hardware, software, and data levels

Output devices and data
Kinds, accuracy, delay in appearance of messages
Reports: range of problems addressed; length, ease of comprehension, structure, accuracy
Explanations: range of questions addressed; length, ease of comprehension, structure, accuracy

Information processor
Intended user functions: how many, how accurately performed, how fast; changes in speed with
    scaling-up of database/coding vocabulary/knowledge base
Unintended functions: bugs, resource crashes, corrupted data
Limitations: numerical precision, data storage capacity, use of national languages

Data and knowledge structures
Speed of retrieval, number and appropriateness of items retrieved

Auxiliary functions
On-line tutorial or help: number of functions covered
Installation time and skills required, subjective ease of process
Ability to tailor or extend the resource: user dictionaries, macros, tailored reports, embedded
    programming language
Ease of maintenance and extension
Time taken to back up data

General
Adherence to standards: hardware, software, clinical coding, user interfaces

(because of limited evaluation facilities and to mimimize distorting the clinical environment by their activity). Appendix B lists some potential measures of the impact of various information resources on health care itself, providers of care, and organizations. As an example of studying resource impact, we consider below how to measure user performance in a situation where improvement due to the introduction of a clinical decision-aid is to be evaluated.

Every medical intervention carries some risk, which must be judged in comparison to the risks of doing nothing or of providing an alternative intervention. It is difficult to decide whether an information resource is an improvement unless the performance of the current decision-takers is also measured[27] in a comparison-based evaluation. For example, if physicians' decisions are to become more accurate following introduction of a decision-support resource, the resource's error rate must be lower than that of the physician, its errors must be in different cases, or they should be of a different kind or less serious than those of the physician.

Thus it is important to know how well clinicians currently make decisions. Suitable measures include the accuracy, timing, and confidence level of their decisions and the amount of clinical data they require before making a decision. Although data for such a study can be collected by giving abstracts of cases to physicians in a laboratory setting (Fig. 3.2), these studies inevitably raise ques-

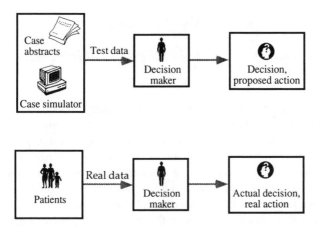

FIGURE 3.2. Two methods for measuring the quality of clinical decisions.

tions of generalization to the real world of health care. We observe here one of many trade-offs that occur in the design of evaluation studies. Although control over the mix of cases possible in a laboratory study can lead to a more precise estimate of clinicians' decision making, ultimately it may prove better to conduct a baseline study while the doctors are making decisions about real patients in a real clinical setting. Such a baseline study can be subject to a Hawthorne effect (see Chapter 7), so it is important to minimize the intrusiveness of the study team. Often this audit of the current decision-taking process provides useful input to the design process for the resource,[1, 26] and provides a reference against which resource performance may later be compared. If the evaluators collect copies of the relevant clinical data while they are studying the decisions taken by the clinicians who managed these cases, they are in a strong position to assess the potential of their resource to improve these decisions.

When conducting impact studies, evaluators can sometimes save themselves much time and effort without sacrificing validity by measuring impact in terms of certain health care processes rather than patient outcomes.[28] For example, measuring the mortality or complication rate in patients with heart attacks requires data collection from hundreds of patients, as complications and death are (fortunately) rare events. However, as long as large, rigorous clinical trials or meta-analyses have determined that a certain procedure (e.g., giving heart attack patients streptokinase within 24 hours) correlates closely with patient outcome, it is perfectly valid to measure the rate of performing this procedure as a valid "surrogate" for outcome. Mant and Hicks demonstrated that measuring the quality of care by quantifying a key process in this way may require one tenth as many patients as measuring outcomes.[28]

Deciding What and How Much to Study

Matching What Is Evaluated to the Type of Information Resource

There are many information resources, with many functional components. Clearly, it is impossible to generate an exhaustive list of everything that can be studied for every kind of resource, but as previously mentioned Appendix A gives samples of some of the issues that can be addressed for a range of information resource components and complete resources. Appendix B lists potential measures of the impact of various resources on health care providers and organizations. Not all of these attributes can or should be measured for every component or resource, and it often requires much thought about the purpose of the evaluation itself to produce a relevant list of issues to pursue. Because facilities for evaluation are always limited, it may be helpful to rank the items listed in the appendices in the order of their likely contribution to answering the questions the evaluation is intended to resolve. Often, as discussed in Chapter 2, priorities are set not by the evaluators but by the stakeholders in the evaluation. The evaluators' role is then to initiate a process that leads to a consensus about what the priority issues should be.

Matching How Much Is Evaluated to the Stage in the Life Cycle

Evaluation, defined broadly, takes place throughout the resource development cycle: from defining the need to monitoring the continuing impact of a resource once it is disseminated. This extended role is hardly surprising, as the development of information resources itself is not an exact science but requires iterative design and test cycles. The place of evaluation in the various developmental phases is illustrated in Figure 3.3. Different issues are explored, at different degrees of intensity, at each stage of resource development.

During the early phases of development, informal feedback and exploration of prototypes is associated with debugging and close user involvement, as discussed earlier in the section about evaluating the need for the information resource. A single prototype is then chosen for more formal testing, with problems being fed back to the development team. Eventually, it passes preset criteria of adequacy, and its effects on users can be tested in a more formal way—though often still under controlled, "laboratory" conditions. Once safety is ensured and there is reason to believe that the information resource is likely to benefit clinicians and patients, its impact can be studied in a limited field test prior to wider dissemination. Once disseminated, it is valuable to monitor the effects of the resource on the institutions that have installed it and evaluate for potential hazards that may only come to light when it is in widespread use—a direct analogy with postmarketing surveillance of drugs for rare side effects.

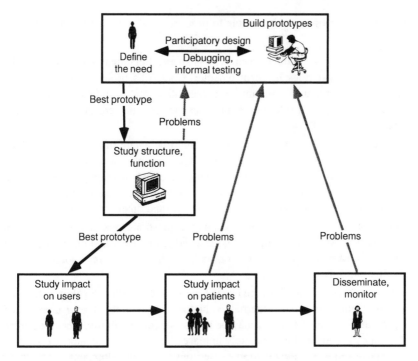

FIGURE 3.3. Changing evaluation issues during development of a clinical information resource.

Evaluation is integral to information resource development, and adequate resources must be allocated for it when time and money are budgeted for a development effort. Evaluation cannot be left to the end of a project. However, it is also clear that the intensity of the evaluation effort should be closely matched to the resource's maturity.[29] For example, one would not wish to conduct an expensive field trial of an information resource that is barely complete, is still in prototype form, may evolve considerably before taking its final shape (such as the ACORN system described earlier), or is so early in its development that it may fail because simple programming bugs have not been eliminated. Equally, once information resources are firmly established in clinical practice, it may take hard work to convince funding organizations that a rigorous evaluation is still necessary. This problem has been the case with MEDLINE.[30, 31]

Organizing Clinical Resource Development Projects to Facilitate Evaluation

We have already discussed the need for evaluation to become a pervasive component of resource development projects. What follows is a list of steps that should ensure that evaluation activity is able to proceed hand in hand with the development process.

- At the first stage of planning a study, it is an excellent idea to make a list of the potential project roles listed in Chapter 2, such as project funder, resource developer, users, and community representative, and to indicate which stakeholders occupy each role. Sometimes this task requires educated guesses, but the exercise is still useful.

- Those planning development projects should be aware of the need to include balanced membership on the evaluation team: many evaluation projects need access to the specialist skills of a computer scientist, an ethnographer, a statistician, a medical informatician, clinicians, managers, and a health economist. Some of these personnel are readily available, and others must be recruited.

- A recurrent problem of evaluation is that the questions to be answered are often not defined. Many problems can be averted if the users and developers have defined a list of specific purposes or goals for the information resource and the evaluation activity.

- Although many evaluations are carried out by the resource development team, placing some reliance on external evaluators may help to uncover unexpected problems—or benefits—and may be necessary for credibility. Recalling from Chapter 2 the ideal of a completely unbiased "goal free" evaluator, we see that excessive reliance on evaluation carried out by the development team can be problematical.

- Parkinson's law (tasks and organizations tend to expand to consume the resources available) can apply to resource development and evaluation activities. It is important to define the goals, time scale, and budget in advance, though it is difficult to apportion the budget between what is spent on development and what is spent on evaluation activities. A starting point for the evaluation activity should be at least 15% of the total budget, but a larger percentage may be appropriate if it is a demonstrator project or one where reliable and predictable resource function is critical to patient safety, such as a closed-loop drug delivery system. In such systems a syringe containing a drug with potentially toxic side effects is controlled by a computer program that attempts to maintain some body function (e.g., blood glucose, depth of anestheisa) constant or close to preprogrammed levels. Any malfunction or unexpected relations between the input data and the rate of drug delivery could have serious consequences. Thus the proportion of the development budget allocated to evaluation of such systems must be large.

- As has been argued, evaluators need an eclectic approach. Depending on the specific needs of the project, it may include subjectivist methods which are important to (1) elucidate problems, expectations, fears, failures, resource transferability, and effects on job roles; (2) identify how to improve the resource; and (3) understand what else apart from information technology is necessary to make the information resource a success.

Finally, evaluation projects do themselves require management. A project quality assurance team can be appointed to oversee the quality and progress of the overall project from the stakeholders' perspective. Such a team typically has no direct managerial responsibility. This quality assurance team should be composed of appropriate people who can advise the evaluation team about priorities and strategy, indemnify them against accusations of excessive detachment or meddling in the evaluation sites, and monitor progress of the studies. Such a team can satisfy the need for a multidisciplinary advisory group and help to ensure the credibility of the study findings.

Answers to Self-Test 3.1

1. Clinical impact
2. Need validation
3. Structure validation
4. Field function
5. Design validation and need validation
6. Laboratory function
7. Laboratory user impact, laboratory function
8. Clinical impact

References

1. Heathfield HA, Wyatt J: Philosophies for the design and development of clinical decision-support systems. Methods Inf Med 1993;32:1–8.
2. Wyatt JC: Clinical data systems, Part III: Developing and evaluating clinical data systems. Lancet 1994;344:1682–1688.
3. Smith MF: Prototypically topical: software prototyping and delivery of health care information systems. Br J Health Care Comput 1993;10(6):25–27.
4. Smith MF: Software Prototyping. London: McGraw-Hill, 1991.
5. Heathfield HA, Hardiker N, Kirby J, Tallis R, Gonsalkarale M: The PEN and PAD medical record model: development of a nursing record for hospital-based care of the elderly. Methods Inf Med 1994;33:464–472.
6. Sommerville I: Software Engineering. Reading, MA: Addison Wesley 1992
7. Fox J: Decision support systems as safety-critical components: towards a safety culture for medical informatics. Methods Inf Med 1993;32:345–348.
8. Perrault L, Wiederhold G: System design and evaluation. In: Shortliffe E, Perrault L, Wiederhold G, Fagan L (eds) Medical Informatics. Reading, MA: Addison-Wesley 1990:151–177.
9. Wellwood J, Spiegelhalter DJ, Johannessen S: How does computer-aided diagnosis improve the management of acute abdominal pain? Ann R Col Surg Engl 1992;74:140–146.

10. Hart A, Wyatt J: Evaluating black boxes as medical decision-aids: issues arising from a study of neural networks. Med Inf (Lond) 1990;15:229–236.
11. Wyatt J: Nervous about artificial neural networks? Lancet 1995;346:1175–1177.
12. Antman E, Lau J, Kupelnick B, Mosteller F, Chalmers T: A comparison of the results of meta-analysis of randomised controlled trials and recommendations of clinical experts. JAMA 1992;268:240–248.
13. Holbrooke A, Langton K, Haynes R, Mathieu A, Cowan S: PREOP: development of an evidence-based expert system to assist with preoperative assessment. Proc Symp Comput Applications Med Care 1991;15:669–673.
14. Nguyen T, Perkins W, Laffey T, Pecora D: Knowledge base verification. AI Magazine 1987;8:69–75.
15. Suwa M, Scott AC, Shortliffe EH: Completeness and consistency in a rule-based system. In: Buchanan BG, Shortliffe EH (eds) Rule-Based Expert Systems. Reading, MA: Addison-Wesley, 1984:159–170.
16. Heckerman D, Horwitz E: The myth of modularity in rule-based systems. In Lemmer J, Kanal L (eds) Uncertainty in AI 2. Amsterdam: Elsevier, 1988:115–121.
17. Shwe M, Tu S, Fagan L: Validating the knowledge base of a therapy planning system. Methods Inf Med 1989;28:36–50.
18. Miller PL, Sittig DF: The evaluation of clinical decision support systems: what is necessary versus what is interesting. Med Inf (Lond) 1990;15:185–190.
19. Clancey WJ: Viewing knowledge bases as qualitative models. IEEE Expert 1989;4:9–23.
20. Spiegelhalter DJ: Evaluation of medical decision-aids, with an application to a system for dyspepsia. Stat Med 1983;2:207–216.
21. Gaschnig J, Klahr P, Pople H, Shortliffe E, Terry A: Evaluation of expert systems: issues and case studies. In: Hayes-Roth F, Waterman DA, Lenat D (eds) Building Expert Systems. Reading, MA: Addison Wesley, 1983.
22. Wasson JH, Sox HC, Neff RK, Goldman L: Clinical prediction rules: applications and methodological standards. N Engl J Med 1985;313:793–799.
23. Lundsgaarde HP: Evaluating medical expert systems. Soc Sci Med 1987;24:805–819.
24. Miller PL: Evaluating medical expert systems. In: Miller PL (ed) Selected Topics in Medical AI. New York: Springer-Verlag, 1988.
25. Nykanen P (ed): Issues in the Evaluation of Computer-Based Support to Clinical Decision Making. Report of SYDPOL WG5. Denmark: SYDPOL, 1989
26. Wyatt J, Spiegelhalter D: Evaluating medical expert systems: what to test and how? Med Inf (Lond) 1990;15:205–217.
27. de Dombal FT, Leaper DJ, Horrocks JC, et al: Human and computer-aided diagnosis of acute abdominal pain: further report with emphasis on performance of clinicians. BMJ 1974;1:376–380.
28. Mant J, Hicks N: Detecting differences in quality of care: the sensitivity of measures of process and outcome in treating acute myocardial infarction. BMJ 1995;311:793–796.
29. Stead W, Haynes RB, Fuller S, et al: Designing medical informatics research and library projects to increase what is learned. J Am Med Inf Assoc 1994;1:28–34.
30. Haynes R, McKibbon K, Walker C, Ryan N, Fitzgerald D, Ramsden M: Online access to MEDLINE in a clinical setting. Ann Intern Med 1990;112:78–84.
31. Lindberg DA, Siegel ER, Rapp BA, Wallingford KT, Wilson SR: Use of MEDLINE by physicians for clinical problem solving. JAMA 1993;269:3124–3129.

Appendix A: Specific Functions of Computer-Based Information Resources

Database
Data security: methods for backing up patient data, changing user defaults/ settings
Data confidentiality: password control, file encryption
Flexibility of file structure, ability to extend contents of data dictionary
Reliability of hardware/software during power loss
Maximum transaction capacity

Data coding/translation component
Use of coded data, coding accuracy, accuracy of mapping codes to another system; percent of data items possible to code; ease of extending codes

Data retrieval component
Completeness, speed of data retrieval, degradation with 10,000 cases using different search methods (query by example, Boolean, string search)
Fidelity of data output to data input (e.g., rounding errors, use of different synonyms)

Any data input component
Subjective ease, objective accuracy, time taken, number of actions (e.g., key presses) required to enter data items, number of errors correctly detected by resource

Speech input component
Accuracy, speaker invariance, resistance to background noise, directionality, ability to enter words via keyboard, accuracy when used via telephone, size of vocabulary, speed of recognition

Full-text database (passive knowledge-base)
Ease of navigation, retrieval using a standardized vocabulary or synonyms, understanding contents, speed, ease of keeping knowledge up to date

Advice generator
Length, apparent ease of comprehension, structuring, accuracy of advice; calibration of any probability estimates

Critique generator
Length, ease of comprehension, structuring, accuracy of critique comments

Explanation generator
Length, ease of comprehension, structuring, accuracy of explanations; flexibility over domains, range of user questions it can address

Imaging system

Spatial resolution (number of pixels, linear size), linear calibration (use of phantoms or models), contrast range, separation (influence of adjacent features), stability over time, amount of data generated per image, internal data storage capacity, time to capture one image

Teaching system

Time to navigate to required section, accuracy compared to other sources, coverage of topic, ability to tailor to user, ease of maintenance, usage of standard vocabulary

Patient simulation package

Ease of use, accuracy compared to what happens in real cases, number of parameters that can be changed as a percentage of total, how well the system's internal state is communicated to the user, speed, stability over time

Patient monitor

Resistance to electromagnetic interference or patient movement; resolution of A to D converter; sampling rate; internal storage capacity; storage format; accuracy of parameters such as amplitudes; wave duration, rates, trends, alarms; stability of baseline; calibration

Appendix B: Areas of Potential Information Resource Impact on Health Care, Care Providers, and Organizations

Database

Frequency of data loss, breaches of data confidentiality, downtime and its consequences, speed of response (e.g., transaction rates or time per transaction) when database in routine use

Data coding/translation process

Accuracy of coded data following clinical input; problems when coding data (e.g., percentage of data items that users wished to enter that were successfully coded, number of new codes added by users)

Data retrieval process

Ease of searching, which search methods are used; time to formulate a search; user satisfaction with searches

Data retrieval: completeness, time taken for data retrieval; degradation with number of cases stored

Any data input process

Ease of data entry, usage rate, subjective ease of data entry

Objective accuracy of data entry, time taken, number of actions (e.g., key presses) taken to enter data items, number of errors correctly detected by the resource; variation among users, repeatability with same user; learning effect

Speech input system

Ease of use, accuracy in a real environment, number of repetitions needed, deliberate use of restricted subsets of vocabulary, speed of use, speaker invariance, resistance to background noise, directionality, frequency that users enter data or commands via alternate means, percentage of time used via the telephone

Knowledge-base (e.g., as a full-text database, part of an advice generator)

Users' perceptions of coverage, detail, ease of reading output, speed, how much is current, ease of using index, finding synonyms

Searching precision, recall and speed given a citation or a specific question; recall after a fixed time spent browsing without a specific question given in advance; quality and number of references included in paragraphs on a given topic retrieved after free access to resource

Effects on accuracy and timing of users' decisions and actions; effect on users' subjective confidence about a case; effect on users' knowledge or understanding of medicine

Advice generator

Users' perceptions of the length, ease of comprehension, structuring and accuracy of the advice; how well calibrated any probability estimates appear

Effects of correct and incorrect advice on accuracy and timing of users' decisions and actions: to collect patient data, to order investigations of diagnosis or interpretation of test results, to refer or admit a patient, to give or adjust therapy, to give a prognosis

Effect of advice on users' subjective confidence about a case; effect of advice on users' knowledge or understanding of medicine

Critique generator

Users' perceptions of length, ease of comprehension, structuring, accuracy of critique comments; influence of each critique comment on accuracy and timing of users' decisions and actions; effect of critique on users' subjective confidence about a case; effect of critique on users' knowledge or understanding of medicine

Explanation generator

Users' perceptions of length, ease of comprehension, structuring, accuracy; range of user questions it addressed; influence of explanation on user (e.g,. causing them to ignore incorrect advice when their prior intention was right or to take correct advice when their prior intention was wrong); effect of explanation on users' subjective confidence about a case; effect of explanation on users' knowledge or understanding of medicine

Imaging system

User's estimate of adequacy of system; number and types of images stored and communicated; usage rates, times, and sites; times taken to review one image and to review all the images necessary for a decision about a patient; effect on accuracy of users' diagnostic, therapeutic, prognostic decisions and actions; effect on users' subjective confidence about a case; effect on users' knowledge or understanding of medicine

Teaching system

Subjective response to the resource; rate and duration of use of the various components (e.g., graphics, simulation routines); total time spent by users per session; time taken to access and learn a given set of facts; accuracy of recall of learned facts, decrement over time; effect on users' diagnostic, therapeutic, prognostic decisions and actions; effect on users' subjective confidence about similar clinical cases; effect on users' knowledge or understanding of medicine

Patient simulation package

Subjective ease of use; number of parameters adjusted by users (as a percentage of the total number); effect on users' diagnostic, therapeutic, prognostic decisions and actions; effect on users' subjective confidence about similar clinical cases; effect on users' knowledge or understanding of medicine

Patient monitor

Users' response to the alarms and the monitor; alarm rate, false alarm rate, detection rate for true alarm conditions; how much of the time the users disable the alarm; effect on users' diagnostic, therapeutic, prognostic decisions and actions; effect on users' subjective confidence about clinical cases

4

Structure of Objectivist Studies

Important human and clinical phenomena are regularly omitted when patient care is...analyzed in statistical comparisons of therapy. The phenomena are omitted either because they lack formal expressions to identify them or because the available expressions are regarded as scientifically unacceptable.[1]

This chapter begins to explore objectivist studies in detail. In Chapters 4–7 we address how to design studies, how to develop measurement procedures to collect data, and how subsequently to analyze the data. The methods introduced relate directly to the comparison-based, objectives-based, and decision-facilitation approaches to evaluation as introduced in Chapter 2. They are useful for addressing most of the purposes of evaluation in informatics, the specific questions that can be explored, and the types of studies that can be undertaken—all as introduced in Chapter 3.

In this chapter we develop a conceptual framework for thinking about objectivist studies. We introduce some terminology that, once established, is used consistently in the chapters that follow. Much of this terminology is familiar, but we probably use some terms in ways that are novel. Unfortunately, there is no single, accepted terminology for describing objectivist studies. Epidemiologists, behaviorial and social scientists, information scientists, statisticians, and evaluators have developed their own variations. As informatics itself reflects a composite of several fields, so must our language. We emphasize that the terms introduced here are more than just labels. They represent concepts that are central to understanding the structure of objectivist studies and, ultimately, being able to design them.

A major theme of this chapter, and indeed the four chapters on objectivist studies as a group, is the importance of measurement. Two of the four chapters in this group are explicitly devoted to measurement, because we believe that a large proportion of the major problems to be overcome in evaluation study design are, at their core, problems of measurement. We also stress measurement issues here because they tend to be overlooked in research methods training based in other disciplines.

After introducing some measurement terminology, this chapter formally establishes the distinction between *measurement studies* designed to explore with how much error "things of interest" in informatics can be measured, and *demonstration studies,* which apply these measurement procedures to answer evaluation questions of substantive and practical concern. The distinction between measurement and demonstration studies is more than academic. As we define them, pure measurement studies are rarely done in informatics. For example, a review of the literature on attitudes toward clinical information systems, going back to 1984, revealed only 17 articles that could be classified as reporting measurement studies.* In the informatics literature, it appears that measurement issues are usually embedded in, and often confounded with, demonstration issues. Although attitudes pose some notoriously difficult challenges for measurement, similar challenges exist across the full range of variables, as introduced in Chapter 3, that are of concern to informatics researchers. This matter is of substantial significance because deficiencies in measurement can affect profoundly the conclusions drawn from a demonstration study. The quote that begins this chapter alerts us to the fact that our ability to investigate is circumscribed by our ability to measure. Unless we possess or can develop ways to measure what is important to know about our information resources, our ability to conduct evaluation studies—at least those using objectivist approaches—is be substantially limited.

This chapter, then, lays the groundwork for understanding the interplay between measurement and demonstration, a relation that is developed more deeply in the three chapters that follow. The next two chapters explore measurement issues in depth. The final chapter in this series focuses on the design and conduct of demonstration studies.

Measurement Process and Terminology

We begin with some ground rules, definitions, and synonyms that relate to the process of measurement. These definitions may use some familiar words in unfamiliar ways, and we apologize for what may appear to be an exercise in transforming the self-evident into the obscure. The process of measurement and the interrelations of the terms to be defined are illustrated in Figure 4.1.

Measurement: Measurement is the process of assigning a value corresponding to the presence, absence, or degree of a specific attribute in an specific object. The terms "attribute" and "object" are defined below. Measurement in this objectivist sense usually results in either (1) assignment of a numerical score representing the extent to which the attribute of interest is present in the object, or (2) assignment of an object to a specific category. Taking the temperature (attribute) of a patient (object) is an example of the process of measurement.

---

*   The authors express their appreciation to Dr. Randy Cork for his comprehensive review of the literature on measurement in medical informatics.

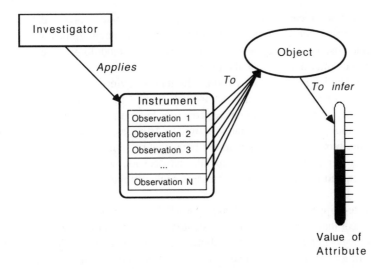

FIGURE 4.1. Process of measurement.

Object and object class: The object is the entity on which the measurement is made, the characteristics of which are being described. Every measurement process begins with the specification of a class of objects. Each act of measurement is taken on an individual object, which is a member of the class. Persons (patients or care providers), clinical cases, information resources, practitioner groups, and health care organizations are important examples of object classes in medical informatics.

The choice of object class is always an important issue in study design. A researcher can, after taking a set of measurements with a particular class of objects, exploit the fact that these objects form natural sets to conduct analyses at a higher level of aggregation. For example, having taken measurements on individual patients, a researcher can combine the measurement results for all patients seen in each clinic, implicitly making the clinic the object class. However, it is impossible to go the other way. If the original measurements are made with clinic as the object class, information about individual patients cannot later be derived.

Attribute: An attribute is a specific characteristic of the object: what is being measured. Information resource speed, blood pressure, the correct diagnosis of a clinical case, the number of new patient admissions per day, and computer literacy are examples of pertinent attributes within medical informatics. It is important to understand that attributes are abstract concepts, often invented by researchers specifically for the purpose of conducting investigations. Over time, each scientific field develops a set of attributes, "things worth measuring," that become part of the culture of the field. Researchers may tend to view the attributes that are part their field's tradition as part of the landscape and fail to recognize that, at some earlier point in history, these concepts were unknown. Blood pressure, for example, had no meaning to mankind until circulation was understood. Computer literacy is a more recent construction stimulated by contemporary technological developments. Indeed, some of the most original research studies are typically those that posit completely new attributes, develop methodology to measure them, and subsequently demonstrate their value.

Many studies in informatics address human behavior and the beliefs that are presumed to motivate this behavior. In such studies, the attributes of interest are usually not physical or physiological properties but, rather, more abstract concepts corresponding to presumed states of mind. Attitudes, knowledge, and performance are broad classes of human attributes that often interest medical informatics researchers. The behavioral, social, and decision sciences have contributed specific methods that enable us to measure such attributes.

Attribute-object class pairs: Having defined an attribute as a quality of a specific object that is a member of a class, it is always possible to view a measurement process in terms of paired attributes and object classes. Table 4.1 illustrates this pairing of attributes and object classes for the examples discussed above. It is important to be able to analyze any given measurement situation by identifying the pertinent attribute and object class. To do this, we might ask ourselves certain questions. To identify the *attribute,* ask: What is being measured? What will we call the result of the measurement? To identify the *object class,* ask: On whom or on what is the measurement made? The reader can use Self-Test 4.1 and the example that precedes it to test his or her understanding of these concepts.

Instruments: The instrument is the technology used for measurement. The "instrument" encodes and embodies the procedures used to determine the presence, absence, or extent of an attribute in an object. For studies in medical informatics, instruments can include self-administered questionnaires, traditional medical devices (e.g., an electrocardiogram or x-ray machine), tests of medical knowledge or skills, performance checklists, and the computer itself through logging software that records elements of resource use. It is apparent from these examples that many measurements in informatics require substantial human interpretation before the value of an attribute is inferred. A radiograph must be interpreted; performance checklists must be completed by observers. In such instances, a human "judge" or perhaps a panel of judges, may be viewed as an essential part of the instrument for a measurement process.

Observations: An observation is a question or other mechanism that elicits one independent element of measurement data. As measurement is customarily carried out, multiple independent observations are employed to estimate the value of an attribute for an object. Use of multiple observations produces a better estimate of the "true" value of the attribute than would be the case for a single observation, and tells us how much variability exists across observations, which is necessary to estimate the error inherent in the measurement. The "speed" of an information resource typically is not assessed via the time taken to perform only one computational task but, rather, by the combined times to perform a variety of appropriately

TABLE 4.1. Attribute–object class pairs

Attribute	Object class
Speed	Information resource
Blood pressure	Patient
Correct diagnosis	Patient
New admissions per day	Hospital ward team
Computer literacy	Person

selected, related tasks. Each task may, for these purposes, be considered an independent observation. When observations are recorded on a form, we often use the term "item" to describe a question or other probe that elicits one element of information on the form.

Example

As part of a study of a computer-based resource for diagnosis, the investigators are interested in how reasonable are the diagnoses suggested by the system, even when these diagnoses are not exactly correct. They conduct a study where the "top five" diagnoses generated by the resource, for a sample of test cases, are referred to a panel of experienced physicians for review.

Focusing on the measurement aspects of this process, name the attribute being measured and the object class. Describe how this measurement process employs multiple independent observations.

To identify the attribute, ask: What is being measured and what do we call the result of the measurement? The result of the measurement is called something like the "reasonableness" of the top five diagnoses, so it is the attribute. To identify the object class, ask: On whom or on what is the actual measurement made? The measurement is made on the diagnosis set generated by the resource for each case, so the case or, more specifically, the "diagnosis set for each case" can be seen as the object class of measurement. The multiple observations are generated by the presumably independent ratings of the expert clinicians.

Self-Test 4.1

1. To determine the performance of a computer-based reminder system, a sample of alerts generated by the system (and the patient record from which each alert was generated) is given to a panel of physicians. Each panelist rates each alert on a four-point scale from "highly appropriate to the clinical situation" to "completely inappropriate." Focusing on the measurement aspects of this process, name the attribute being measured, the class of measurement objects, and the instrument used. Describe how this measurement process employs multiple independent observations.

2. The physicians in a large community hospital undergo training to use a new clinical information system. After the training, each physician completes a test

comprising 30 questions about the system to help the developers understand how much knowledge about the system has been conveyed via the training. Again, name the attribute being measured, the class of measurement objects, the instrument used. Describe how this measurement process employs multiple independent observations.

3. A computer-based resource is created to review patient admission notes and identify pertinent terms to "index" the cases using the institution's controlled clinical vocabulary. As part of a study of this new resource, a panel of judges familiar with the clinical vocabulary reviews a set of cases. The set of terms identified by the system for each case is reviewed to see if the case is correctly indexed. Again from a measurement perspective, name the attribute and object class.

[Answers to these questions are found at the end of the chapter.]

Importance of Measurement

Having introduced some terms and concepts, we can appreciate the importance of measurement in objectivist studies by revisiting the major premises underlying the objectivist approaches. These premises were originally introduced in Chapter 2 but are stated in somewhat revised form to exploit the new terminology. Like all premises, they are based on assumptions that reflect idealized views of the world and our ability to understand it through certain methods of empirical research. Readers who have difficulty accepting these assumptions might find themselves more attracted to the subjectivist approaches discussed in Chapters 8 and 9.

In objectivist studies we assume the following.

- *Attributes* inhere in the *object* under study. Merit and worth are part of the object and can be measured unambiguously. An investigator can measure these attributes without affecting the object's structure or function.
- All rational persons agree (or can be brought to consensus) on what attributes of an object are important to measure and what measurement results would be associated with high merit or worth of the object. In medical informatics, this is tantamount to stating that a "gold standard" of practice can always be identified, and that informed individuals can be brought to consensus on what this gold standard is.
- Because numerical measurement of attributes allows precise statistical comparisons across groups and across time, numerical measurement is prima facie superior to verbal description.
- Through comparisons of measured attributes across selected groups of objects, it is possible to demonstrate at a specific level of confidence, for example, that a particular medical information resource is superior to what it replaced or to some alternative design of that resource.

From these premises, it follows that proper execution of objectivist studies requires careful and specific attention to methods of measurement. It can never be assumed, particularly in informatics, that attributes of interest are measured without error. Accurate and precise measurement must not be an afterthought.* Measurement is of particular importance in medical informatics because, as a relatively young field, informatics does not have a well established tradition of "things worth measuring" or proved instruments for measuring them. By and large, those planning studies are faced with the task of, first, deciding what to measure and then developing their own measurement methods. For most researchers, this task proves more difficult and more time-consuming than initially anticipated. In some cases, informatics investigators can adapt the measures used by other investigators, but they often need to apply these measures to a different setting, where prior experience may not apply.

The choice of what to measure, and how, is an area where there are few prescriptions and where sound judgment, experience, and knowledge of methods come into play. Decisions about *what* and, above all, *how* to measure require knowledge of the study questions, the intervention and setting, and the experience of others who have done similar work. A methodological expert in measurement is of assistance only when teamed with others who know the terrain of informatics. Conversely, all medical informatics researchers should know something about measurement.

Measurement and Demonstration Studies

The importance of measurement can be underscored by establishing a formal distinction between studies undertaken to develop methods for making measurements, which we call *measurement studies,* and the subsequent use of these methods to address questions of direct importance in informatics, which we call *demonstration studies.* Establishing a distinction between these types of studies and lending them approximately equal status in this textbook on methodology are steps intended to ensure that measurement issues are not overlooked by informatics researchers.

Measurement studies, then, seek to determine with how much error an attribute of interest can be measured in a population of objects. In an ideal objectivist measurement, all observers agree on the result of the measurement. Any disagreement is therefore due to error, which should be minimized. The more agreement there is among observers or across observations, the "better" is the measurement. It is also important that the observers are observing what is intended. Measurement procedures developed and validated through measurement studies provide researchers with what they need to conduct demonstration studies. Once it is known with how

---

* Terms such as "accuracy" and "precision" are used loosely in this chapter. They will be defined more rigorously in Chapter 5.

much error an attribute can be measured using a particular procedure, the measured values of this attribute can be employed as a variable in a demonstration study to draw inferences about the performance, perceptions, or effects of an information resource. For example, once a measurement study has established the error inherent in measuring the speed of an information resource, a related demonstration study would explore whether a particular resource has sufficient speed—with speed measured using methods developed in the measurement study—to meet the needs of busy clinicians.

As this discussion unfolds we will see numerous relations between measurement and demonstration study design, but there are also many important distinctions. There are differences in terminology that can become somewhat confusing. For example, measurement studies are concerned with attributes and objects, whereas demonstration studies are concerned with variables and subjects. With measurement we are concerned with differences between individual objects and how accurate the measurement is for each one. With demonstration studies, the primary interest is usually at the level of the group and how accurately we can estimate the mean (or some other indicator of central tendency) of a variable for that group. The two issues are, of course, intertwined. It is impossible to conduct a satisfactory demonstration study using poorly performing measurement methods. As is seen in subsequent chapters, errors in measurement can make differences between groups more difficult to detect or can produce apparent differences when none are truly present.

The bottom line is that investigators must know that their measurement methods are adequate—we define "adequacy" more rigorously in the next chapter—*before* collecting data for their studies. As shown in Figure 4.2, it is necessary to perform a measurement study involving data collection on a small scale to establish the adequacy of all measurement procedures if the measures to be used do not have an established "track record." Even if the measurement procedures of interest have a track record in a particular health care environment and with a specific mix of cases and care providers, they may not perform equally well in a different environment. Therefore measurement studies may still be necessary even when apparently tried-and-true measurement approaches are being employed. Researchers should always ask themselves: How good are my measures in this particular setting? whenever they are planning a study and before proceeding to the demonstration phase. The importance of measurement studies for informatics was signaled in 1990 by Michaelis et al.[2] Examples of published measurement studies in medical informatics are given in Appendix A.

Goals and Structure of Measurement Studies

The overall goal of a measurement study is to estimate with how much error an attribute can be measured for a class of objects, ultimately leading to a viable measurement process for later application to demonstration studies. We develop in Chapter 5 a theory that describes in more detail how measurement errors are esti-

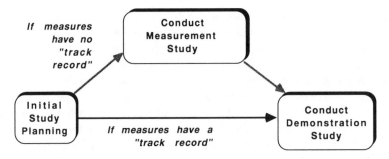

FIGURE 4.2. Measurement and demonstration studies.

mated, and in Chapter 6, building on that theory, we address the design of measurement studies in greater technical detail.

One specific objective of a measurement study is to determine how many independent observations are necessary to reduce error to a level acceptable for the demonstration study to follow. In most situations, the greater the number of independent observations comprising a measurement process, the smaller is the measurement error. This suggests an important trade-off because each independent observation comes at a cost. If the speed of a computer-based resource is to be tested over a range of computationally demanding tasks, each task must be carefully constructed or selected by the research team. Similarly, if persons are the objects of measurement, the time required to complete the multiple observations may be greater than these individuals are willing to provide. For example, a questionnaire requiring 100 answers from each respondent may be a more precise instrument than a questionnaire of half that length; but no one, especially a busy health professional, has the time available to complete it. In this case an investigator may be willing to trade off greater measurement error for a higher rate of participation in a demonstration study. Without a measurement study conducted in advance, however, there is no way to quantify this trade-off and determine the optimal balance point.

Another objective of measurement studies is to verify that measurement instruments are well designed and functioning as intended. Even a measurement process with an ample number of independent observations has a high error rate if there are fundamental flaws in the way the process is conducted. For example, if human judges are involved in a rating task and the judges are not trained to use the same criteria for the ratings, the results reveal unacceptably high error. Fatigue may be a factor if the judges are asked to do too much, too fast. Also, consider a computer program developed to compute a measure of medication costs directly from a computer-based patient record. If this program has a bug that causes it to fail to include certain classes of medications, it cannot return accurate results. An appropriate measurement study can detect these kinds of problems.

The researcher designing a measurement study should also try to build into the study features that challenge the measurement process in ways that might be expected to occur in the demonstration study to follow. Only in this way is it possible to determine if the results of the measurement study will apply when the measurement process is put to use. For example, in the rating task mentioned above, the judges should be challenged in the measurement study with a range of cases typical of those expected in the demonstration study. An algorithm to compute medication costs should be tested with a representative sample of cases from a variety of clinical services in the hospital where the demonstration study will ultimately be conducted. A related issue is that a measurement technique may perform well with individuals from one particular culture but perform poorly when transferred to a different culture. In informatics, this problem could arise when a study moves from a hospital that is growing and where employees have a great deal of autonomy to one where task performance is more rigidly prescribed. The same questionnaire administered in the two settings may yield different results because respondents are interpreting the questions differently. This issue too can be explored via a measurement study.

Measurement studies are planned in advance. The researcher conducting a measurement study creates a set of experimental conditions, applies the measurement technique under development to a set of objects, often makes other measurements on the objects, studies the results, and makes modifications in the measurement technique as suggested by the results. Measurement studies are sometimes conducted more informally than demonstration studies. Samples of convenience are often employed instead of systematically selected samples of objects, although there is clearly some risk involved in this practice. As a practical matter, measurement studies are often undertaken outside the specific setting where the demonstration study will later be performed. This is done because the investigator does not want to presensitize the setting in which the demonstration study will be conducted and thus introduce bias into the demonstration study. Also as a practical matter, in some situations where proved measurement methods do not exist, it is not possible to conduct measurement studies in advance of the demonstration studies. In these situations, researchers use the data collected in the demonstration study as the basis for statistical analyses that are customarily done as part as a measurement study.

As an example, consider a study of a new admission–discharge–transfer (ADT) system for hospitals. The attribute of "time to process a new admission" might be important for this study. Although on the surface this factor might seem trivial to measure, many potential difficulties arise on closer scrutiny. To cite a few: When did the admission process for a patient begin and end? Were there interruptions, and when did each of these begin and end? (Note that "patients" are the object class for this measurement process.) It was decided that human observers would be the instruments. In a measurement study, three or four observers might simultaneously observe the same set of admissions. The observers' level disagreement about the time to process these admissions would be used to determine how many observers (whose individual results are averaged) are necessary to obtain an acceptable error rate. If the error rate is too high, the measurement study might reveal that it is because the form on which the observers are recording their observations is flawed in some way, or because the observers had not been provided with adequate instuctions about how to deal with interruptions. The measurement study might be performed in the admissions suite of a hospital similar in many respects to the one in which the demonstration study will later be performed. The demonstration study, once the measurement methods were established, would explore whether the hospital processes admissions faster with the new system than with the preexisting system.

Self-Test 4.2

Clarke and colleagues developed the TraumAID system[3] to advise on initial treatment of patients with penetrating injuries to the chest and abdomen. Measurement studies of the utility of TraumAID's advice required panels of judges, for a set of "test cases," to rate the adequacy of management of these cases—as recommended by TraumAID and as carried out by care providers. To perform this study, case data were fed into TraumAID to generate a treatment plan for each case. TraumAID's plans were carefully edited, so judges performing subsequent ratings would have no way of knowing whether the described care was peformed by a human or recommended by computer. Two groups of judges were employed in the measurement studies: one group from the medical center where the resource was developed, the other a group of senior physicians from across the country.

For this measurement situation, name the attribute of interest and the object class; describe the instrumentation. List some issues that might be clarified by this measurement study. [Answers are found at the end of the chapter.]

Gold Standards and Informatics

A final issue before we leave the topic of measurement is the often-used term "gold standard" and its relation to measurement in informatics. In medical informatics we often bemoan the lack of so-called gold standards.[4] As we embark on an exploration of objectivist methods, it is timely to ask: What exactly is a gold standard? By traditional definition a gold standard is a composite of two notions. In the first sense a gold standard is an expression of practice carried out perfectly: the optimal therapy for a given medical problem or the best differential diagnosis to be entertaining at a particular point in the evolution of a case. In the second sense a gold standard implies complete acceptance or consensus. For a given situation, everyone qualified to render a judgment would agree to what the gold standard is. These two aspects of a gold standard are tightly interrelated. If there exists only one standard of care, it is a standard everyone would endorse completely.

The lack of gold standards in medicine has led some to adopt a view that in the absence of perfect gold standards it is not useful to conduct formal studies of medical information resources, because these studies would always be tainted by the fuzziness of whatever comparative standard is employed. Such individuals might further argue that we should, instead, rely on instinctive, marketplace, or political interpretations of the value of these resources. Other, less nihilistic researchers might still conduct empirical studies, but their studies are designed to bypass the gold standard issue. For example, instead of comparing the performance of an information resource against an imperfect standard of health care, about which there is necessarily disagreement among human experts, such studies seek to show that the resource agrees with the experts to the same extent that experts agree with each other.[5]

In the chapters to follow we take the position that gold standards, even if unattainable, are worth approximating. That is, "tarnished" or "fuzzy" standards are better than no standards at all. As we develop a theory of measurement, we develop a methodology for addressing the fuzziness of gold standards, joining others who have engaged in similar efforts.[6, 7] Perfect gold standards do not exist, in medical informatics or in any other domain of empirical research, but the extent to which these standards are less than perfect can be estimated and expressed as forms of measurement error. Knowledge of the magnitude and origin of this error enables the researcher to, in many cases, take the error into account in statistical analyses and thereby draw stronger conclusions than otherwise would be possible. Although zero measurement error is always the best situation, a good estimate of the magnitude of the error is sufficient to allow rigorous studies to be conducted. Thus we also argue that studies comparing the performance of information resources against imperfect standards, so long as the degree of imperfection has been estimated, represent a stronger approach than studies that bypass the issue of a standard altogether.

With this position as a backdrop (and with apologies for the colorfully mixed metaphor), the gold standard becomes a sort of red herring. More pragmatically we can view any standard employed in a study as the *measured* value of a chosen attribute, which we *accept* as an expedient knowing that the standard approximates but is not necessarily equal to the true "gold standard." For example, a patient's discharge diagnosis might be the imperfect standard in a study of a diagnostic system.[8] Even though we know that a discharge diagnosis sometimes proves later to have been incorrect, this is the best measure available, so we accept it. The alternative to accepting a less than perfect standard would be not to do the study, as an error-free appraisal of the patient's diagnosis may not be available until the patient's death—and may never be available if the patient fully recovers from his or her illness. Consistent with this view, the researcher's obligation is to develop the best possible ways to measure a standard suited to the context of the research, conduct measurement studies to estimate the error associated with measurement of the standard, and then, in demonstration studies, incorporate this error estimate appropriately into statistical analyses and interpretation of the results.

Each domain of clinical care creates its own challenges for researchers who inevitably find themselves in the role of developers and measurers of standards. Some domains make this task more challenging than others. We can speak of the "carat level" of a standard as a heuristic estimate of its level of error: the accuracy and precision with which its true value can be known. Table 4.2 lists some of the

TABLE 4.2. Prototypical "carat scale" of gold standards

Carats	Criteria
23+	Diagnosis of a patient who underwent a definitive test
20	Diagnosis of a patient about whom a great deal is known but for whom there is no definitive diagnosis
18	Appropriateness of a therapy plan for a patient with a specific diagnosis
15	Correctness of a critique issued by an advisory system
13	Adequacy of a diagnostic workup plan
10	Quality of a substance-abuse screening interview

domains that are addressed in medical informatics studies as well as a heuristic "carat level" reflecting the intrinsic difficulty of making precise measurements in that domain. (Table 4.2 is offered for illustrative purposes only, and no specific interpretation should be attached to the numbers provided.)

According to Table 4.2, there is no absolute 24-carat gold standard for any problem in medicine. Even a pathological process identified on autopsy might be erroneously identified or might be unrelated to the patient's symptoms. As seen later in our theory of error, the carat level of a standard can be estimated but cannot be determined precisely. Precise determination would require, for each member of a class of objects, knowledge of the true value of an attribute against which the purported standard can be compared; and if we knew the true value, it would by definition become the 24-carat standard. There are, in addition, some clinical situations where an almost-perfect standard can be known, but only through studies that are too expensive or dangerous to conduct. In such cases, we accept the more approximate, lower carat standard. For example, electrocardiography plus a thallium scan is a currently accepted protocol to evaluate coronary artery disease because an arteriogram involves too much risk in patients with minimal symptoms.

Structure of Demonstration Studies

We move now from a discussion of measurement to a discussion of demonstration. Demonstration studies differ from measurement studies in several respects. First, they aim to say something meaningful about the utility of an information resource in health care or to answer some other question of substantive interest in informatics. With measurement studies the concern is with the error inherent in assigning a value of an attribute to each individual object, whereas with demonstration studies the concern is redirected toward determining the magnitude of that attribute or if groups of objects differ in terms of the magnitude of that attribute. For example, in a study of an information resource to support management of patients in the intensive care unit, a measurement study would be concerned with how accurately and precisely the "optimal care" (attribute) for a patient (object) can be determined. The demonstration study might explore whether care providers supported by the resource deliver care more closely approximating optimal care.

The terminology of demonstration studies also changes from that used for measurement studies. Most notable are the following points:

- The *object* of measurement in a measurement study is typically referred to as a *subject* in a demonstration study.
- An *attribute* in a measurement study is typically referred to as a *variable* in a demonstration study.

In theory, these terminology differences are disconcerting, but in practice they seldom cause confusion.

When designing objectivist studies, variables are divided into two categories: dependent and independent. The *dependent variables* are a subset of the variables in the study that capture outcomes of interest to the investigator. For this reason, dependent variables are also called "outcome variables." The *independent variables* are those included in a study to explain the measured values of the dependent variables.

Demonstration studies can be descriptive, comparative, or correlational in design, as illustrated in Figure 4.3. A study falls into one of these categories largely based on its intents.

Descriptive Studies

A *descriptive* design seeks only to estimate the value of a dependent variable or set of dependent variables in a selected sample of subjects. Descriptive designs have no independent variable. If a group of nurses were given a rating form (previously validated through a measurement study) to ascertain the "ease of use" of a nursing information system, the mean value of this variable would be the key result of a demonstration study. If this value were found to be toward the low end of the scale, the researchers might conclude from this descriptive study that the system was in need of substantial revision. Even though they seem deceptively simple, descriptive studies can be highly informative. The often-cited study by Teach and Shortliffe[9] of physicians' attitudes toward medical decision support is an example of a descriptive study that has had substantial impact. Descriptive studies can be tied to the "objectives-based" approach to evaluation described in Chapter 2. When an investigator seeks to determine whether a resource has met a predetermined set of performance objectives, the logic and design of the resulting study may be seen as descriptive. The objections themselves are external to the empirical study.

Comparative Studies

In a *comparative* study, the investigator typically creates a contrasting set of conditions. After identifying a sample of subjects for the study, the researcher assigns

(A)

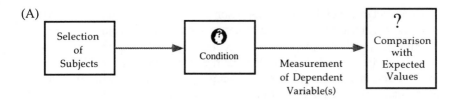

(B)

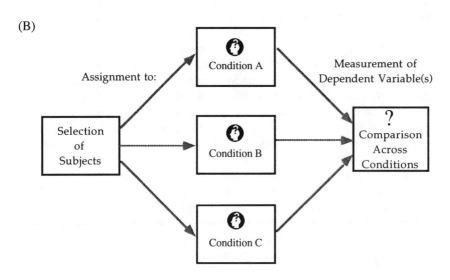

(C)

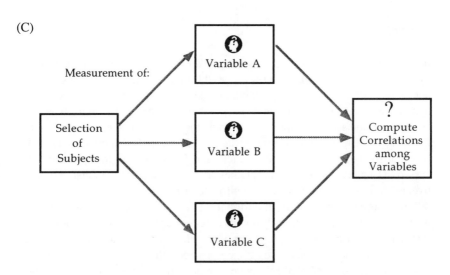

FIGURE 4.3. (A) Descriptive study design. (B) Comparative study design. (C) Correlational study design.

each subject to one of these conditions. Some variable of interest is then measured for each subject, and the measured values of this variable are compared across the conditions. The contrasting conditions comprise the independent variable for the study, and the "variable of interest" comprises the dependent variable. The study by MacDonald et al.[10] of the effects of reminder systems is a classic example of a comparative study applied to informatics. In this study, groups of clinicians (subjects) either received or did not receive computer-generated reminders about their patients (conditions comprising the independent variable), and the investigators measured the extent to which clinicians took clinical actions consistent with the reminders (dependent variable). Comparative studies are aligned with the "comparison-based" approach to evaluation introduced in Chapter 2.

When the contrasting experimental conditions are created by the investigator, and all other differences are eliminated by random assignment of subjects, it is possible to explore the effect due solely to the difference between the conditions. This also allows the researcher to assert that these effects are causal, rather than merely coincidental. Under such controlled conditions, a comparative study can approach the ideal of the randomized clinical trial as described in the literature of clinical epidemiology.[11] However, it is not always possible to manipulate the environment to the extent required to conduct such a pure experiment. In some of these cases, the investigator might forego random assignment of subjects to groups and thus conduct what is called a "quasi-experiment." Even when the results of a quasi-experiment reveal a difference between groups on the dependent measure, the source of the effect cannot be isolated as the independent variable because some unknown difference between the groups themselves may be the causal factor.

Correlational Studies

In other cases, researchers conduct *correlational* studies, which explore the hypothesized relations among a set of variables the researcher measures but does not manipulate in any way. Correlational studies are guided by the researcher's hypotheses, which direct the choice of variables included in the study. The independent variables are the hypothesized predictors of an outcome of interest, which is the dependent variable. Correlational studies are linked most closely to the "comparison-based" and "decision-facilitation" approaches to evaluation discussed in Chapter 2. Correlational studies are also called observational, retrospective, or ex post facto studies. Case-control studies in epidemiology can be seen to fall into this category as well. In informatics, an example of a correlational study is one where the researcher analyzes the extent of use of an information resource (the dependent variable) as a function of the clinical workload and the seniority (two independent variables) of each care provider (the subjects) in a hospital. In this study, the values of all the variables are properties of the subjects that cannot be manipulated and are studied retrospectively. As another example of a correlational study, the number of physicians in a hospital who enter their own medication orders may be followed over time. If an increase is seen soon after a new user interface is implemented, the investigator would be led to argue that the change in user interface was the cause of the increase. Although such an uncontrolled study cannot be the basis of a strong inference of cause and effect, correlational studies can be highly persuasive when carefully conducted.

Laboratory studies of information resources, as discussed in Chapter 3, tend to be comparative in nature because they include variables that are manipulated by the experimenter. Field studies tend to be more correlational in nature. Although it is possible with great effort and at substantial expense to conduct a carefully controlled, comparative study in the field, in many settings it is difficult, and sometimes even unethical, to manipulate variables and impose statistical controls where ongoing health care is delivered. Such a dilemma may arise, for example, with an alerting system that warns clinicians of drug interactions. If laboratory studies that have already been conducted suggest that the advice of this resource is accurate, a human subjects review committee (also known as an Institutional Review Board, or IRB) might disallow a randomized trial of the resource because it is considered unethical to withhold this advice from the care of any patient. To cite one example, a clinical trial of the MEDIPHOR system at Stanford University was disallowed on these grounds (S.N. Cohen, personal communication, 1996).

Shared Features of Objectivist Studies

By comparing Figures 4.3A, B, and C, it can be seen that these different study designs share several features. They all entail a deliberate selection of subjects, an explicit identification of variables, and a process of measurement yielding data for analysis. They differ, as discussed above, in their general aims, the degree of imposed control or manipulation, and the logic of data analysis.

It is important, as a prerequisite to undertaking the design of studies to understand the distinctions offered in this section. The distinction between independent and dependent variables is central.

Self-Test 4.3

Classify each of the following demonstration study designs as descriptive, comparative, or correlational. In each study, who or what are the subjects? Identify the independent and dependent variables.

1. In Chapter 2, we discussed the T-HELPER system. One of this resource's goals is to identify patients who are eligible for specific clinical protocols. A demonstration study of T-HELPER is implemented to examine protocol enrollment rates at sites where T-HELPER was and was not installed.

2. A new clinical workstation is introduced into a network of medical offices. Logs of 1 week of resource use by nurses are studied. The report enumerates sessions on the workstation, broken down into logical categories.

3. A number of computer-based information resources have been installed to support care on an inpatient service. The information resources log the identity of the patients about whom inquiries are made. By chart audit, the investigators identify a number of clinical characteristics of each patient's clinical problems. The investigators then study which characteristics of patients are predictive of the use of resources to obtain further information about that patient.

4. Students are given access to a database to help them solve problems in a biomedical domain. By random assignment, half of the students use a version of the database emphasizing hypertext browsing capabilities; half use a version emphasizing Boolean queries for information. The proficiency of these students at solving problems is assessed at the beginning and end of the second year of medical school.

Planning Demonstration Studies

We close this chapter with a description of the steps required to develop a demonstration study. This discussion is a preview of the much more complete exploration of designs for demonstration studies in Chapter 7. It is included to alert the reader to the complexities of demonstration studies, particularly those carried out in ongoing patient care or educational settings. Planning a demonstration study can be seen as a three-stage process, as shown in Figure 4.4. First, one must define the problem the study is intended to address. This means eliciting the aim of the study and the main questions to be answered. It is then useful to classify the study, as clearly as possible, using the distinctions offered in Chapter 3 and summarized in Table 3.1. A study may emphasize structure, function, or impact; and it may be seen as occurring primarily in a laboratory or field setting. From this information a general design for the study—descriptive, comparative, correlational—can be inferred. The needs of studies that address resource stucture and function are often satisfied by an objectives-based approach (Is the resource performing up to the level the designers expected?), which would recommend a descriptive study design. If a study addresses impact (Does the resource make a difference in health care?), a comparative or correlational design must be employed, depending on the amount of control that can be imposed on the study setting. Comparative designs are also employed in studies where the investigators seek to show that the information resource is an improvement over what it replaced. Once the general design has been determined, evaluators can go on to define the dependent and independent variables and consider how these factors might be measured. If the measurement instruments and procedures proposed for use do not have a "track record" (Fig. 4.2), it may be necessary to undertake measurement studies before the demonstration study itself can be completed.

The second stage of planning a study is to propose a more specific design. As suggested in Figure 4.4, a study design consists of three parts. There must be a statement of the setting in which the study will be conducted and of the source, kind, and number of subjects. The conditions of the study must be established if

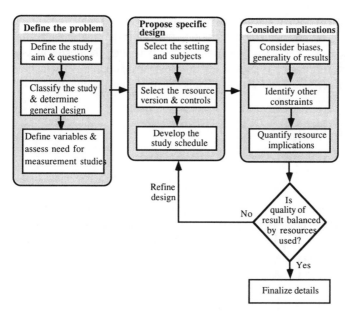

FIGURE 4.4. Three stages of study planning.

the study is comparative in nature. The version of the resource and any "control" resource to be tested must be selected. The final part is to outline the study schedule. In the case of evaluations of resource function (see Chapter 3), the schedule may be simple, but in studies concerned with the impact of the resource on users or on health care the schedule may be complex because the study must be embedded in an organized routine of health care that usually cannot be altered substantially to suit the needs of the study. The schedule must clarify which subjects have access to which version of the resource at each phase of the study.

The third stage of planning an evaluation is to consider the possible implications of the proposed study design. The most important of these implications are biases that threaten the study's scientific validity. Specific biases to consider are discussed in detail in Chapter 7. Even if there are no significant biases, there may be limits to the generalizability of the study results or other constraints (related to ethics, time, or other factors) that make certain study plans not feasible. Each plan also has resource implications that may require careful examination.

Once the implications of the proposed plan have been listed, evaluators can balance the probable quality of the intended results with the kind and quantity of resources necessary to obtain them. If this balance proves initially to be unsatisfactory, it becomes necessary to refine the proposed plan and reconsider its implications several times before a promising plan emerges. Finally, evaluators must clarify the details of the study plan and express it in a study contract before the study is started to ensure that as many problems as possible are anticipated and defused. Every investigator designing a study must do so with the realization that every study is in some way a compromise, balancing the desire to assess many variables with many subjects under the most ideal conditions against the realities of limited resources and what is permissible in the environment.

Answers to Self-Tests

Self-Test 4.1

1. The attribute is "appropriateness" of each alert. "Alerts" comprise the object class. (Note that cases are *not* the object class here because each alert is what is directly rated—the attribute of "appropriateness" is a characteristic of each alert—and because each case may have generated multiple alerts related to different clinical aspects of the case.) The instrument is the rating form as completed by a human judge. Each individual judge's rating of the appropriateness of an alert constitutes an independent observation.
2. The attribute is "knowledge of the clinical information system." Physicians comprise the object class. The instrument is the written test. Each question on the test constitutes an independent observation.
3. The attribute is "correctness" of the indexing. "Cases" comprise the object class.

Self-Test 4.2

The attribute is "adequacy of management"; cases (trauma patients) comprise the object class; the instrumentation includes the judges and the form used to record their ratings.

The measurement study could elucidate (1) whether there is a difference between local and national judges, which may be embodied in practice norms that are part of the institutional culture; (2) how many judges are needed to rate each case with an acceptable error rate; (3) if the training for the task and forms used for the task need improvement; (4) if the test cases show sufficient difficulty as a set to be useful in demonstration studies. If all cases are managed perfectly by both TraumAID and the care providers, they are not challenging enough to be used in the demonstration study.

Self-Test 4.3

1. It is a comparative study because the investigators presumably had some control over where the resource was or was not installed. The site is the "subject"

for this study. (Note that this point is a bit ambiguous. Patients could possibly be seen as the subjects in the study; but as the question is phrased, the enrollment rates at the sites are going to the basis of comparison. Because the enrollment rate must be computed for a *site,* then site must be the "subject.") It follows that the dependent variable is the protocol enrollment rates; the independent variable is the presence or absence of T-HELPER.

2. It is a descriptive study. Sessions on the workstation are the "subjects." There is no independent variable. Dependent variables are the extent of workstation use in each category.

3. It is a correlational study. The patients on the service are the subjects. The independent variables are the clinical characteristics of the patients; the dependent variable is the extent of use of information resources.

4. Comparative study. Students are the subjects. Independent variable(s) are the version of the database and time of assessment. The dependent variable is the score on the problem-solving assessment.

References

1. Feinstein AR: Clinimetrics. New Haven: Yale University Press, 1987:viii.
2. Michaelis J, Wellek S, Willems JL: Reference standards for software evaluation. Methods Inf Med 1990;29:289–297.
3. Clarke JR, Webber BL, Gertner A, Rymon KJ: On-line decision support for emergency trauma management. Proc Symp Comput Applications Med Care 1994;18:1028.
4. Shortliffe E: Computer programs to support medical decisions. JAMA 1987; 258:61–66.
5. Quaglini S, Stefanelli M, Barosi G, Berzuini A: A performance evaluation of the expert system ANAEMIA. Comp Biomed Res 1987;21:307–323.
6. Walter SD, Irwig LM: Estimation of test error rates, disease prevalence and relative risk from misclassified data: a review. J Clin Epidemiol 1988;41:923–937.
7. Phelps CD, Hutson A: Estimating diagnostic test accuracy using a "fuzzy gold standard." Med Decis Making 1995;15:44–57.
8. Bankowitz RA, McNeil MA, Challinor SM, Parker RC, Kapoor WN, Miller RA: A computer-assisted medical diagnostic consultation service: implementation and prospective evaluation of a prototype. Ann Intern Med 1989;110:824–832.
9. Teach RL, Shortliffe EH: An analysis of physician attitudes regarding computer-based clinical consultation systems. Comput Biomed Res 1981;14:542–558.
10. McDonald CJ, Hui SL, Smith DM, et al.: Reminders to physicians from an introspective computer medical record: a two-year randomized trial. Ann Intern Med 1984;100:130–138.
11. Sackett DL, Haynes RB, Guyatt GH, Tugwell P: Clinical Epidemiology: A Basic Science for Clinical Medicine. Boston: Little Brown, 1991.

Appendix A: Compendium of Measurement Studies

This list was compiled by Randy Cork, a medical informatics fellow at the University of North Carolina, 1994–1996. The list is divided into two sections. The first section offers a set of studies that are purely measurement studies; the second section offers a set of studies that include demonstration study results but that also explicitly address measurement issues. The focus of this compendium is studies of attitudes and other psychological states that relate directly to the use of information technology in health care.

Measurement Studies

Baggs JG: Two instruments to measure interdisciplinary bioethical decision making. Heart Lung 1993;22(6):542–547.

Bailey JE: Development of an instrument for the management of computer user attitudes in hospitals. Methods Inf Med 1990;29:51–56.

Cohen BA, Waugh GW: Assessing computer anxiety. Psychol Rep 1989; 65:735–738.

Cohen S, Kamarck T, Mermelstein R: A global measure of perceived stress. J Health Soc Behav 1983;24:385–396.

Jette AM, Davies AR, Cleary PD, et al: The functional status questionnaire reliability and validity when used in primary care. J Gen Intern Med 1986; 1:143–149.

Kernan MC, Howard GS: Computer anxiety and computer attitudes: an investigation of construct and predictive validity issues. Educ Psychol Meas 1990; 50:681–90.

Loyd BH, Gressard C: Reliability and factorial validity of computer attitude scales. Educ Psychol Meas 1984;44:501–505.

Meadows KA, Fromson B, Gillespie C, et al: Development, validation, and application of compter-linked knowledge questionnaires in diabetes education. Diabetic Med 1988;5:61–67.

Moore GC, Benbasat I: Development of an instrument to measure the perceptions of adopting an information technology innovation. Inf Syst Res 1991;2: 192–222.

Nickell GS, Pinto JN: The computer attitude scale. Comput Hum Behav 1986;2:301–306.

Pillar B: The measurement of technology anxiety. Proc Symp Comput Applications Med Care 1985;9:570–574.

Reece MJ, Gable RK: The development and validation of a measure of general attitudes toward computers. Educ Psychol Meas 1982;42:913–916.

Shore BE, Franks P: Physician satisfaction with patient encounters: reliability and validity of an encounter-specific questionnaire. Med Care 1986;24:580–589.

Shortell SM, Rousseau DM, Gillies RR, Devers KJ, Simons TL: Organizational assessment in intensive care units (ICUs): construct development, reliability, and validity of the ICU nurse-physician questionnaire. Med Care 1991; 29:709–726.

Staggers N: The Staggers nursing computer experience questionnaire. Appl Nurs Res 1994;7:97–106.

Stronge JH, Brodt A: Assessment of nurses' attitudes towards computerization. Comput Nurs 1985;3:154–158.

Thomas B: Development of an instrument to assess attitudes toward computing in nursing. Comput Nurs 1988;6:122–127.

Demonstration and Measurement Issue Studies

Anderson RM, Donnelly MB, Hess GE: An assessment of computer use, knowledge, and attitudes of diabetes educators. Diab Educ 1992;18:40–46.

Anderson JG, Jay SJ, Schweer HM, Anderson MM: Perceptions of the impact of computers on medical practice and physician use of a hospital information system. Proc Symp Comput Applications Med Care 1985;9:565–570.

Anderson JG, Jay SJ, Schweer HM, et al: Physician utilization of computers in medical practice: policy implications based on a structural model. Soc Sci Med 1986;23:259–267.

Anderson JG, Jay SJ, Schweer HM, et al: Why doctors don't use computers: some empirical findings. J R Soc Med 1986;79:142–144.

Brown SH, Coney RD: Changes in computer anxiety and attitudes related to clinical information system use. J Am Med Inf Assoc 1994;1:381–394.

Burkes M: Identifying and relating nurses' attitudes toward computer use. Comput Nurs 1991;9:190–201.

Dixon DR, Dixon BJ: Adoption of information technology enabled innovations by primary care physicians: model and questionnaire development. Proc Symp Comput Applications Med Care 1994;18:631–635.

Farrell AD, Cuseo-Ott L, Fenerty M: Development and evaluation of a scale for measuring practitioners' attitudes toward computer applications. Comput Hum Behav 1988;4:207–220.

Gerritty MS, DeVellis RF, Earp JA: Physicians' reactions to uncertainty in patient care: a new measure and new insights. Med Care 1990;28:724–736.

Koohang AA: A study of attitudes towards computers: anxiety, confidence, liking, and perception of usefulness. J Res Comput Educ 1989;2:137–150.

Melhorn JM, Legler WK, Clark GM: Current attitudes of medical personnel towards computers. Comput Biomed Res 1979;2:327–334.

Murphy CA, Maynard M, Morgan G: Pretest and post-test attitudes of nursing personnel toward a patient care information system. Comput Nurs 1994;12:239–244.

Reznikoff M, Holland CH, Stroebel CF: Attittudes toward computers among employees of a psychiatric hospital. Ment Hyg 1967;51:419–425.

Scarpa R, Smeltzer SC, Jaison B: Attitudes of nurses toward computerization: a replication. Comput Nurs 1992;10:72–80.

Schwirian PA, Malone JA, Stone VJ, et al: Computers in nursing practice: a comparison of the attitudes of nurses and nursing students. Comput Nurs 1989;7:168–177.

Startsman TS, Robinson RE: The attitudes of medical and paramedical personnel toward computers. Comput Biomed Res 1982;5:218–227.

Teach RL, Shortliffe EH: An analysis of physician attitudes regarding computer-based clinical consultation systems. Comput Biomed Res 1981; 4:542–548.

Thomas B: Development of a measure to assess attitudes toward computing in nursing. Proc Symp Comput Applications Med Care 1988;12:355-357.

5

Basics of Measurement

There is growing understanding that all measuring instruments must be critically and empirically examined for their reliability and validity. The day of tolerance of inadequate measurement has ended.[1]

In Chapter 4 we established a strong distinction between *measurement studies* to determine how well (with how much error) we can measure an attribute of interest and *demonstration studies*, which use these measures to make descriptive or comparative assertions. Whereas we might conclude from a measurement study that a certain process makes it possible to measure the "speed" of a resource in executing a certain family of tasks to a precision of ±10%, we would conclude from a demonstration study that a hospital where resource A is deployed completes this task with greater speed than a hospital using resource B. Demonstration studies are the focus of Chapter 7; measurement and measurement studies are the foci of this chapter and the next.

Recall from Chapter 4 that measurement studies are, ideally, always conducted before demonstration studies exploring the same issues. All measurement studies have a common general structure and employ an established family of analytical techniques, which are introduced in this chapter. In such a study the measurement of interest is undertaken with a sample of objects under conditions similar to those expected in the demonstration study, to the extent that those conditions can be created or simulated. The data generated by a measurement study are analyzed to estimate the error inherent in the measurement process. The error estimate—which is indeed an estimate because it derives from a *sample* of objects and perhaps also from a sample of circumstances under which the measurement will be made—is the primary result. In general, the greater the sample size in a measurement study, the greater the confidence the researcher can place in the estimate of the size of the measurement error. Sometimes the results of a measurement study suggest that measurement methods must be further refined before the demonstration study can be undertaken with confidence. After the refinements are made, the researcher may wish to repeat the measurement study to verify that the expected reduction in error has occurred.

A demonstration study usually yields, as a by-product, data that can be analyzed to estimate some kinds of measurement error. It is good to carry out these analyses to confirm that errors are in accord with expected levels. However, orthodox measurement studies conducted fully in advance of demonstration studies are always preferable. If error estimates derived from a demonstration study reveal unacceptable levels of measurement error, it can invalidate the demonstration study and all the time and effort that went into it. Of course, the researcher conducting the demonstration study does *not* have to conduct a measurement study if results of measurement studies previously conducted by other researchers, using the same instruments under similar circumstances, provide credible error estimates. For this reason, carefully designed and conducted measurement studies are themselves important contributions to the literature, as they can enable future researchers to choose measurement methods with greater confidence and without having to conduct measurement studies of their own.

Error: Reliability and Validity of Measurement

Nothing is perfect. All measurements have errors. Much of the work in measurement is devoted to (1) estimating the magnitude of the error and (2) minimizing the error. We initially develop the notion of error according to a classical theory of measurement within which the two central concepts are reliability and validity.[1,2]

In classical theory, reliability is the degree to which measurement is consistent or reproducible. A measurement that is reasonably reliable is measuring *something*. Validity is the degree to which that *something* is what the investigator wants to measure. Reliability is a logical and pragmatic precursor to validity. We cannot even discuss the validity of a measurement process until we demonstrate it to be reasonably reliable. Note that reliability and validity are not properties solely of the measurement instrument but, rather, of the total measurement process. Changing any aspect of the total measurement process may introduce error or change the nature of the error. A classic example is a simple altimeter, which becomes invalid if the barometric pressure changes. A questionnaire written using technical computer language and shown to be reliable when administered to a sophisticated group of computer users may be much less reliable when administered to a group untrained in the technology.

Classical theory makes the assumption that an observed score for any object can be represented as the sum of the unknowable result of a perfectly reproducible measurement (the "true" score) and measurement error. This point is illustrated in Figure 5.1.

The "true" score, in addition to being unknowable, is also something of a misnomer because it still may not be fully accurate. Although perfectly reproducible for each object and therefore totally reliable, the true score is not necessarily accurate because it may be invalid. The true score may be measuring a composite of the attribute of interest and some other attributes. The true score thus has two components: a valid component capturing the extent to which it reflects the desired attribute and an invalid component reflecting the extent to which it reflects some other attribute(s). In classical theory, the errors that contribute to unreliabil-

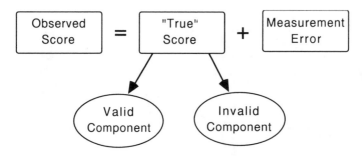

FIGURE 5.1. Components of an observed (measured) score in classical theory. (Note that the "true score" is not all that its name implies!)

ity are unsystematic. They are assumed to be normally distributed about a mean of zero and to be uncorrelated with true scores and any other sources of error. In effect, these errors introduce noise into the result of a set of measurements. They affect the results of measurements in ways that are estimable in magnitude, over a set of measurements, but unpredictable in detail as they affect the results of measurements on individual objects. By contrast, the errors that contribute to invalidity tend to affect measurement results in ways that can potentially be explained.

The analogy to an archer shooting at an irregularly shaped target, as shown in Figure 5.2, may be instructive. Each target corresponds to an object with a fuzzy "bull's-eye" corresponding to a completely accurate result of the measurement. Each arrow corresponds to a single observation, the result of one act of measurement. The bull's-eye is fuzzy because the archer knows that the target has a bull's-eye but does not know exactly where the bull's-eye is. The irregularly shaped target gives only imprecise cues as to the location of the bull's-eye, and each target has its bull's-eye in a different location. So for each target the archer aims at where he *thinks* the bull's-eye is. If there is enough coherence to the archer's shooting to speak meaningfully of a central point about which the arrows cluster, the archer has enough reliability to prompt a meaningful discussion of validity. The reliability is inversely related to the amount of scatter of the arrows about the central point. The central point, even if no arrows strike it exactly, estimates the result for which the archer was aiming. If the archer shoots an infinite number of arrows, the central point about which these arrows would cluster would be exactly equal to the point the archer was aiming for. This central point is analogous to the true score. The smaller the distance between this central point—for which the archer was aiming—and the bull's-eye on the target, the greater is the archer's validity. We can estimate the reliability of a measurement process through the relatively easy task of measuring the scatter of the arrows; determining the validity of the measurement entails a much more complicated and uncertain process of trying to determine the real location of the bull's-eye.

In other disciplines, terms equivalent to reliability and validity are used to describe and quantify measurement error. Of greatest importance to medical

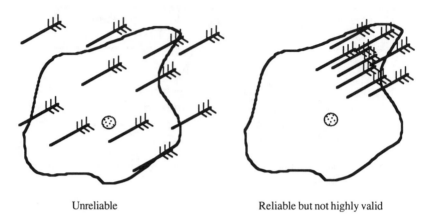

Unreliable   Reliable but not highly valid

FIGURE 5.2. Measurement as archery.

informatics, some clinical epidemiologists use "precision" as a synonym for reliability and "accuracy" as a synonym for validity.[3] Feinstein suggested that "consistency" may be a preferable substitute for both reliability and precision.[4]

Method of Multiple Simultaneous Observations

In general, the reliability of a measurement can be improved by increasing the
number of observations for each object and averaging the results. In this way, the
observed score more closely approximates the true score. Using the archery
metaphor, the more arrows the archer shoots, the more precisely do the results
estimate the point at which the archer is aiming.

Moving from the world of archers, how do we undertake multiple measurements in our world? One logical, often useful way is to repeat them over time.
This method provides an estimate of what is known as *test–retest reliability*. This
approach is conceptually elegant and works well in the laboratory where the
objects of study are nonhuman and relatively stable over time, as with measurements of machine performance. However, the repeated measurements technique
often does not work well when studying the attributes of humans or of humans in
interaction with machines, as is often the case in medical informatics. When
humans are involved in test–retest studies, it is necessary to bring them back for
the repeat study at just the right time and recreate precisely the circumstances of
the initial measurement. The timing is critical. If too little time has elapsed, perhaps only 1 day, humans remember what they did the last time and just do it again,
which overestimates the reliability of the measurement. If too much time has
elapsed, perhaps as little as 1 month, the values of the objects' true scores may
have changed owing to some experience in the world, which then underestimates

the reliability of the measurement. The test–retest approach to reliability, then, can have two limitations—because it is difficult to convince people to do anything again and even more difficult to get them back after what is considered to be the correct interval for the particular measurement under study.

An alternative approach, often necessary for studies of human behavior, employs multiple observations conducted on the *same occasion*. These simultaneous observations cannot be carried out identically, of course. In that case, humans would respond identically to each one. *The observations can be crafted in ways that are different enough for each observation to create a unique challenge for the object yet similar enough that they all measure essentially the same attribute.* The agreement between the results of these multiple simultaneous observations provides an estimate of *internal consistency reliability.* Using the archery metaphor, it is roughly analogous to having a set of archers, each placed at a slightly different angle so each has a slightly different view of the target. On command, each archer shoots one arrow simultaneously with the others (Fig. 5.3).

To see the contrast, consider the TraumAID system to advise on the care of patients with penetrating injuries of the chest and abdomen.[5] This resource might be studied by asking expert judges to rate the procedures suggested by the system over a series of cases. Thus the objects are the cases (and more specifically the set of procedures within each case), the judges' ratings comprise the observations, and the attribute is the "appropriateness" of the recommended care for each case. If each judge rated each case and then, 3 months later, rated the same set of cases again, the agreement of each judge with himself or herself from one time to the next would assess test–retest reliability. If each judge rated each case only once, the agreement across judges would be a measure of internal consistency reliability. The appeal of the test–retest approach is limited because the judges may remember the cases even after an interval as long as three months, or they may be unwilling to carry out the ratings twice. Lengthening the time interval between ratings increases the risk that the standard of care would change. Disagreements between test and retest judgments, then, might be attributable to sources other than measurement error.

A set of differing observations taken at approximately the same time, each purporting to measure the same attribute, may be called a *scale* or an *index*.* Thinking of measurement problems in terms of multiple observations to measure a common attribute is useful for several reasons. First, without these multiple observations we may have no way of estimating the reliability of a measurement process, as the test–retest approach is often impractical. Second, a one-observa-

---

* Technically, there is a difference between a scale and an index,[6] but for purposes of this discussion the terms can be used interchangeably. Also note that the term "scale" has two uses in measurement. In addition to the definition given above, "scale" can also refer to the set of response options from which one chooses when completing a rating form or questionnaire. In popular parlance, one might say "respond on a one to ten scale" how satisfied you are with this information system. We often move freely, and without too much damage, between these two senses of the term.

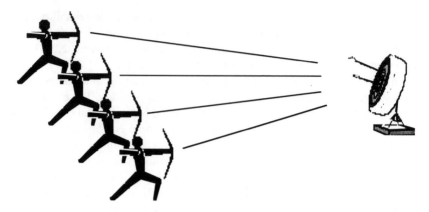

FIGURE 5.3. Archery and the method of multiple simultaneous observations.

tion measurement rarely is sufficiently reliable for use in research: How can we possibly determine, based on one arrow, at what an archer was aiming? Hence multiple observations are necessary to produce a functioning research instrument. One shortcoming of the multiple observations approach is that the observations we believe to be equivalent (and thus to comprise a scale) may not in fact be equivalent. To address this problem, there is a well-codified methodology for constructing scales (discussed in Chapter 6).

Whether we use the test–retest method or the multiple simultaneous observation approach, the best estimate of the true value of the attribute for each object is the average of the independent observations. If we know the reliability of a measurement process, we can then estimate the error due to random or unsystematic sources in any individual object's score. This error estimate is known as the standard error of measurement and is defined more precisely in the next section. Also, knowledge of the reliability of a measurement process can help us understand to what degree errors of measurement are contributing to a possible underestimate of group differences in demonstration studies. Lack of measurement reliability may erode estimates of the accuracy of a decision support system.

Estimating Reliability and Measurement Errors

One important goal of a measurement study is to quantify the reliability of a measurement process. We have seen that it can be accomplished by two general methods. Using a representative sample of objects we can employ a measurement process using multiple simultaneous observations to estimate internal consistency reliability, or we can repeat a measurement process on separate occasions, which enables estimation of test–retest reliability. From the results of both of these studies we can compute a reliability coefficient with a maximum value of 1.0. The reliability coefficient (ρ) is defined, somewhat abstractly, as the fraction of the total variability in the scores of all objects attributable to differences in the true scores of the objects themselves. That is:

$$\rho = \frac{V_{\infty}}{V_{total}}$$

where: V_{∞} = variability due to true score differences
V_{total} = total variability in the measurements

This formula, as it stands, is not helpful. The true score variability cannot be observed directly from the results of a measurement process. However, by using the assumptions of classical measurement theory and performing some algebra not shown here, we can put this formula in a more useful form. Using the assumption that the errors that reduce reliability of measurement are unsystematic and thus uncorrelated with true scores, we can conclude that the true score variability is equal to the total variability minus the variability due to error. We may thus write:

$$\rho = \frac{V_{total} - V_{error}}{V_{total}}$$

This formula is more helpful because both quantities on the right side of the formula can be computed directly from the data generated by a measurement study. The total variability is the statistical variance of all observations over all objects used in the measurement study, and the variability due to error can be estimated as the extent to which object scores vary across observations. Returning to the archery metaphor, V_{error} can be likened to the observable scatter of the arrows about the point the archer was aiming for. The greater the scatter, the lower the reliability.

As a first example, consider the following result of a measurement study, a result rarely seen in nature. Each object displays an identical result for all five observations thought to comprise a scale. The objects in this example could be clinical cases, and the observations could be the ratings by expert judges of the quality of care provided in each case. Alternatively, the objects could be people, and the observations could be their responses to a set of questions that address a specific issue on a questionnaire. Table 5.1 is the first example of an objects-by-observations matrix, which is the way results of measurement studies are typically portrayed. Because scores for each object are identical across observations, the best estimate of the error is 0 and the best estimate of the reliability is 1.0. (In this situation each arrow always lands in the same place on each target!) Because the average of the observations is the result of the measurement, object A's score would be 3, object B's score would be 4, and so forth. There is no scatter or variability in the results from the individual observations, so we place high confidence in these results as a measurement of *something*. (A separate issue is whether this *something* is in fact what the investigator thinks it is. This is the issue of validity, discussed later.) If the matrix in Table 5.1 were the result of a measurement study,

TABLE 5.1. Perfectly reliable measurement

Object	Observations					Object score
	1	2	3	4	5	
A	3	3	3	3	3	3
B	4	4	4	4	4	4
C	2	2	2	2	2	2
D	5	5	5	5	5	5

TABLE 5.2. More typical measurement result

Object	Observations					Object score
	1	2	3	4	5	
A	4	5	3	5	5	4.4
B	3	5	5	3	4	4.0
C	4	4	4	4	5	4.2
D	3	2	3	2	3	2.6

this estimate of perfect reliability would be limited to the set of objects and obser-vation methods employed in the study. For a hypothetical object E added to the study, the results of all five observations might not be identical, which would lower the estimated value of the reliability.

In a more typical example (Table 5.2), the observations vary in terms of their values for each object. Each object's score is now the average of observations whose results are not identical. The total variability has a component due to error, the magnitude of which can be estimated from the amount of disagreement among the observations for each object. The reliability coefficient in this particular case is 0.81. We still place high credence in the results as a measurement of *something*, but the measurement is now associated with an error whose magnitude we can estimate.

The details of the reliability computation are beyond this discussion. A variety of statistical packages perform this reliability calculation, or it can be readily pro-grammed on a spreadsheet using formulas provided in Appendix A. The reliabil-ity coefficient generated by these methods is known as Cronbach's alpha (α).[7] Other reliability coefficients exist, but α is commonly used and is applicable to a wide range of situations.

To the extent that a measurement lacks reliability, the results of the measure-ments on each object are associated with greater error. We cannot specify the magnitude or direction of this error precisely—if we could, we could correct it—but using the classical theory of measurement, we can compute the *standard error of measurement* (SE) as:

$$SE_{meas} = SD\sqrt{1 - \rho}$$

where SD is the standard deviation of all measurement results: the standard deviation of the "object scores" in Table 5.2.

The standard error of measurement allows us to place an error bracket around the result of a measurement for each object. The standard error of measurement is the estimated value of the standard deviation for a series of measurements made on the same object. The mean of a series of measurements estimates the "true score." Recall that measurement errors are assumed to be normally distributed and that, for a normally distributed variable, 68% of the observations fall within one standard deviation of the mean. It follows that 68% of the observations of an object fall within one standard error of measurement on either side of the true score, as illustrated in Figure 5.4. In Table 5.1, the standard deviation of the scores for the four objects is 1.29, but because the reliability is unity the standard error of measurement is 0. In the more realistic example of Table 5.2, the standard deviation of the results is 0.82, and the standard error of measurement (applying the above formula) is 0.36. For object 1, then, the measured score of 4.4 should be roughly interpreted as 4.4 ± 0.4.

This classical approach to measurement is limited in that only one source of error, which we have generically called "observations," can be considered at a time. Using a more sophisticated approach, known as the generalizability theory, it is possible to base a reliability estimate on multiple facets of a measurement process, taking multiple sources of error simultaneously into account. Nonetheless, measurement problems with one important source of error arise frequently in informatics, and we can often split more complex measurement problems into a sequence of problems each having one source of error. For example, if the diagnostic accuracy of several expert systems is ultimately the matter of interest, our first measurement concern might be how accurately we can determine a standard of care, as measured by judgments of expert clinicians, for each of a set of test cases. Here the reliability can be estimated using judges for the observations and cases for objects. The attribute of interest is "standard of care." Once the error

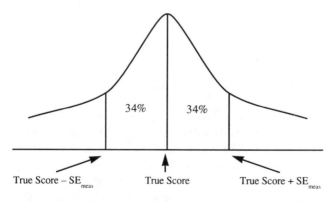

FIGURE 5.4. Distribution of measurement results illustrating the standard error of measurement.

inherent in this measurement process is established, the next measurement problem is assessment of the accuracy of the system over a series of test cases. For this second measurement problem, the objects are the expert systems and the observations are the test cases. The attribute of interest is the conformity to the standard of care for each system on each case.

Self-Test 5.1

1. What are the effects on the standard error of measurement of (a) adding a constant to each measurement result and (b) multiplying each measurement result by a constant?
2. The measurement result given below has a reliability of 0.88.

	Observations			
Object	1	2	3	4
1	2	4	4	3
2	3	3	3	4
3	2	3	3	2
4	4	3	4	4
5	1	2	1	2
6	2	2	2	2

a. Compute the score for each object and the standard deviation of these scores. (Standard deviations can be computed by most spreadsheet programs. The formula can be found in any basic statistics text.)
b. Compute the standard error of measurement.
c. Would changing the result of observation 1 on object 1 from 2 to 4 increase or decrease the reliability?

Reliability and Measurement Studies

Let us assume that the data in Table 5.2 are the results of a measurement study, conducted with four objects and five observations, to estimate the error when measuring some attribute. The first aspect of these results to note is that the reliability estimate must be interpreted much like the results of any study. The study results can be generalized only with great care. If the objects were sampled in some representative way from a larger population of objects, the result can be generalized only to that population. The estimate of measurement error might be different if objects were sampled from a different group. For example, assume that Table 5.2 gives the results of a measurement study where the attribute to be measured was speed, the objects were clinical information systems, and the observations were execution times (in tenths of a second) for a selected set of clinical information processing tasks. The measurement study results, with $\rho = 0.81$, suggest that the tasks are measuring an attribute of the objects with some appreciable consistency, but it cannot be assumed that these same tasks, when applied to a new generation of information systems designed on different software principles, can yield the same reliability when the speed of these new systems is assessed using the same set of tasks.

As illustrated in Tables 5.1 and 5.2, the results of a measurement study take the form of an objects-by-observations matrix, we now discuss the effects of changing the dimensions of this matrix. We begin with the horizontal (observations) dimension.

Effects of Changing the Number of Observations

Increasing the number of observations typically increases the magnitude of the estimated reliability. We offer this result without proof, but it can be seen intuitively by returning to the archery metaphor. If, for each target, the archer is aiming at a particular point, the greater the number of arrows he shoots, the more accurately the central point of where the arrows land estimates the location of the point of aim. More rigorously, the Spearman-Brown prophecy formula provides a way to estimate the effect on reliability of adding observations to or deleting observations from a measurement process. If one knows the reliability with k observations, its reliability with n observations is given by:

$$\rho_n = \frac{q\rho_k}{1+(q-1)\rho_k}$$

where: ρ_n = reliability with n observations
ρ_k = reliability with k observations
q = n/k

This formula assumes that the observations added perform equivalently to the observations already in the process. So the prophecy formula is just what its name implies. One never knows, in advance of the experience, what the effect of changing the number of observations will be. It is a huge assumption, often ignored as such in research practice. To illustrate the effect of changing the number of observations, consider a hypothetical situation where four judges are asked to assess the quality of care for each of a set of 30 cases. In this situation, judges are the observations, cases are the objects, and "quality of care" is the attribute. If the reliability of the four judges is calculated to be 0.65, Table 5.3 shows the prophesied effects, using the above formula, of adding or deleting judges who perform equivalently to those already in the study. The result in boldface is the result of the measurement study. All other values were derived by the prophecy formula.

TABLE 5.3. Application of the prophecy formula

	Number of judges							
	1	2	**4**	6	8	10	20	100
Adjustment factor	0.25	0.5	**1.0**	1.5	2.0	2.5	5.0	25.0
Reliability	0.317	0.481	**0.650**	0.736	0.788	0.823	0.903	0.979

Table 5.3 raises the question of how much reliability is "good enough." It is difficult to precisely interpret reliability coefficients. How much reliability is necessary depends primarily on how the results of the measurement are to be used. If the measurement results are to be used for demonstration studies where the focus is comparisons of groups of objects, a reliability coefficient of 0.7 or above is usually adequate, although higher reliability is always desirable. By contrast, a reliability coefficient of 0.9 or above is often necessary when the concern is assignment of scores to individual objects with a high degree of precision. In these situations researchers often set a target level of the standard error of measurement and seek to attain a reliability that allows them to reach their target. The question of how much reliability is enough is often answered with: "enough to make the standard error of measurement as small as we need it to be to draw the conclusions we need to draw." Measurements with reliabilities of 0.5 or less are rarely adequate for anything but preliminary research. *As a general rule, the reliability of measures used in any research effort should be estimated and reported by the investigators.*

Again with reference to Table 5.3, if our concern is a demonstration study where we compare the quality of care for groups of cases, the collective opinions of at least six judges would be adequate to achieve a reliability of more than 0.7. However, if our concern is to assign a precise "quality of care" score to each case, more than 20 judges would be needed to reach a reliability of 0.9. The reliability of one or two judges, for this hypothetical study, would therefore be less than acceptable.

Effects of Changing the Number of Objects

Increasing the number of objects typically increases the accuracy of the estimate of the reliability. It is also important to note that the result of a measurement study provides an *estimate* of the reliability. In general, the greater the number of objects in the measurement study, the greater is the accuracy of this estimate. We can see intuitively from Tables 5.1 and 5.2, which portray measurement studies with four objects each, that addition of a fifth object on which the observations were highly discrepant would have a dramatic effect on the reliability estimate. However, if the measurement study included 25 objects, the incremental effect of a discrepant 26th object would be less profound. Reliability estimates based on large numbers of object are thus more stable. For measurement study design where an almost unlimited number of objects is available, at least 100 objects should be employed for stable estimates of reliability. For example, in a measurement study of a questionnaire to be completed by nurses, the number of objects (nurses in this case) is large. When the total number of objects is limited, the designer of a measurement study should use a dense sample of the objects available. For example, if patients with a rare disease were the objects of measurement, and a total of 100 cases were in existence, a measurement study using 50 of these cases would provide a reasonably stable estimate of reliability. Our examples in Tables 5.1 and 5.2 were purposely flawed to enable concise presentation. Both examples contain too few objects for stable estimation of reliability unless the four objects used in the study were all that exist.

Self-Test 5.2

For the data in question 2 of Self-Test 5.1, what is the prognosticated reliability if the number of observations were (a) increased to 10 or (b) decreased to 1.

Measurement Error and Demonstration Studies

Up to this point, we have discussed the effect of measurement error (random errors that erode reliability) on the result of a measurement for each object. What about the effects of such errors on the estimate of the mean of some attribute for a *group* of objects, which is the main concern of a demonstration study? For any sample of size N, the mean of a variable is associated with a standard error of the mean computed as:

$$SE_{mean} = \frac{SD}{\sqrt{N}}$$

As a general rule, random measurement error adds variability to the results of a measurement process. The greater the error, the greater the standard deviation (SD in the formula above) of the scores for each object; and as the standard deviation increases, so does the standard error of the mean. Thus measurement error contributes to the uncertainty with which we can know the mean value of some attribute in a sample. Random errors do not bias the estimates of the means of a group; they affect only the scatter or variability of measured values around the mean.

In demonstration studies we are often interested in whether the mean of some attribute differs in two groups or samples of objects. Because measurement error adds imprecision to the estimates of the means for each sample, the lack of reliability decreases the probability that a true difference between the mean values in the samples, if such a difference exists, can be detected by the study. So measurement error reduces the statistical power of demonstration studies. For example, we might compare the costs of management of hypertensive patients with and without support from a computer-based advisor. With samples of 100 patients in each group, the mean ($\pm\,SE_{mean}$) of these costs might be $595 ($\pm$ $2) per patient per year with the advisor and $600 ($\pm$ $2) without it. This difference is not statistically significant. Suppose, however, it was found that the measurement methods used to determine these costs were so unreliable that measurement error was contributing a substantial part of the variability reflected in the standard error of the mean. Through use of improved measurement methods, it may be possible to reduce the standard error of the mean by 25%. If this were done, the most likely results of a hypothetical replication of the study would then be $595 ($\pm$ $1.60) for the advisor group and $600 ($\pm$ $1.60) for the control group. This difference *is* statistically significant.[*]

In other types of demonstration studies, we are not interested in the values of the means across various samples, but, rather, in the correlations between two attributes in a single sample. For example, we might want to compare, for a sample of health care providers, the extent of use of a clinical workstation with each provider's score on a knowledge test administered at the end of a training session. In this type of study, the effect of measurement error is to reduce the observed magnitude of the correlation. The "true" level of correlation between the extent of use and test score is higher than that suggested by the results of the study. This effect of measurement errors on correlations is known as *attenuation*. An approximate correction for attenuation can be used if the reliabilities of the measures are known.

$$r_{corrected} = \frac{r_{observed}}{\sqrt{\rho_1 \rho_2}}$$

where: $r_{corrected}$ = correlation corrected for attenuation
$r_{observed}$ = observed or actually measured correlation
ρ_1 = reliability of measure 1
ρ_2 = reliability of measure 2

Because the reliability of any measure cannot exceed unity, the absolute magnitude of the corrected correlation is always equal to or exceeds the absolute magnitude of the observed value. This correction must be applied with caution because it makes the standard assumptions of classical measurement theory: that all measurement errors are uncorrelated with anything else. If this assumption is violated, it is possible to obtain corrected correlations that are dramatically inflated and in some cases more than 1.0.[8] Nonetheless, the attenuation phenomenon is important in medical informatics, and an example is discussed in detail later in the chapter.

To see why this attenuation happens, first consider two variables (Y_{true} and X_{true}), each measured with perfect reliability ($\rho = 1$) and between which the correlation is high. The relation between Y_{true} and X_{true} is shown in the upper part of Fig-

---

[*] For those experienced in inferential statistics, a *t*-test performed on the case with the larger standard errors reveals $t = 1.77$, $df = 198$, $p = 0.08$. With the reduced standard errors, $t = 2.21$, $df = 198$, $p = 0.03$.

ure 5.5. The values of Y_{true} and X_{true} fall nearly on a straight line and the correlation coefficient is 0.95. By applying a small, normally distributed error function to Y_{true} and X_{true}, we generate representative values of these variables as they might be measured with error: Y_{error} and X_{error}. The plot of Y_{error} versus X_{error} in the lower part of Figure 5.5 shows the degradation of the relations and the corresponding attenuation of the correlation coefficient from 0.95 to 0.68. The variance in the data added by the measurement error is observed in part from the increased range of values for Y_{error} and X_{error}, which is greater than the range for Y_{true} and X_{true}. (Y_{error} ranges from 6 to 14, and Y_{true} ranges from 7 to 13; X_{error} ranges from 1.3 to 6.8, and X_{true} ranges from 2 to 6.)

Self Test 5.3

Assume that the assumptions underlying the correction for attenuation hold. Use the correction formula to show that $r_{observed} \leq \sqrt{\rho_1 \rho_2}$. (*Hint:* Use the fact that the corrected correlation must be ≤ 1.0.) This equation is important because it points out that the reliability of a measure sets an upper bound on the correlation that can be measured between it and other measures.

Validity and Its Estimation

Reliability estimates indicate the degree of random "noise" in a measurement, and validity indicates the degree of "misdirection" in the measurement. To the extent that a measurement is reliable the results are meaningful, but to the extent that a measurement process is invalid the results mean something different from what the researcher believes them to mean. More rigorously, the validity of a measurement process is the fraction of the perfectly reliable true scores that reflects the attribute of interest (see Figure 5.1). Returning to the archery metaphor, the validity is the extent of concordance, over a series of targets, between the point at which the archer was aiming on each target and the location of the bull's-eye, which is unknown to her.

We previously saw that a measurement process, if conducted appropriately so it includes multiple observations, can reveal its own reliability through analysis of the consistency of the results of the observations. Estimation of validity is a different process requiring the collection of additional information. Whereas the reliability of our archer can be determined from the scatter of her arrows on each target, we need to collect additional information if we want to know how close to the bulls-eye her point of aim really was. One way to do this is to collect additional information by asking her, but in so doing we would have to recognize that her perceptions, though providing some useful information, may not be completely credible. This analogy illustrates the fundamental dilemma of measurement as it applies to validity. Although we can collect additional information to establish validity, no single source of information is completely credible, and often multiple sources must be used.

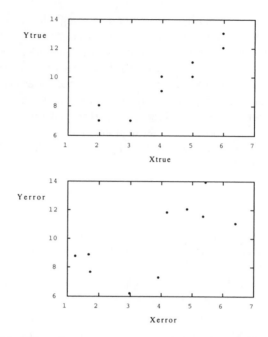

FIGURE 5.5. Effect of measurement error on the correlation between two variables.

Complete measurement studies seek to establish the validity of a measurement process as well as its reliability. In real measurement activities, we can estimate validity by asking people to examine the instruments used and opine as to what attribute the process appears to be addressing, or we can estimate validity by conducting statistical studies. Such studies might examine, for a set of objects, the relation between the results of the measurement process under study and the results of other measurement processes whose validity has been previously established. These results are typically expressed as correlations between the new process and the processes selected as standards. If the results of such studies are in accord with expectations, a strong case can be made for the validity of the measurement process.

There are many more ways to estimate validity than there are to study reliability. Often multiple approaches are used, and the strongest case for the validity of a measurement process is made by accumulating evidence across a series of studies. More rigorously, studies of validity are of three general types: content, criterion-related, and construct.[9]

Content Validity

Regarding content validity, certain questions pertain: By inspection of the instruments, do the observations appear to address the attribute that is the measurement target? Does the process make sense? This is the most basic notion of validity, otherwise more loosely known as "face" validity. Content validity can be determined by seeking opinions from informed individuals, for example by asking panels to review the observations purported to constitute a scale. Assessment of content validity requires the instrument to be inspected rather than administered.

Although it should be expected that most measurement processes have content validity, the issues involved can become subtle. For example, a researcher may be constructing a checklist to measure a resource's "ease of use." Using the method of multiple simultaneous observations, the checklist would contain several observations hypothesized to comprise a scale, each item purporting to measure "ease of use" from a slightly different perspective. In a content validity study, a group of judges may be asked: Which of the following items belong on the "ease of use" scale?

- Accessibility of help
- System response time
- Format of displayed information
- Clarity of user interface

There might be little disagreement about the items addressing user interface and information displays, but some judges might argue that the "system response time" item addresses the attribute of "performance" rather than "ease of use," and that "accessibility of help" is not a characteristic of the system itself but, rather, the environment in which the resource is installed. In sum, content validity of a measurement process cannot be assumed and must be verified through appropriately designed studies.

Criterion-Related Validity

For criterion-related validity the question is different: Do the results of a measurement process correlate with some external standard or predict an outcome of particular interest? For example, do those who score highly on a scale purported to measure computer literacy also learn more quickly to navigate an unfamiliar piece of software? Does a scale that prospectively rates the quality of radiotherapy treatment plans identify treatment plans associated with longer patient survival? Determination of criterion-related validity depends on the identification of criteria that are generally accepted. If the measurement process under study is to be considered valid, the correlation with a criterion would be expected to be moderately high, with coefficients of at least 0.4 and preferably higher. Unlike the content validity, which can be assessed through inspection of the measurement instruments themselves, determination of criterion-related validity requires a study where the measurement process is conducted with a representative sample of objects. For this sample, measurements are made using the instrument being validated as well as the instruments needed to assess the criterion. Returning to the above example, study of the criterion-related validity of a computer literacy scale requires that the scale be completed by a sample of health professionals who also try their hand at using an unfamilar piece of software.

Construct Validity

Construct validity resembles criterion-related validity in that the concern is also with how scores generated by the instrument to be validated correlate with other measures, but the approach is more sophisticated. When exploring construct validity, we ask: Do results of this measurement correlate highly with other measures (constructs) that, theoretically, would be expected to be closely related to this one? Do they also correlate poorly with other constructs that, again theoretically, would be expected to be unrelated to this one? This method is the most complex, but in many ways the most compelling, way to estimate validity.

Construct validity estimation, like criterion validity estimation, requires specific studies using multiple instruments on a representative sample of objects. Consider as an example the development of an instrument to assess the attribute of "user satisfaction" for a medical information system (Fig. 5.6). The attribute of "user satisfaction" might be expected to correlate highly, but not perfectly, with other attributes, such as "experience with computers." Satisfaction would *not* be expected to correlate highly with the specific health profession of the completer of the form. To assess construct validity, data on experience with computers and health professional training would be collected, using already validated procedures, along with the user satisfaction data using the measurement process to be validated. The correlation between user satisfaction and computer experience should be neither too low nor too high. If too high, the two instruments are measuring the same construct; if too low, the new instrument is not valid. In sum, by collecting data addressing a set of attributes and comparing the observed correlations with those that might be expected on theoretical and logical grounds, the construct validity of a scale can be inferred.

Concern about validity of measurement extends throughout all of science. When astrophysicists detect a signal in their radiotelescopes and try to determine what it means, their concern is with validity. In general, concern with validity increases when the attributes are more abstract and only indirectly observable, but this concern never vanishes. For example, the notion of computer speed is relatively concrete, and there exists a relatively robust consensus about what the concept of speed means. Yet if a study is undertaken whereby a computer is put through a series of tasks, how can the researcher be sure that the result of the measurement solely reflects speed, uncorrupted by some other characteristic of the machine? The picture becomes more complex as one moves into the realm of attributes hosted by the behavioral sciences. When attitudes and other states of mind, such as "satisfaction," become the focus of measurement, the need for validity studies becomes self-evident.

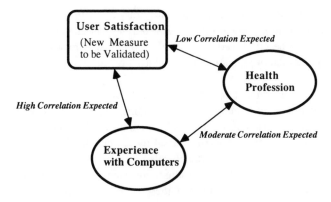

FIGURE 5.6. Construct validity study.

Self-Test 5.4

Is each of the following studies primarily concerned with content, criterion-related, or construct validity?

1. A researcher develops a rating form to ascertain the "quality" of a differential diagnosis for patients with illnesses of unknown cause. The ratings for a set of test cases are studied in relation to the time until a definitive diagnosis is established.
2. A researcher developing a computer literacy questionnaire convenes a panel of experts to identify the core competencies defining computer literacy.
3. A researcher develops a measure of the speed of a medical information system using a set of benchmark information processing tasks. For a set of information systems, the results of the new measure are studied in relation to the overall satisfaction with each system, as judged by samples of clinician-users in health care settings where the systems have been installed.

Levels of Measurement

We mentioned earlier that measurement often, but not always, leads to a quantitative result in the form of a continuous variable. The level of measurement of a set of observations determines how the result of the measurement can be represented quantitatively. Level of measurement also directs the statistical analyses that can be applied to the results. There are four such levels of measurement

1. *Nominal:* Measurement on a nominal scale results in the assignment of each object to a specific category. The categories themselves do not form a continuum or have a meaningful order. Examples of nominal measurements are ethnicity and medical specialty. To represent the results of a nominal measurement

quantitatively, the results must be assigned arbitrary codes (e.g., 1 for internists, 2 for surgeons, 3 for family practitioners). The only aspect of importance for such codes is that they be employed consistently to represent measurement results. Their actual numerical or alphanumerical values have no significance.

2. *Ordinal:* Measurement on an ordinal scale also results in assignment of objects to categories, but the categories have some meaningful order or ranking. For example, some physicians use a "plus" system of recording clinical signs ("2+ pitting edema"), which represents an ordinal measurement. The classification of computers as micro, mini, or mainframe is also measurement on an ordinal scale. When coding the results of ordinal measurements, we typically assign a numerical code to each category, but no aspect of these codes except for their numerical order contains any interpretable information.

Note that both nominal and ordinal measurements can be termed "categorical" and are often referenced that way. Using "categorical" as a descriptor for nominal and ordinal measures conceals the important difference between them.

3. *Interval:* Results of interval measurements are continuous variables that have an arbitrarily chosen zero point. The classic examples are the Fahrenheit and centigrade scales of temperature. This level of measurement derives its name from the "equal interval" assumption, which all interval measures must satisfy. To satisfy this assumption, equal differences between two measurements must have the same meaning irrespective of where on the scale they occur. On the Fahrenheit scale, a difference of 50 and 40 degrees has the same meaning, in terms of thermal energy, as a difference of 20 and 10 degrees. An "interval" of 10 degrees is interpreted similarly all along the scale. Investigators often assume that the measures employed in their studies have interval properties when, in fact, there is reason to question this belief. In medical informatics we often use the average response of a group of judges—each of whom responds using a set of ordinal options ("excellent," "good," "fair," "poor")—to produce a measured result for each object. We typically assume that the average of these ordinal judgments has interval properties. This assumption is controversial and is explored in Chapter 6.

4. *Ratio:* Ratio measures are interval measures with the additional property of a true zero point. The kelvin scale of temperature, with a zero point that is not arbitrarily chosen, is a ratio scale, whereas the other temperature scales are not. Most physiological and physical measures have ratio properties. This level of measurement is so named because one can assign meaning not only to the interval between, but also to the ratio of, two measurement results.

In any study, it is almost always desirable to use the highest possible level of measurement, with ratio measurement being the highest of the levels. In this way the measured results contain the maximum amount of information; and for demonstration studies statistical tests with greater power can usually be employed. A common mistake of researchers is to make measurements at a lower level than the attribute allows. For example, in a survey of health care providers, the researcher may want to know each respondent's years of professional experience, naturally a ratio measure. Frequently, such measures are assessed using discrete response categories, each containing a range of years. Although this measurement strategy provides some convenience for the respondent, it reduces what is naturally a ratio variable to ordinal status, with inevitable loss of information.

Self-Test 5.5

Determine the level of measurement of each of the following

1. Serum potassium level
2. "Stage" of a neoplastic illness
3. Internal medicine service to which each of a set of patients is assigned

Study Results and Measurement Error: An Example

In demonstration studies, failing to take measurement error properly into account can have several detrimental effects. We have argued that researchers should carry out measurement studies, preferably in advance of demonstration studies, to estimate the nature and degree of measurement error. If the measurement error is not known, researchers are literally at its mercy. They must act as if the measurements were without error but knowing this is not the case.

If the performance of a resource is compared to a standard whose carat level is taken to be a perfect "24" but in fact is less, we have seen that the effect of the measurement error is to underestimate the true value of the correlation between the resource and the standard. To see how it develops in practice, we examine the work of van der Lei and colleagues,[10] who studied the performance of Hypercritic, a knowledge-based system that offers critiques of the treatment of hypertensive patients by scanning the electronic records of these patients.[*] For illustrative purposes, we present a somewhat simplified version of the original study as well as a different approach to analysis of the data. The reader is encouraged to read the original paper.

In the simplified version, we assume that Hypercritic and each member of a panel of eight physicians have independently "reviewed" the records of a set of hypertensive patients for the purpose of generating comments about the care of each patient. As a result of this initial review, a set of 298 comments was generated. Each comment in the set was generated either by Hypercritic or by one or more of the physician panelists. Subsequently, each physician independently reviewed all 298 comments and judged each to be either "correct" or "incorrect." If Hypercritic generated a comment as it scanned the patient records during the initial review, it may be assumed that Hypercritic considered the comment to be correct. The structure of the study is illustrated in Figure 5.7.

---

[*] The authors are grateful to Johan van der Lei and his colleagues for sharing the original data from their study and allowing us to develop this example.

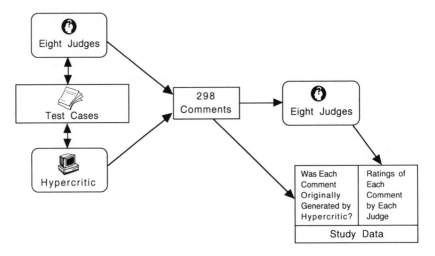

FIGURE 5.7. Hypercritic study.

The results of the study can be portrayed in a table, with each comment comprising a row, one column reflecting the ratings of that comment by each judge, and a separate column indicating whether each comment was generated by Hypercritic during the initial record review. Table 5.4 presents the study results for a subset of 12 comments. Judges are labeled A through H, and judges' ratings of comments are coded as "1" for correct and "0" for incorrect. With reference to Table 5.4, it is evident that Hypercritic and the judges did not always agree, and that the judges did not always agree among themselves. Comment 1 was generated by Hypercritic (and perhaps by one or more judges as well) on the initial review and was subsequently rated as correct by judges A, B, and D. Comment 2 was not generated by Hypercritic—on the initial review it was generated by one or more of the judges—and it was subsequently endorsed by judges B, C, D, and G. A demonstration study exploring the accuracy of Hypercritic's advice would seek to correlate the level of judges' endorsement of these comments on the second review with Hypercritic's "endorsement," as inferred from whether Hypercritic generated the comment on the initial review. We can consider the pooled ratings of the judges to be a less-than-perfect standard against which Hypercritic may be tested, but the extent of a disagreement among the judges can provide an estimate of measurement error in, or the carat level of, this standard. A measurement study can estimate this carat level, helping us determine if the judges' ratings are measuring something meaningful.

Measurement Study

The measurement study is concerned only with the ratings of the judges (A through H in Table 5.4). Hypercritic's performance is irrelevant at this point.

TABLE 5.4. Results from a subset of 12 comments in the Hypercritic study

Comment no.	Generated by Hypercritic?	Ratings by each judge								Judges' "correctness" score
		A	B	C	D	E	F	G	H	
1	Yes	1	1	0	1	0	0	0	0	3
2	No	0	1	1	1	0	0	1	0	4
3	No	1	1	1	1	0	0	1	0	5
4	Yes	1	1	0	1	0	0	1	1	5
5	No	1	1	1	1	1	0	0	1	6
6	No	0	1	1	1	0	0	1	1	5
7	No	1	1	1	1	0	0	1	1	6
8	No	1	1	1	1	0	0	1	1	6
9	Yes	1	1	0	1	1	1	1	1	7
10	Yes	1	1	1	1	1	0	1	1	7
11	No	1	1	1	1	1	1	0	1	7
12	Yes	1	1	0	1	1	1	1	1	7

Casting the judges' ratings more precisely in terms of our measurement theory, the objects of measurement are the comments, and the attribute of primary interest may be seen as the "correctness" of these comments. We may consider each judge's rating to be an assessment of the "correctness" attribute for each comment. Each rating by a judge is thus an independent observation. Classical measurement theory then enjoins us to sum or average these independent judgments to obtain the best estimate of the correctness of each comment. (*Note:* If you do not follow this conceptualization, you should review the earlier section on "Method of Multiple Simultaneous Observations" before proceeding further .)

Applying this approach generates for each comment a correctness score equal to the number of judges who considered that comment to be correct. The correctness score is shown in the rightmost column of Table 5.4. From Table 5.4, comment 1 would have a correctness score of 3 and comment 11 would have a correctness score of 7. For the complete data in this study, we can estimate the reliability of these correctness scores by using the matrix of judges' ratings across all 298 comments. The full set of 298 correctness scores has a mean of 5.2 and a standard deviation of 2.0. The reliability coefficient, when computed for all 298 cases, is 0.65. The standard error of measurement of each correctness score is 1.2.[*]

The results of this measurement study allow us to conclude that the ratings by the judges are measuring something meaningful, although a higher reliability obtainable using more judges would be desirable. To complete the measurement study, we would also need to consider the validity of these ratings: whether the

---

[*] Readers familiar with theories of reliability might observe that coefficient α, which does not take into account rater stringency or leniency as a source of error, might overestimate the reliability in this example. In this case, however, use of an alternate coefficient[11] has a negligible effect.

ratings represented the attribute of "correctness" or some other attribute. Content or face validity of the ratings might be explored by examining the credentials of the judges. The ratings of senior physicians experienced in hypertension management would have higher content validity than those of inexperienced physicians. A measure of criterion-related validity might be obtained by examining the incidence of hypertension-related complications for the patients included in the study in relation to the correctness scores of the comments about their care, for cases where the corrective action recommended by the comment was *not* taken. A positive correlation between complication rates and correctness scores would be an indication of validity.

Demonstration Study

Having computed the reliability of the correctness scores, we are in a strong position to analyze the complete data using the logic of a demonstration study where we are interested in estimating the accuracy of Hypercritic. One measure of the accuracy of Hypercritic is the correlation between Hypercritic's "assessment" of each comment —determined by whether Hypercritic generated the comment on its review of the patients' charts—and the correctness score obtained by pooling the eight judges' comments. The correlation coefficient based on all 298 comments is 0.50, which signals a moderate and statistically significant relation. We might also suspect that this observed correlation is an underestimate of the magnitude of the relation between Hypercritic's output and the correctness scores because the observed correlation has been attenuated by measurement error. To estimate the effects of error on the observed correlation, we might apply the correction for attenuation (see page 102) and obtain a corrected value of 0.62. By comparing the corrected correlation of 0.62 with the observed correlation of 0.50, we see that measurement error may be eroding the estimate of Hypercritic's accuracy by approximately 24%.

As we will discover later when demonstration studies are discussed in detail, the correlation coefficient is a measure of system accuracy that has useful statistical meaning but says little about the nature of the disagreement between Hypercritic and the pooled ratings of the judges. For the purpose of a comprehensive evaluation of a system such as Hypercritic, additional analyses would therefore be performed. Contingency table methods, discussed in detail in Chapter 7, might be used to look at the number and nature of the disagreements between the resource and the judges. Such an analysis would require the investigators to choose a threshold level corresponding to the number of endorsements a comment would require from the judges to be considered valid. Doing this reduces the level of measurement from interval to ordinal and, as such, results in some loss of information. (All comments taken as correct are considered to be equally correct, and all comments taken as incorrect are equally incorrect.) The original authors of the study used endorsement of a comment by five or more judges as a criterion for overall correctness. Using this same criterion, the data may be mapped into a contingency table (Table 5.5).

TABLE 5.5. Hypercritic demonstration study results in contingency table format

	Pooled rating by judges		
Hypercritic	Comment valid (≥ 5 judges)	Comment not valid (< 5 judges)	Total
Comment generated	145	24	169
Comment not generated	55	74	129
Total	200	98	298

This analysis is useful because it shows that false-negative and false-positive errors occur in roughly equal proportion if endorsement by five or more judges is taken as the threshold. That is, Hypercritic had a false-negative rate of 28% because it failed to generate 55 of the 200 comments that were endorsed by five or more judges. Hypercritic had a false positive error rate of 25%, reflecting its generation of 24 of 98 comments that were subsequently rated invalid by the judges. Note that the false-positive and false-negative rates depend on the researcher's choice of a threshold. The design and analysis of demonstration studies, including the analysis of contingency tables, are considered in more detail in Chapter 7.

Self-Test 5.6

Assume that the data in Table 5.4, based only on 12 comments, constitute a complete pilot study. The reliability of these data, based on 12 comments (objects) and eight judges (observations) is 0.29. (Note that this illustrates the danger of conducting measurement studies with small samples of objects, as the reliability estimated from this small sample is different from that obtained with the full sample of 298 comments.)

1. What is the standard error of measurement of the "correctness of a comment" as determined by these eight judges?
2. If there were four judges instead of eight, what would the estimated standard error of measurement be? What if there were 10 judges?
3. Using the pooled ratings of all eight judges as the standard for accuracy, express the accuracy of Hypercritic's relevance judgments as a contingency table using endorsement by six or more judges as the threshold for assuming a comment to be correct.
4. For these data, the correlation between Hypercritic's judgments and the pooled ratings is 0.09. What effect does the correction for attenuation have on this correlation?
5. Optional: Using the formulas in Appendix A, verify that the reliability is 0.29 and compute the various sums of squares that are part of the computation.

References

1. Kerlinger F: Foundations of Behavioral Research. New York: Holt, Rinehart and Winston, 1986.
2. Thorndike RL, Hagen E: Measurement and Evaluation in Psychology and Education. New York: Wiley, 1977.
3. Weinstein MC, Fineberg HV, Elstein AS, et al: Clinical Decision Analysis. Philadelphia: Saunders, 1980.
4. Feinstein AR: Clinimetrics. New Haven, CT: Yale University Press, 1987.
5. Clarke JR, Cebula, DP, Webber BL: Artificial intelligence: a computerized decision aid for trauma. J Trauma 1988;28:1250–1254.
6. Babbie ER: The Practice of Social Research. Belmont, CA: Wadsworth, 1992.
7. Cronbach L: Coefficient alpha and the internal structure of tests. Psychometrika 1951;16:297–334.
8. Phelps CD, Hutson A: Estimating diagnostic test accuracy using a "fuzzy gold standard." Med Decis Making 1995;15: 44–57.
9. Standards for Educational and Psychological Tests. Washington, DC: American Psychological Association, 1974.
10. Van der Lei J, Musen MA, van der Does E, Man in 't Veld AJ, van Bemmel JH: Comparison of computer-aided and human review of general practitioners' management of hypertension. Lancet 1991;338:1504–1508.
11. Shrout PE, Fleiss JL: Intraclass correlations: uses in assessing rater reliability. Psychol Bull 1979;86: 420–428.

Answers to Self-Tests

Self-Test 5.1

1. a. Adding a constant has no effect on the standard error of measurement, as it affects neither the standard deviation nor the reliability.
   b. Multiplication by a constant increases the standard error by that same constant.
2. a. The scores are 13, 13, 10, 15, 6, 8 for objects 1–6. The standard deviation of the six scores is 3.43.
   b. 1.19.
   c. The reliability would increase because the scores for object 1, across observations, become more consistent. The reliability in fact increases to 0.92.

Self-Test 5.2

a. 0.95
b. 0.65

Self-Test 5.3

The answer may be obtained by substituting $r_{corrected} \leq 1$ into the formula:

$$r_{corrected} = \frac{r_{observed}}{\sqrt{\rho_1 \rho_2}}$$

to obtain the inequality:

$$1 \geq \frac{r_{observed}}{\sqrt{\rho_1 \rho_2}}$$

Self-Test 5.4

1. Criterion-related validity. The time until a definitive diagnosis is established might be viewed as a universally accepted standard.
2. Content validity.
3. Construct validity. The relation between system speed and user satisfaction is complex, and the correlation would not be expected to be perfect.

Self-Test 5.5

1. Ratio
2. Ordinal
3. Nominal

Self-Test 5.6

1. SE_{meas} (eight judges) = 1.10
2. SE_{meas} (four judges) = 1.19; SE_{meas} (10 judges) = 1.07
3.

Hypercritic	Judges	
	Valid	Not valid
Generated	3	2
Not generated	4	3

4. Corrected correlation is 0.17.
5. Total sum of squares (SS) = 19.84; judges (observations) SS = 5.84; comments (objects) SS = 2.33; error SS = 11.67.

Appendix A: Computing Reliability Coefficients

The computation of reliability coefficients is based on a matrix of objects by observations as shown in Table 5.6. This calculation is presented without proof. It

TABLE 5.6. Sample data for reliability calculation

Object	Data, by no. of observations					Object sums
	1	2	3	4	5	
A	4	5	3	5	5	22
B	3	5	5	3	4	20
C	4	4	4	4	5	21
D	3	2	3	2	3	13
Observation						
sums	14	16	15	14	17	

is familiar to those experienced with analysis of variance. We use standard matrix notation, so each observation is given by $X_{i,j}$ where i denotes the object and j denotes the observation. In the matrix in Table 5.6, $X_{2,3}$ is the value of the third observation on object B, with a value of 5. The total number of objects is therefore n_i, and the total number of observations is n_j.

We begin by calculating three "sums of squares": total sum of squares (SS_{total}), the sum of squares for objects ($SS_{objects}$), and the sum of squares for observations ($SS_{observations}$). The total sum of squares is given by:

$$SS_{total} = \sum_{i,j} X_{i,j}^2 - \frac{(\sum_{i,j} X_{i,j})^2}{n_i n_j}$$

Note that $\sum_{i,j} X_{i,j}$ equals the sum of all observations for all objects, and $\sum_{i,j} X_{i,j}^2$ equals the sum of the squared values of all observations for all objects.

The sum of squares for objects is given by:

$$SS_{objects} = \frac{\sum_{i=1}^{n_i} (\sum_{j=1}^{n_j} X_{i,j})^2}{n_j} - \frac{(\sum_{i,j} X_{i,j})^2}{n_i n_j}$$

The sum of squares for observations is given by:

$$SS_{observations} = \frac{\sum_{j=1}^{n_j} (\sum_{i=1}^{n_i} X_{i,j})^2}{n_i} - \frac{(\sum_{i,j} X_{i,j})^2}{n_i n_j}$$

From these three quantities, we can compute the sum of squares for error as:

$$SS_{error} = SS_{total} - SS_{objects} - SS_{observations}$$

Now the reliability can be computed using the formula:

$$\rho = 1 - \left[\frac{SS_{error}/(n_i - 1)(n_j - 1)}{SS_{objects}/(n_i - 1)} \right]$$

In the sample matrix in Table 5.6, using these formulas, we obtain:

Total sum of squares = 19.2
Sum of squares for objects = 10.0
Sum of squares for observations = 1.7
Error sum of squares = 7.5
Reliability = 0.81

6

Developing Measurement Technique

This chapter applies the theoretical material of Chapter 5 to actual practice. In Chapter 5 we introduced theories of measurement that were, in effect, theories of error. In this chapter we address specific procedures for estimating and minimizing error. We discuss the structure of measurement studies, the mechanics of conducting them, and how to use the results of these studies to improve measurement techniques. We consider how to develop measurement methods that yield results that are acceptably reliable and valid. We discuss in detail three specific situations that arise frequently in informatics: first, when the repeated observations in a measurement process are tasks completed by either persons or information resources; second, when the repeated observations are the opinions of judges about clinical cases; and third, when the repeated observations are items or questions on forms. Although the same overall measurement issues apply in all three instances, there are issues of implementation and technique specific to each.

Structure of Measurement Studies: Objects, Observations, and Scales

Recall from Chapter 5 that in measurement studies we typically make multiple independent observations on each of a sample of objects. These observations are not carried out identically but are similar enough to measure essentially the same attribute. The data of a measurement study take the form of an objects-by-observation matrix (Fig. 6.1). In the objectivist world view, all independent observations of the same phenomenon should yield the same result. The closer the observations approach agreement for each object, the more reliable and therefore "objective" the measurement process can be considered to be. Disagreement reflects "subjectivity" on the part of the instruments, be they human, mechanical, electronic, or some combination thereof.

In Chapter 5, we developed quantitative methods for estimating errors of measurement, enabling the researcher to draw conclusions to engineer the measurement process for optimal performance. We saw that the variability due to objects contributes to "true score" variability which should be maximized relative to vari-

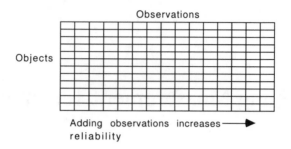

FIGURE 6.1. Objects-by-observations matrix.

ability from other sources. The variability due to all other sources contributes to errors that erode reliability and so should be minimized. The reliability can be increased and the standard error of measurement decreased by increasing the number of independent observations. The methods for estimating reliability introduced in Chapter 5 allow us to quantify measurement error directly from the objects-by-observations matrix using data generated by the measurement process itself.

We also saw in Chapter 5 that reducing to zero the errors that are estimable from the measurement process itself does not guarantee a perfect measurement of the desired attribute. Even if the measurement is perfectly reliable, the results may be invalid. Human judges in near-perfect agreement about the accuracy of a decision support system's advice may still be incorrect if the judges share a fund of medical knowledge that is obsolete. Separate validity studies, which typically require use of external standards, are needed to explore these additional issues. Because the conduct of a complete set of measurement studies, exploring both reliability and validity, is complex and time-consuming, it is vitally important that results of measurement studies be published so other informatics researchers can reuse the measurement methods developed and calibrated by their colleagues.

With this brief review as background, we now can describe the specific steps for conducting a measurement study.

1. Design the measurement process to be studied. Precisely define the attribute(s), object class, instrumentation, measurement procedures, and what will constitute the multiple independent observations. Recall that the object class is an expression of who or what the measurements are "made on."
2. Decide from which hypothetical population the objects will be sampled. It may also be necessary to decide from which population the observations will derive. (For example, if the observations are to be made by human judges, what real or hypothetical group do they represent?) This step is key because the results of the measurement study cannot be generalized beyond these populations.
3. Decide how many objects and and how many independent observations will be included in the measurement study. This point determines the dimensionality of the objects-by-observations matrix for the data collected.

4. Collect data using the measurement procedures as designed and any additional data that may be used to explore validity.
5. Analyze the objects-by-observations matrix to estimate reliability. Cronbach's α can be computed using any of several computer programs for statistical analysis. Alternatively, the formulas in Appendix A of Chapter 5 can be used to create a spreadsheet that computes reliability coefficients.
6. Conduct any validity studies that are part of the measurement study.
7. If the reliability or validity is too low, attempt to diagnose the problem. Recall that the Spearman-Brown formula can be used to estimate the effects on reliability of changing the number of independent observations.
8. Decide whether the results of the measurement study are sufficiently favorable to proceed directly to a demonstration study, or if a repeat of the measurement study, with revised measurement procedures, is needed.

Example

In a realistic but hypothetical situation, suppose that a reseacher is interested in the performance of a decision support system and so seeks to assess the attribute of "accuracy of advice" for each patient (case) evaluated by this information resource. "Patients" are the object class of measurement. Human judges, abstracts of each patient's history, a report of the system's advice, and the form used to elicit the ratings comprise the instrumentation. For the measurement study, the investigator elects to use 30 patients and 6 judges, each of whom will rate the accuracy of advice for each of the patients, to generate the multiple repeated observations. The dimensions of the matrix to be analyzed are 30 by 6. The choice of patients and judges is nontrivial because the results of the study cannot be generalized beyond the characteristics of populations from which these individuals are selected. To increase the generalizability, the investigator chooses 30 patients from a citywide network of hospitals and 6 expert clinician judges from across the country. Conducting the study requires the resource to generate its advice for all 30 patients, and for each of the judges to review and rate the advice for all of the patients. The reliability of the ratings is estimated from the resulting objects-by-observations matrix to be 0.82. Using the Spearman-Brown formula, it is predicted that four judges will exhibit a reliability of 0.75. Given the time and effort required for the demonstration study to follow, the investigator decides to use four judges in the demonstration study.

When a measurement study reveals a low reliability (typically a coefficient of less than 0.70), the investigator can improve it by increasing the number of independent observations drawn from the same population. Had the estimated reliability been too low in our example, the investigator could have added more judges chosen from the same national group, but it would have come at a cost. Increasing the number of observations increases the work involved in conducting each measurement, increasing the time and expense incurred when conducting the study, and often creating logistical challenges. In some other situations, as we saw above, a measurement study can yield higher-than-needed reliability, and the results of the measurement study can lead the investigator to streamline the study by reducing the number of independent observations per object. Increasing or decreasing the number of observations, *so long as they represent the same population,* can be assumed to affect reliability only.

Alternatively, the investigator can try to improve the mechanics or instrumentation of the measurement. In our example, he or she might try better training of the judges, replacing a judge whose ratings seem unrelated to the ratings of his or her colleagues, or giving the judges an improved form on which to record the ratings. This approach, which addresses the substance of the measurement process, often yields better results than merely increasing the number of observations. It is important to understand, however, that such changes can affect *what* is being measured and thus can affect both reliability and validity. When an investigator responds to a measurement study by changing the number of observations, it is typically not necessary to repeat the study because the impact of the change can be predicted from the Spearman-Brown prophecy formula. When the changes are more fundamental (e.g., a change in the format of a rating instrument or a change in the population from which judges are selected) it may be necessary to repeat the measurement study, possibly going through several iterations until the process reaches the required level of performance.

Self-Test 6.1

With reference to the example described above:

1. What is the predicted reliability of this measurement process using one judge only? Would you consider this figure acceptable?
2. In the measurement study, the ratings were generated on a "1 to 4" response scale and had a mean of 2.3 with a standard deviation of 0.8. What was the magnitude of the standard error of measurement?
3. How might validity be explored in this hypothetical measurement study?

[Answers are found at the end of the chapter.]

Using Measurement Studies to Diagnose Measurement Problems

Two basic courses of action exist for an investigator if a measurement study reveals suboptimal reliability or validity: (1) modify the number of independent observations in the measurement process (typically affects reliability only); or (2) modify in more substantive ways the mechanics of the measurement (typically affects both reliability and validity). In this section we discuss how the investigator can use measurement study results to decide which of these strategies to pursue. Recall that we are referring here to observations in the most generic sense. The observations can be human judgments, items on a questionnaire, or data recorded by an automated process.

Analyzing the Objects-by-Observations Matrix

The diagnostic process entails some further analysis of the objects-by-observations matrix to determine which of the observations, if any, is eroding the reliability. Recall that each independent observation in the measurement process is hypothesized to assess the same attribute. If these observations do assess the same attribute, their means and standard deviations are approximately equal, and the results of each pair of observations across a sample of objects tend to be at least modestly correlated. That is, an object with a high score on one observation tends to also have a high score for the other observations. Observations that assess different attributes tend to be uncorrelated. So the key to the diagnostic process is to, first, inspect the means and standard deviations of each observation for gross nonuniformity and then compute and inspect the matrix of correlations among the observations. This matrix of intercorrelations may be computed directly from the objects-by-observations matrix generated by the measurement study. Pearson product-moment correlations are customarily used for this purpose.[*] Each correlation may be computed using the following for two attributes, denoted x and y, with measurements of both attributes performed on i objects:

$$r = \frac{\sum_i (x_i - \bar{x})(y_i - \bar{y})}{\sqrt{\sum_i (x_i - \bar{x})^2 \sum_i (y_i - \bar{y})^2}}$$

where x_i and y_i are values of the individual observations of x and y, and $\bar{x}$ and $\bar{y}$ are the mean values of x and y over all objects in the study sample. This formula looks imposing but is a built-in function in almost all spreadsheet programs.

Observations that are "well behaved" should be similarly distributed and at least modestly intercorrelated (correlations as low as 0.2 can be acceptable) with all other observations. These observations should be retained in the measurement process, as each observation works to increase the reliability of the measurement of the attribute. (As discussed in Chapter 5, a set of observations that is well behaved as a group can be said to comprise an index, or scale.) When a measurement study reveals that a specific observation is not well behaved, and thus does not belong with the others in the group of observations, it should be revised or deleted from the measurement process.

In practice, computing all of the correlations among observations is cumbersome, as a set of N observations has $N(N-1)/2$ unique correlation coefficients that

---

[*] When the purpose of computing the coefficients is to inspect them to determine if the observations are "well behaved," the Pearson coefficient is widely used and is the only coefficient discussed explicitly here. The Pearson coefficient assumes that the variables are both measured with interval properties and normally distributed. Even though both assumptions are frequently violated, the Pearson coefficient provides useful guidance to the investigator performing measurement studies. A helpful discussion of the various correlation coefficients and their use in measurement is found in a concise book by Issac and Michael.[1]

must be inspected, and the pattern among these correlations inferred. Analysis of 10 items, for example, involves inspection of 45 coefficients. There are some shortcuts that make the process more tractable. The most common shortcut is to compute and then inspect the "corrected part–whole" correlation coefficients for each observation. This correlation is between an observation and the total score excluding that observation. The process for computing this correlation is described below. Using corrected part–whole correlations, only N correlations need be inspected for N observations to determine if the observations are well behaved. Typically, an observation exhibiting a corrected part–whole correlation below 0.4 should be modified or deleted. Always keep in mind that modifying an observation or eliminating it from a set can change what the scale is assessing and can affect the validity of the measurement.

To see how this works computationally, examine Table 6.1, which portrays the "typical measurement result" previously shown in Table 5.2. Recall that the reliability coefficient for these measurement results is 0.81.

To compute the corrected part–whole correlation for each observation, it is necessary to create ordered pairs of numbers representing the score for each observation and the total score for each object, excluding that observation. Table 6.2 illustrates computation of the corrected part–whole correlation for observation 1 from Table 6.1. The ordered pairs used to compute the correlation consist of each object's score for observation 1 paired with the object's total score summed across all observations but excluding observation 1. Because object A has a total score of 22, excluding observation 1 yields a corrected total score of 18. The correlation coefficient of 0.62, as shown in the bottom row of Table 6.1, is computed from these four ordered pairs.

The other corrected part–whole correlations are computed by creating analogous ordered pairs for each of the other observations: the scores on observation 2 paired with the total scores excluding observation 2, which yields a correlation of 0.83; the scores on observation 3 paired with the total scores excluding observation 3, which yields a correlation of 0.11; and so on. These calculations are relatively straightforward on a spreadsheet.

TABLE 6.1. "Typical measurement result" with corrected part–whole correlations

| Object | Results of five observations | | | | | Total score |
	1	2	3	4	5	
A	4	5	3	5	5	22
B	3	5	5	3	4	20
C	4	4	4	4	5	21
D	3	2	3	2	3	13
Corrected part-whole correlation	0.62	0.83	0.11	0.77	0.90	

TABLE 6.2. Computing the corrected part–whole correlation for observation 1

Object	Score for observation 1	Corrected total score, excluding observation 1
A	4	18
B	3	17
C	4	17
D	3	10

Having seen how the "short-cut" method of part–whole correlations works in practice, we now explore the full matrix of correlations among all pairs of observations. Table 6.3 displays these correlations for the measurement results given in Table 6.1. Overall, there are $5(5 - 1)/2$, or 10, correlation coefficients to inspect. The correlation between observations i and j is found at the intersection of the ith row and jth column. Because this matrix of intercorrelations is symmetrical about the diagonal and the diagonal elements are equal to 1.0, only the values of elements above the diagonal are shown.

In this example, observation 3 is not well behaved, which is seen several ways. From Table 6.1, it can be seen that an object with the highest total score (A) has a relatively low score on observation 3. The object with the second lowest total score (B) has the highest score on observation 3. We also see evidence of observation 3's misbehavior because the corrected part–whole coefficient is less than 0.4. whereas the others are high. In Table 6.3 the correlations between observation 3 and the other observations, seen in boldface type, show no consistent pattern: Two are negative, and two are positive. Deleting observation 3 increases the reliability of measurement (in this case, from 0.81 to 0.89), even though the number of observations in the measurement process is decreased. Observations can also fail to be well behaved if their mean values (across all objects observed) are close to either the high or low extremes, or if they display no variability across objects. Such observations add no useful information to the measurement process and should be modified or deleted.

What Corrected Part–Whole Correlations Can Reveal

In later sections of this chapter we discuss specific ways to improve measurement technique for specific situations that arise frequently in informatics studies. Here we consider general strategies that may be followed from a diagnostic process using part–whole correlations computed from the objects-by-observations matrix. For brevity's sake, we refer to corrected part–whole correlations simply as part–whole correlations.

1. *If all part–whole correlations are reasonably large but the reliability is too low:* Add equivalent observations to the measurement process.

TABLE 6.3. Correlations between observations for the "typical measurement result"

Item	1	2	3	4	5
1	—	0.41	**−0.30**	0.89	0.91
2		—	**0.49**	0.73	0.74
3			—	**−0.13**	**0.09**
4				—	0.94

2. *If many part–whole correlations are low:* Something affecting all observations is fundamentally amiss. There are likely to be only small differences in the scores among objects. Check aspects of the measurement process that relate to all observations; for example, if human judges are using a rating form, the items on the form may be phrased misleadingly.

3. *If one (or perhaps two) observations display low part–whole correlations:* First try deleting the misbehaving observation(s). The reliability may be higher and the entire measurement process more efficient if so pruned. Alternatively, try modifying or replacing the misbehaving observation(s).

4. *If two or more observations display modest part–whole correlations and the others are high:* This situation is ambiguous and may indicate that the observations as a group are measuring two or more different attributes. In this case, each subset displays high intercorrelation of its member observations, but the observations from different subsets are not correlated with each other. This possibility cannot be fully explored using part–whole correlations and requires either careful inspection of the full intercorrelation matrix or use of more advanced statistical techniques. If the investigator expected the observations to address a single attribute and in fact they address multiple discrete attributes, it is not a satisfactory result and requires modification of the measurement process. (To play out an example in detail, perform Self-Test 6.2.)

If a specific observation is not well behaved (outcome 3, above), several things may be happening; and it may be necessary pinpoint the problem in order to fix it. For example, consider items on a questionnaire as a set of observations. A misbehaving item may be so poorly phrased that it is not assessing anything at all; or perhaps the particular objects—in this case, questionnaire respondents used for the measurement study—lack some specific knowledge that enables them to respond to the item. In this case an improved part–whole correlation may be observed if the item is tested on a different sample of objects. Alternatively, the item may be well phrased but, on logical grounds, does not "belong" with the other items on the scale. This situation can be determined by inspecting the content of the item, or, if possible, talking to the individuals who completed it to see how it was interpreted.

Because it is necessary to collect new measurement data after making major revisions to any set of observations, developing measurement procedures is an iterative and time-consuming process. As a rule, an investigator should borrow from other investigators and other studies whenever possible, particularly if data exist to suggest that the scales have good measurement properties; that is, they have been demonstrated to be reliable and valid when used with objects (people or resources) similar to those proposed for the investigator's own study. Also, these examples, by using unrealistically few objects, may have underrepresented the work required to conduct a rigorous measurement study. As discussed later in the chapter, measurement studies that generate stable and thus credible results typically include many more than four objects.

In addition to computation of part–whole correlations, the data resulting from measurement studies may be analyzed using one of the many statistical techniques for grouping of observations. The most popular is exploratory factor analysis and its many close relatives.[2, 3] These techniques suggest which of the observations are well behaved, in a way that is more precise and informative than inspecting part–whole correlations or values of correlations between observations. The mechanics of these methods are beyond this discussion. The reader is advised to consult his or her local statistician or psychometrician or to read one of the books, cited above, on these techniques.

Self Test 6.2

1. Consider the following measurement result, with a reliability of 0.61. What is your diagnosis of this result? What would you do to improve it?

Object	Results of six observations					
	1	2	3	4	5	6
A	4	3	5	2	1	4
B	2	4	5	3	2	2
C	3	4	3	4	4	3
D	2	3	1	2	1	2
E	3	3	2	2	4	3
Part–whole correlation	0.49	0.37	0.32	0.37	0.32	0.49

2. Consider the following measurement result, for which the reliability is 0.72.

Object	Results of six observations					
	1	2	3	4	5	6
A	4	5	4	2	2	3
B	3	3	3	2	2	2
C	4	4	4	4	5	4
D	5	5	4	2	2	1
Part–whole correlation	0.21	0.13	0.71	0.76	0.68	0.51

The matrix of correlations among items for these observations is as follows.

Item	1	2	3	4	5	6
1	—	0.85	0.82	0	0	−0.32
2			0.87	−0.17	−0.17	−0.13
3				0.33	0.33	0.26
4					1	0.78
5						0.78

How would you interpret these results? What would you do to improve this measurement process?

3. Refer to the data in Table 5.4. Using corrected part–whole coefficients, determine who is the best judge in terms of agreement with his or her colleagues. Who is the worst? What would happen to the reliability if the worst judge's ratings were removed from the set?

New Terminology: Facets and Levels

Until now, we have considered measurement situations where only one source of error—one type of independent observation—is under explicit consideration. In a more general case, multiple sources of error may be identified by the investigator.

Consider a more complicated version of the example earlier in the chapter, where the investigator is interested not only in the effects on the measurement of the number of judges employed but also the effects of the way the patient history is abstracted for purposes of generating the ratings. The investigator divides the judges into two groups. The judges in the first group are assigned to rate all patients using a long abstract, whereas the other group of judges uses a shorter version. In this situation the measurement study is doing double-duty. Two sources of error (due to judges and abstracting methods) are being investigated simultaneously. The objects-by-observations matrix takes on a third dimension, as two characteristics of the observation have been purposefully included in the measurement study. From this more complex study, the investigator can draw conclusions not only about the necessary number of judges for accurate measurement but also about the adequacy of abstracts of varying lengths.

In the language of measurement, each source of error that is purposefully explored in a measurement study is called a facet.[4] In our example as originally developed, "judges" is the single facet of the measurement study. In the more complex version of the example, there are two facets: "judges" and "abstract length." Each facet has a number of levels corresponding to the number of independent observations that facet contributes to the measurement process. In the two-facet example, with six judges used in the measurement study, the "judges" facet is said to have six levels; and with two abstract lengths, the facet "abstract

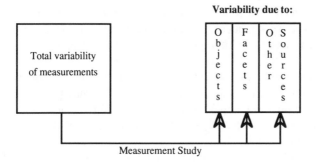

FIGURE 6.2. Analytical process of a measurement study.

length" is said to have two levels. Note that the object class ("patients" in our example) is not considered a facet of the measurement study.

As shown in Figure 6.2, the analytical process in a measurement study determines how much of the total variability of the measurement result is statistically attributable to the objects, to the facets purposefully included in the study, and to other factors including random errors. Using this new terminology, the specific methods developed in Chapter 5 and in earlier sections of this chapter allow us to analyze the results of measurement studies that have one facet, where all observations are made on all objects. These methods also tell us how to prognosticate the effects on reliability of changing the number of levels of that facet. These techniques serve the needs of many investigators. We introduce in the next section more complex measurement situations that employ multiple facets simultaneously. Appendix A briefly introduces the methods of generalizability theory as a way to treat these more complex problems.

Self-Test 6.3

In Chapter 4 we introduced as an example a study of a new admission–discharge–transfer (ADT) system for hospitals and the challenge of measuring the attribute of "time to process a new admission," with human observers completing a paper rating form as the "instruments." A measurement study may be designed with measurements taken simultaneously by five observers, at three different times of day, in each of four hospitals. The same five observers are employed for the entire measurement study. What is the object class for this measurement? What are the facets of the measurement study? How many levels does each facet have?

Key Objects and Facets of Measurement in Informatics

We turn now to the range of measurement issues encountered in the real world of informatics. Four specific categories of object classes—care providers or decision makers, care recipients (often called patients or cases), information resources themselves, and work groups or organizations that provide health care—are usually of primary interest in informatics research and evaluation studies. Similarly, four types of facets—tasks, judges, items, logistical factors—arise frequently in our work. A specific measurement process can involve one and only one class of objects. By contrast, a measurement process may have multiple facets. The investigator can choose how many facets to include in a formal measurement study. In many situations a one-facet study suffices because the effect of one source of error is often of dominant interest.

Among the classes of objects, health care providers and decision makers are important in informatics because attributes of these individuals influence whether and how information resources are used.[5, 6] Important attributes of care providers include their domain-specific biomedical knowledge; their attitudes toward information technology, work environment, and change itself; their experience with information technology; and many others.

Care recipients (patients) emerge as objects of interest because their medical problems are complex and the attributes of these problems, central to evaluation studies, are difficult to assess. Important attributes of patients that often require measurement are diagnosis, prognosis, appropriateness of actual or recommended management, and typicality of disease presentation.

Information resources have many attributes (e.g., speed of task execution, ease of use, reliability, and degradation at the limits of their domain) that are of vital interest to informatics investigators.

Finally, work groups and organizations have many attributes (e.g., mission, age, size, budget structure, complexity, and integration) that determine how rapidly they adopt new technology and, once they do, how they use it. Chapter 10 discusses evaluation issues focusing on organizations.

The four facets of frequent interest in informatics are defined as follows.

1. *Tasks:* In many studies, measurement is made by challenging the object with something to do. An information resource may be challenged to process a set of patient records, or a care provider may be asked to provide diagnoses for sets of clinical findings. With these kinds of performance-based assessment, which occur often in informatics, the problems assigned to objects can be generically referred to as tasks.
2. *Judges:* Many measurement processes in informatics employ judges: humans with particular expertise who provide their informed opinions, usually by completing a rating form, about behavior they observe directly or review, in retrospect, from some record of that behavior. Chart audit is a common example of retrospective review.
3. *Items:* They are the individual elements of a form used to record ratings, opinions, or perceptions. On an attitude questionnaire, for example, the individual questions would be considered a type of item.
4. *Logistical factors:* Many measurement processes are strongly influenced by procedural, temporal, or geographic factors, such as the places where and times when observations take place.

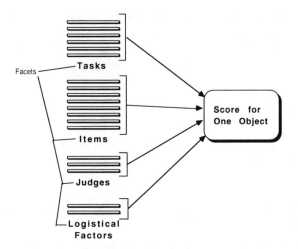

Figure 6.3. General (four-facet) measurement problem. A score for one object is obtained by averaging over all levels of each facet and then averaging across the facets. Note that in this example the task facet has five levels, the items facet eight levels, the judges' facet three levels, and the logistical factors facet two levels

The most general measurement process in informatics includes simultaneously all four of the key facets, as illustrated in Figure 6.3. Recalling that each facet usually has multiple levels, this general process entails multiple judges completing a rating form with multiple items to rate each object completing multiple tasks under differing logistical conditions. To assign each object a single score for the attribute of interest, we would average across judges, items, tasks, and conditions (thus averaging across each level of each facet), as shown in Figure 6.3. For a correspondingly general measurement study, we would conduct the complete measurement process with a selected set of objects and determine how much variability is attributable to each of the four facets. We would also learn from such a study how many levels of each facet would be necessary to achieve an adequate level of reliability. The methods of generalizability theory (see Appendix A) are required to work analytically with a multifacet measurement problem.

We discuss in the following section the practical aspects of the three facets that arise most frequently in measurement studies: tasks, judges, and items. Although we do not discuss logistical factors explicitly, they may be important facets of some measurement processes. As seen in the earlier example of an ADT system, the accuracy with which one can measure the time to process a patient admission could depend on logistical factors, such as the general state of the clinic, which in turn could depend on the time of day, time of year, and other factors. We emphasize that the choice of specific facets to include in a measurement study rests completely with the investigator. If a facet is included, the amount of error it contributes to the measurement process can be quantified. If a facet is excluded, its contribution to measurement error is combined with all "other sources," as illustrated in Figure 6.2, and cannot be separately identified.

For each facet, we explore the following: (1) in studies, why the results for a given object vary from observation to observation and how much variation to expect; (2) in practice, how many levels of the facet are needed for reliable measurement; and (3) what can be done to improve this aspect of measurement.

Self-Test 6.4

For the measurement problem and study described in Self-Test 6.3, to what category does each facet belong?

Pragmatics of Measurement Using Tasks, Judges, and Items

In this section, we decompose the multifacet general measurement problem and focus separately on each key facet of measurement in informatics. We focus first on tasks as the key facet of interest, then on judges, and then on items. The three decomposed measurement problems are illustrated in Figure 6.4.

Task Facet

Many evaluation studies in informatics are performed using real-world tasks or laboratory simulations of these tasks. In medical informatics, the task facet is of primary importance when the quality of performance of some important clinical activity is the attribute of interest. The object classes are usually care providers, information resources, or both. The tasks themselves are usually clinical problems (equivalently called test cases) used to challenge these care providers or "intelligent" information resources. How these persons or resources are asked to perform these tasks depends on the goals of the study. They may be asked to diagnose, interpret, explain etiology, retrieve pertinent information, propose management, or critique the performance of others. For many reasons, selection and design of these tasks, for measurement as well as demonstration studies, is perhaps the most perplexing aspect of objectivist study design.

Sources of Variation Among Tasks

The performance of human care providers and information resources is highly dependent on the content of the clinical material with which they are challenged. For information resources, which are programmed to perform specific tasks within specific domains, this statement is hardly surprising. However, in studies involving human problem-solvers the extent of this "task-dependence" of performance is far greater than was believed as recently as the late 1970s, prior to the appearance of the classic study of medical problem solving by Elstein and colleagues.[7] Suppose a sample of persons is given two diagnostic problems to work.

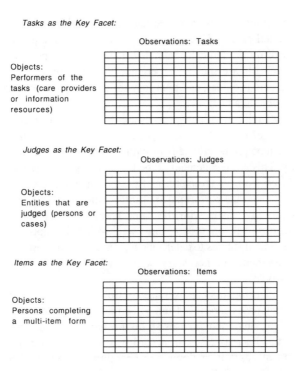

FIGURE 6.4. Three important one-facet measurement problems.

If we compute the correlation between performance on the first problem with performance on the second, the magnitude of these correlations is typically small. High performance on one problem does not strongly imply a high performance on another. For this reason, "task dependence" or "case specificity" of medical expertise is now a central issue in research and evaluation, and the clinical cases used in any study are a key feature of that study's design.

It follows that studies employing only one task are intrinsically weak because the results are an artifact of the features of that task, and the measurement error attributable to task specificity cannot be estimated. To make a statement in a demonstration study that one group of subjects performs better than another group, it is necessary to challenge each member of each group with a large number of carefully selected tasks. Determining how many tasks are required for acceptable measurement is, of course, the major goal of a measurement study.

Whether the objects of measurement are persons or machines, the interobservation correlation for tasks increases in proportion to the "similarity" of the tasks themselves. However, the features that make tasks "similar" are highly idiosyncratic to the task and objects and are often not predictable in advance. This point is particularly true with humans as objects because humans vary enormously in their personal knowledge and how that knowledge is organized. Human ability to diagnose or manage a clinical problem is best predicted by each individual's experience with cases of exactly that type and only weakly predicted by individual traits such as intelligence.[8] Therefore two care providers of equal intelligence and seniority may differ dramatically in their performance on the same case, according to their levels of case-specific experience. The features of a case that make it "familiar" to a care provider, and thus easy for him or her to address, are also not readily predictable in advance.

Similarly, when information resources are the objects of measurement, neither the performance of the system on a specific task nor the intertask variability in performance can be predicted in advance once these systems reach a certain level of complexity. This is a restatement of the fact that system function cannot in general be predicted from its structure, as first introduced in Chapter 3. Typically, generalizations about the performance of information resources and human problem solvers must be made with the same care. The fact that an information resource performs well on task A only weakly implies good performance on task B. Measurement studies to determine how many tasks (cases) are required for reliable measurement are necessary when the objects are either information resources or people.

In practice, investigators can exercise control over the task facet in two ways: first, by selecting cases carefully from some real or hypothetical population; and second, by employing enough cases so high reliability is seen when the performance is averaged across cases. In accord with our measurement theory, use of large numbers of cases is analogous to shooting a large number of arrows to ensure that the effects of idiosyncratic factors "average out."

Number of Tasks Needed

Much research on medical problem-solving has clarified the number of cases necessary for reliable measurement of human performance in clinical medicine. The best controlled research has been performed using standardized patient-actors. To reach a reliability of 0.70, 6–24 cases within a specific domain appear to be required depending on the aspect of performance under study. For diagnostic problems, 24 cases may be required.[9] This requirement creates a challenge for researchers to include relatively large numbers of time-consuming tasks in their studies, but there are some ways to streamline the process, which are addressed in the following section. Although it is not always clear what makes cases similar, the more similar the cases that comprise a test set, the higher are the intercorrelations between them and thus the reliability for a set comprising a given number of cases. For some situations, a highly homogeneous mix, such as differing presentations of the same disease, might be appropriate and fewer such cases may be required. In general, the choice of the test set of tasks should follow logically from the purposes of the study.

For studies of information resource performance, it is difficult to give an analogous figure because few measurement studies have been performed. Swets, for example, pointed to the need for "large and representative samples" but did not quantify "large."[10] In domains other than medicine, for example weather forecasting, it is common to test prognostic systems with thousands of cases. Jain's otherwise thorough discussion of "workloads" for computer system performance testing did not directly address the size of the workload necessary for reliable measurement.[11] Lacking guidelines for the number of tasks to use for studying information resource performance in medical domains, the most sensible approach is to conduct measurement studies in advance.

Improving Measurement Using Tasks

When humans, and especially care providers, are the objects of measurement, it is important to challenge them with a set of tasks large enough for reliable measurement, but no larger than necessary. The longer the task set, the greater the risk of fatigue, noncompliance, or half-hearted effort; data loss through failure to complete the task set; or expense if the individuals are compensated for their work. The inherent task-to-task variability in performance cannot be circumvented, but many other steps can be taken to ensure that every task in a set is adding useful information to a study. The approaches to improve measurement in this domain are multiple: (1) careful abstracting of case data; (2) sampling a large number of tasks from a known population; and (3) systematic assignment of tasks to objects.

1. *Abstracting:* Much of the published research in informatics is based on case abstractions of various types to provide a representation of a case that is completely consistent wherever and whenever it is employed. Typically, a subset of findings from a case is extracted from the patient's chart and summarized in a concise written document, creating the ubiquitous "paper cases" that embody the tasks for a study. Yet care providers in the real world work with live patients who provide verbal and nonverbal cues about their condition. These cues are revealed over time in a way that a paper abstract cannot capture. The effects of these abstractions on medical informatics studies are largely unexplored, but it is clear that inconsistent abstracting diminishes the intercorrelations between cases comprising a set. To address this problem, the rules to select findings for inclusion in the summary should be clearly stated, even if the same person is doing all of the abstracting. These rules should also be carefully reviewed to ensure that they are free of an evident bias, such as omission of the clinical information key to successful completion of the task by person or machine. Otherwise, abstracters' judgments about what is "important" could substantially skew the results of a study. The need for consistency goes beyond the choice of which findings to include. These findings must be represented in a consistent fashion, so that, for example, a laboratory value that is normal in one case is normal in all other cases in the set. The abstracters must also decide how much interpretation of findings to provide and take steps to ensure that they do it consistently.

There are, of course, alternatives to the paper representations of cases, but they are time-consuming and expensive. At the extreme of high fidelity is the simulated patient, an actor trained to sound, look, and feel like the actual patient with a particular disease. A lower-fidelity compromise is representation via computer simulation of a case, which could allow access to all clinical findings via a natural language interface, visual representation of the patient, and access to many clinical findings such as radiographs in uninterpreted form. Computer simulations themselves vary in ornateness,[12] and the simplest simulation that meets the needs of a study should be selected. Although possibly expensive to set up initially, the recurring cost of using a computer simulation is low. In both of these formats, the abstraction problem remains. The actor is trained to know a finite set of clinical information, and a computer simulation cannot present more than it is programmed to present.

2. *Sampling:* Case selection can be addressed by two major strategies. One strategy builds controlled variability into the set. Assuming that the investigator knows which case features are important for determining performance, he or she maps these features into a sampling grid and subsequently selects cases to ensure balanced representation of these features. With this approach the investigator can control the amount of variability in the case set but must do so with recognition that it involves a compromise. On the one hand, constraining the variability too much (making the cases too similar) leads to high reliability of measures but does not allow generalization beyond that homogeneous set. On the other hand, purposeful building of a highly diverse case set inevitably requires a larger number of cases for reliable measurement.

Although building a case set from such a blueprint gives the investigator a great deal of control, it generates a population that is hypothetical. With the second strategy, the investigator selects cases based on natural occurrence; for example using consecutive admissions to a hospital as the criterion. The resulting set of cases has a clear reference population, but the variability in the case mix is not under the investigator's control. In a study of a diagnostic decision support system, for example, the diagnoses of interest to the system may not occur with sufficient frequency in a naturally occurring sequence of cases. Whichever strategy is followed, the key to this process is to have a defensible selection plan that follows from the purposes of the study and in turn allows the investigator to identify the population from which the cases were selected. The implications of these strategies for demonstration study design are discussed in Chapter 7.

3. *Assignment:* Many techniques can be used to assign tasks to objects in measurement studies, but whenever possible this assignment should be done by preordained design rather than chance encounter. As shown in Figure 6.5, two common assignment modes include the "fully crossed" approach, where every object is challenged by every case in the sample, and a "nested" approach, where specific subsamples of objects are assigned specific subsamples of cases. The nested approach is especially helpful when the investigator is studying persons as objects, wishes to include a large number of cases in the full study, but does not want to burden any single person with the entire case set. In informatics, the persons employed in studies are typically busy trainees or care providers; their time is scarce or expensive (or both). Using a nested approach, 15 cases can be randomly divided into three groups. If each person is assigned to work one group of cases, each works only five cases (a more manageable task than 15), and the investigator

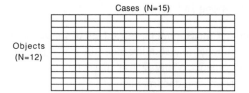

Fully Crossed Design: All Cases Assigned to All Objects

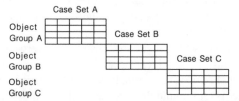

Nested Design: Sets of 5 Cases Assigned to Groups of Objects

FIGURE 6.5. Assignment of tasks (cases) to objects.

is not seriously limited in the conclusions he or she can draw from the study. Nested designs are useful in both measurement and demonstration studies. In situations where large numbers of cases are available, nested designs should be considered a way to take advantage of the ability to generalize from that large number of cases without having to expose every object to every case. In measurement studies, generalizability theory (see Appendix A) provides a way to estimate sources of measurement errors for nested designs.

Judges Facet

The judges facet enters into a measurement problem whenever informed human judges assess the quality (or some other important aspect) of an activity or a product they are observing. A typical study might employ expert clinicians to judge the appropriateness of the clinical advice generated by a computer-based resource. Because advice is generated for each of a set of cases, cases may be seen as the object class of measurement. In other examples, observers may assess some aspect of the interaction of end-users with a new information resource during a beta test. Here, the end-users, usually care providers, comprise the object class of measurement. As in all facets of measurement, a key issue is the correlation among the observations—in this situation, the judges—and the resulting number of judges required to obtain a reliable measurement. A set of "well-behaved" judges, all of whom agree with one another to an acceptable extent when rating a representative sample of objects, can be said to form a scale. A large literature on performance assessment speaks in more detail to many of the issues addressed here.[13, 14]

Sources of Variation Among Judges

With an ideal objectivist measurement, all judges of the same object, using the same criteria and instrumentation, should render the same judgment. All variation should then be among objects. Many factors that erode interjudge agreement are well known and have been well documented.[15]

1. *Interpretation or logical effects:* Judges may differ in their interpretations of the attributes to be rated and the meanings of the items on the forms on which they record their judgments. They may give similar ratings to attributes that are logically related in their own minds.
2. *Judge tendency effects:* Some judges are consistently overgenerous or lenient; others are consistently hypercritical or stringent. Others do not employ the whole set of response options or a form, locating all of their ratings in a narrow region, which may be at the middle or toward either end of the set. This phenomenon is known as a "central tendency" effect.
3. *Insufficient exposure:* Sometimes the logistics of a study require that judges base their judgments on less exposure to the object than is necessary to come to an informed conclusion.
4. *Inconsistent conditions:* Unless multiple judges make their observations simultaneously, the phenomena observed can vary from judge to judge.

Number of Judges Needed

Although steps can be taken to reduce the effects of the factors listed above, interjudge variability cannot be eliminated; and as with the other facets of measurement, multiple observations (in this case multiple judges) are necessary. The maximum reliability that can be expected from a one judge study is on the order of 0.5.[16] In Chapter 5 we saw that van der Lei and colleagues obtained a reliability of 0.65 when using eight judges in the study of Hypercritic. In the self-test below, we see that three judges are sufficient for some situations. There is, however, no precise way to determine this number in advance. A measurement study is necessary to verify that acceptable reliability is obtained for any particular situation.

Improving Measurement Using Judges

The general approach is to increase the number of judges or improve the quality of the measurement process by training the judges or designing better instruments for them to use. Increasing the number of judges helps only if the judges added perform equivalently to, or better than, the judges already included. If they do, the Spearman-Brown prophecy formula illustrates how much improvement can be obtained. What makes a human judge intrinsically "good" is perhaps less clear than for other facets of measurement.

To improve the quality of the measurement process, a major factor under the investigator's direct control is to ensure that each judge observes a representative sample of the phenomena of interest. A nested design can be helpful when there is danger of asking each judge to do more observation than is reasonable. The phenomena to be observed can be sectioned by time (judge 1 observes on Monday the first week, Tuesday the second week, and so on), or by other natural subdivisions. Other benefits of the nested design include economy of effort, as each judge does less work, and the potential for a greater range of phenomena to form the basis of the ratings, leading to greater generalizability of the results.

Additional benefit can derive from formal training or orientation of the judges.[15] Many strategies can be useful here. A meeting where the judges discuss their personal interpretations of the attributes to be rated and the meaning of the responses can increase reliability. A more formal training activity where the judges watch a videotaped or live sample of the phenomenon to be rated can also be helpful. Here judges first observe the phenomenon, which might be a representative interaction of a user with an information resource, and make their ratings independently. Then the individual ratings are collected and summarized in a table, so all can see the aggregate performance of the group. This step is followed by a discussion among the judges, where they share their reasons for rating as they did.

Some simple logistical and practical steps, often overlooked, can also improve measurement using judges. First, eliminate judges who, for a variety of reasons, are inappropriate participants in the study. An individual with a certain role relative to a study, such as director of the clinic where a resource is under test, should not participate as a judge. Do not use unwilling conscripts, who might have been "asked" by their supervisors to participate. Second, make the work of the judges as straightforward as possible, with a minimum of complications. Most judges have a fixed amount of time to devote to their task. The more time they devote to administrative aspects, such as making their own copies of forms to record their judgments, the less time they devote to the substantive task at hand. For laboratory studies, where the conditions are controllable, it may not be necessary for multiple judges to work at the same time, and the judges can be accommodated by allowing them to work as their time permits.

Judges are often used with "patients" ("cases") as the object class of measurement, for example to obtain the closest approximation to the gold standard diagnosis for each patient. This is a key measurement problem in informatics because, clinically, it is essential to assess the accuracy of an information resource against the closest possible approximation to the "truth" about each patient. In these situations, the patients should be followed for as long as is ethically and practically possible so the judges have a large amount of information on which to base their ratings. To increase the reliability and validity of measurement, several domain experts, preferably from different medical centers, should be recruited. To reduce the influence of unusually persuasive judges and to obtain a true estimate of their agreement on each case, judges should review case data independently. In many instances the attribute to be assessed has interval or ratio properties, such as a rating of the quality of care provided to the patient. In these instances the best approximation to the true value of the attribute is obtained by averaging the judges' ratings. In other situations the attribute to be assessed has nominal properties—for example, the final diagnosis of a case. In these cases it may be necessary to first obtain a shortlist of possible diagnoses from a set of judges and then ask these judges or others to rate each member of the list. If the disagreement is too great among the judges, it may be that a sufficiently good approximation to a gold standard is unobtainable for this case and it should be omitted from any subsequent demonstration study. In cases where judges disagree, the case can be referred to a "senior" judge for a deciding vote.[17] Although it is a useful expedient, there is no guarantee that the truth resides with this individual. Also, once the final decision is vested in a single individual and not the mean of a set of independent judges, the error in the measurement process is no longer estimable.

Self-Test 6.5

The TraumAID system[18] was developed to provide minute-by-minute advice to trauma surgeons in the management of patients with penetrating wounds to the chest and abdomen. As part of a laboratory study of the accuracy of TraumAID's advice, Clarke and colleagues asked a panel of three judges—all experienced surgeons from the institution where TraumAID was developed—to rate the appropriateness of management for each of a series of cases that had been abstracted to paper descriptions. Ratings were on a scale of 1 to 4, where 4 indicated essentially flawless care and 1 was indicative of serious deficiencies. Each case appeared twice in the set: (1) as the patient was treated, and (2) as TraumAID would have treated the patient. The abstracts were carefully written to eliminate any cues as to whether the described care was computer-generated or actually administered.

Overall, 111 cases were rated by three judges, with the following results.

| Condition | Corrected part–whole correlations | | | |
	Judge A	Judge B	Judge C	Reliability of ratings
Actual care	0.57	0.52	0.55	0.72
TraumAID	0.57	0.59	0.47	0.71

| Condition | Mean ± SD ratings | | |
	Judge A	Judge B	Judge C
Actual care	2.35 ± 1.03	2.42 ± 0.80	2.25 ± 1.01
TraumAID	3.12 ± 1.12	2.71 ± 0.83	2.67 ± 0.95

1. What are the dimensions (number of rows and number of columns) of the two objects-by-observations matrices used to compute these results?
2. Is there any evidence of rater tendency errors (leniency, stringency, or central tendency) in these data?
3. Viewing it as a measurement study, what would you be inclined to conclude about the measurement process? Consider reliability and validity issues.
4. Viewing it as a demonstration study, what would you be inclined to conclude about the accuracy of TraumAID's advice?

Items Facet

As defined earlier, items are the individual elements of an instrument used to record ratings, opinions, knowledge, or perceptions of an individual we generically call a "respondent." Items usually take the form of questions. The instruments containing the items can be self-administered, read to the respondent in a highly structured interview, or completed interactively at a computer. Attitude surveys, rating forms used by judges, and tests of knowledge are examples of instruments containing multiple items. For the same reason that a single task cannot be the basis for reliable assessment of performance of an information resource, a single item cannot be used to measure reliably an individual's beliefs or degree of knowledge. The measurement strategy to obtain accurate measurement is always the same: Use multiple independent observations (in this case, items) and pool the results for each object to obtain the best estimate of the value of the attribute for that object. If the items forming a set are shown to be "well behaved" in an appropriate measurement study, we can say that they comprise a scale.

When people (care providers or patients) are the object class of interest, we use multi-item forms to assess the personal attitudes, beliefs, or knowledge of those people. This technique generates a basic one-facet measurement problem with items as the observations and persons as the objects. Items can also form a facet of a more complex measurement problem when, for example, multiple judges complete a multi-item form to render their opinions about multiple medical cases. There is a vast array of item types and formats commonly in use. In settings where items are used to elicit beliefs or attitudes, there is no "correct answer" to the items; in tests of knowledge, a particular response is identified by the item developer as "correct." We explore a few of the more common formats here and discuss some general principles of item design that work to reduce measurement error.

Almost all items consist of two parts, whether they are used to assess personal beliefs or judge performance. The first part is a stem, which elicits a response; the second provides a structured format for the individual completing the instrument to respond to the stem. Reponses can be elicited using graphic scales, as shown in Figure 6.6. Alternatively, responses can be elicited via a discrete set of options, as shown in Table 6.4. The response options themselves may form a semantic axis, which can be unipolar ("never" to "always") or bipolar ("strongly agree" to "strongly disagree"). The literature does not reveal a great deal of difference

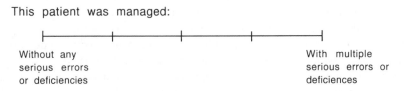

FIGURE 6.6. Rating item with a graphic response scale.

TABLE 6.4. An "optimism" scale for medical informatics

Effect of computers on	Highly detrimental	Detrimental on the whole	Neither detrimental nor beneficial	Beneficial on the whole	Highly beneficial
Cost of health care	1	2	3	4	5
Clinician autonomy	1	2	3	4	5
Quality of health care	1	2	3	4	5
Interactions within the health care team	1	2	3	4	5
Role of the government in health care	1	2	3	4	5
Access to health care in remote or rural areas	1	2	3	4	5
Management of medical/ ethical dilemmas	1	2	3	4	5
Enjoyment of the practice of medicine	1	2	3	4	5
Status of medicine as a profession	1	2	3	4	5
Continuing medical education	1	2	3	4	5
Self-image of clinicians	1	2	3	4	5
Humaneness of the practice of medicine	1	2	3	4	5
Rapport between clinicians and patients	1	2	3	4	5
Personal and professional privacy	1	2	3	4	5
Clinicians' access to up-to-date knowledge	1	2	3	4	5
Patients' satisfaction with the quality of care they receive	1	2	3	4	5
Generalists' ability to manage more complex problems	1	2	3	4	5

among these formats in terms of the quality of the measurement information obtained.[16, 19]

We now explore how multiple items can be used to form a scale. Table 6.4 contains an excerpt from a longer questionnaire that assesses the attitudes of academic physicians toward information technology.[20] Each of the items in Table 6.4 addresses the perceived effects of computers on a particular aspect of health care, but the items can be seen as having something deeper in common. Each item reflects, in part, a sense of "optimism" about the future role of information technology in health care. The response options form a bipolar axis. We might expect an individual who responds favorably to one item to have a tendency to respond favorably to the other items in the set because of this general belief or outlook. In this sense, each item can be seen as an observation of the attribute "optimism." The assumption can be tested via an appropriate measurement study; and if the assumption holds, a person's level of optimism may be assessed using the sum (or average) of the responses to the set of items. Across a set of items that address the same underlying attribute, it is assumed that the idiosyncratic reactions to the individual items cancel out and the average reflects the individual's "true" level of belief.

We already know how to test such an assumption using a measurement study, by examining the distributions of the responses to the individual items, and the correlations among them, as generated by administering the items to a representative sample of individuals. As for all other measurement facets, perfect correlation among the different items is not expected. With this particular set of items, all but one of the items was found to be well behaved (R.D. Cork, C.P. Friedman, and W.M. Detmer, unpublished observations) The reliability of the scale with this item removed was 0.86. Of course, showing that the items form a well-behaved cluster does not demonstrate that they combine to assess "optimism." Additional studies of the validity of the scale are required for this purpose.

Scales to measure attitudes and beliefs are typically developed through an iterative process where the investigators first clearly identify the attribute to be assessed and the kinds of objects (in this case, kinds of persons) who will be completing the scale. They then create an initial set of items. To do this, they might conduct open-ended interviews or develop a initial set from their own personal experience. The scale developers then conduct measurement studies, administering the scale to samples of objects and identifying, revising, or replacing items that are not well behaved. Over successive measurement studies, the reliability of the scale usually improves to acceptable levels. The validity of the scale—content, criterion-related, construct—must then be established using methods discussed in Chapter 5.

Similar challenges are presented by other measurement situations requiring the use of multiple items to measure some underlying attribute. For example, a knowledge test might contain individual items that appear different but share the attribute of knowledge of the specific subject area addressed by the test. By the same token, the multiple items addressing different aspects of a clinical task have in common the attribute of competence in performing that particular task.

Sources of Variation Among Items

Variability from item to item is built into the way beliefs are measured because the respondents are being asked different questions that have something fundamental in common. However, as with all measurement processes, this variability can and should be minimized via careful item design. If items are ambiguously phrased, if the stems and response options are not logically matched, or if the response options do not accurately mirror the range of beliefs the respondents hold, measurement error seen as high levels of inter-item variability will result. Specific ways to address these problems are described below.

The halo effect is a well known problem that manifests when items are the key facet of measurement. When completers of an instrument are asked to render a belief that is elicited in the form of responses to multiple items, they may form an overall impression that affects the way they respond to the entire set of items. If the overall impression is positive, all items are completed positively regardless of the completer's "true" beliefs about each item. If the overall impression is negative, the opposite occurs. Halo effects result in artificially reduced inter-item variability. Ways to reduce halo effects are also discussed below.

Number of Items Needed

Typically, a minimum of eight to ten items is needed to measure a belief or an attitude. The 16-item computer optimism scale (Table 6.4) had a reliability of 0.86. The Spearman-Brown formula suggests that an eight-item version of the same scale would still have a reliability of 0.75, but removal of some of the items would raise concerns about validity. In extreme cases such as high-stakes standardized tests, where high reliability is necessary to make decisions about each individual's competence, more than 100 items are routinely used within a knowledge domain. In this situation, large numbers of items are required both to attain the high reliability necessary to generate a small standard error of measurement and to sample adequately a broad domain of knowledge. For ratings of performance by expert judges, fewer items on a form may be necessary because the attribute to be rated is often specific. For any particular measurement situation, a measurement study can determine how many items are necessary and which items should be deleted or modified to improve the performance of the item set comprising a scale.

Improving Measurement with Items

We offer here several practical suggestions to minimize measurement errors through attention to item design. We focus here on ratings and other elicitations of attitudes and beliefs because these applications arise more frequently during the evaluations that are the focus of this book.

1. *Make items specific.* Perhaps the single most important way to improve items is to make them as specific as possible. The more information the respondents get from the form itself, about what exactly is being asked for and what the response options mean, the greater is the consistency of the results. Consider a basic item that may be part of a multi-item rating form (Fig. 6.7A). As a first step toward specificity, the item should offer a definition of the attribute to be rated, as shown in Figure 6.7B. The next step is to change the response categories from broad qualitative judgments to behavior or events that might be observed. Response categories that are purely quantitative should be avoided, unless the respondent is being asked specifically to estimate a quantity. As shown in Figure 6.7C, we might change the logic of the responses by specifically asking for the opinion as to how frequently the explanations were clear.

2. *Match the logic of the response to that of the stem.* This step is vitally important. If the stem—the part of the item that elicits a reponse—requests an estimate of a quantity, the response formats must offer a range of reasonable quantities from which to choose. If the stem requests a strength of belief, the response for-

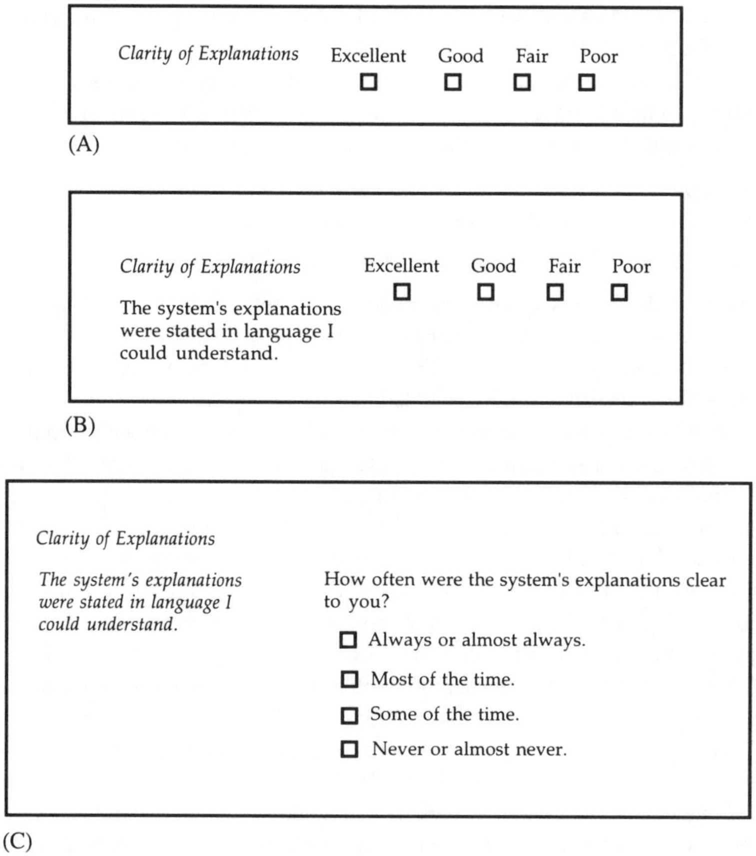

(A)

(B)

(C)

FIGURE 6.7. (A) Basic rating item. (B) One improvement: define the attribute. (C) Second improvement: make the response categories correspond to what is directly observable.

mats must offer an appropriate way to express the strength of belief, such as the familiar "strongly agree" to "strongly disagree" format.

3. *Provide a range of semantically and logically distinct response options.* Be certain that the categories span the range of possible responses and do not overlap. When response categories are given as quantitative ranges, novice item developers often overlap the edges of the response ranges, as follows.

Bad Example 1
In your opinion, with what fraction of your clinic patients this month has the system offered useful advice?

☐ 0–25%   ☐ 25–50%   ☐ 50–75%   ☐ 75–100%

Clearly it is necessary to begin the second option with 26%, the third with 51%, and the fourth with 76%.

Similarly, when response categories are stated verbally, the terms used should be carefully chosen so the categories are as equally spaced, in a semantic sense, as possible. Consider another mistake commonly made by novice item writers.

Bad Example II
How satisfied are you with the new system, overall?

☐ Extremely   ☐ Very   ☐ Generally   ☐ Not at all

In this example, there is too much semantic space between "generally" and "not at all." There are three response options that reflect positive views of the system and only one option that is negative. To rectify this problem, a response option of "slightly" or "modestly" might be added to the existing set.

4. *Include an appropriate number of response options.* Although it may seem tempting to use a large number of response options to obtain a "precise" measurement, the results might prove illusory. In general, the number of response options should be limited to a maximum of seven.[19]* For most purposes, four to six discrete options suffice. Using a five-option response format with a bipolar semantic axis allows a neutral response. We can offer arguments for and against neutral responses. A potential benefit is that a respondent whose true belief is neutral has a response option reflective of that belief. In the opposing view, a neutral response option plays to the "central tendency" problem. It provides a way to respond that is safe and noncommittal, even though it may not be accurate.

5. *Invite a nonresponse.* Giving respondents permission to decline to respond to each item is also highly functional. When using rating forms, for example, raters may be reluctant to admit they have not had sufficient experience or do not "know enough" to offer an informed rating. If an "unable to respond" category is explicitly available, it may assuage such concerns. If an "unable to respond" category is offered, it should be in a different typeface or otherwise visually apart from the continuum of informed responses. In this way, an "unable to rate" response is not intepreted as a negative response to the stem.

6. *Request elaborations.* Asking the respondent specifically for verbal elaborations or justifications of his or her responses can serve multiple purposes. It often forces the respondent to be more thoughtful. A respondent may "check off" a specific option and then, when trying to elaborate on it, realize that his or her deeper beliefs differ from what a first impression suggested. Elaborations are also a source of valuable data, particularly helpful when the items are part of a rating form that is in the early stages of development, to help validate the forms. Elaboration can also be informative as a source of evaluation data. If the purpose of a study is to understand "why," in addition to "how much," these verbal elabora-

---

* It is generally known that humans can process about seven (plus or minus two) items of disparate information at any one time.[21] The practical upper limit of seven response options may be attributable to this feature of human cognition.

tions may even be essential. Chapters 8 and 9, where we discuss subjectivist approaches to evaluation, indicate that these verbal comments can become the data of primary interest to the investigator.

7. *Address halo effects.* There are two major ways to minimize halo effects through item design. The first is to include, within a set of items comprising a scale, some that are phrased positively and some negatively. For example, the set might include both of the following (although not back-to back).

My ability to be productive in my job was enhanced by the new computer system.

☐ Strongly agree   ☐ Agree   ☐ Neither agree nor disagree   ☐ Disagree   ☐ Strongly disagree

The new system slowed the rate at which I could complete routine tasks.

☐ Strongly agree   ☐ Agree   ☐ Neither agree nor disagree   ☐ Disagree   ☐ Strongly disagree

In this example, the co-presence of items that can be both endorsed and not endorsed if the repondent feels positively about the system forces the respondent to attend more closely to the content of the items themselves. This strategy increases the chance that the respondent will evaluate each item on its own terms, rather than responding to a global impression.

A second stategy, useful in situations where one instrument is being used to assess multiple attributes, is to intermix items that measure different attributes. This practice is common on psychological instruments to conceal the attributes measured by the instrument so respondents respond more honestly and spontaneously. It may not, however, be an advisable strategy when, for example, an instrument comprising a set of items is used to rate performance. In this case the rating form should be organized to make the rating process as easy as possible, and items addressing the same attribute should be clustered together. If a form is being used to rate some behavior occurring in real time, it is particularly important that the form be arrayed as logically as possible so respondents do not have to search for the items they wish to complete.

The Ratings Paradox

On rating forms there are profound trade-offs involved in making the items more specific. The greater the specificity of the items on a form, the less judgment the raters exercise when offering their opinions. Rating forms that are highly specific in the interest of generating interrater consistency can become almost mechanical. Raters are merely observing the occurrence of atomic events, and there would be little reason for them to disagree. A major part of the art of ratings is to identify the right level of granularity. As attributes rated by individual items become more global, agreement among raters is difficult to achieve; as they become more atomic, the process becomes mechanical and, possibly, trivial. It can also be viewed as a trade-off between reliability and validity. The more global the ratings, the more valid they are likely to be, in the sense that the world believes that the attributes being rated are important and what should be measured. This comes at a price of low (possibly unacceptably low) inter-rater agreement and thus low reliability.

Self-Test 6.6

Using the guidelines offered in the previous section, find and fix the problems with each of the following items.

Item 1:
Accuracy of system's advice

☐ Excellent   ☐ Good   ☐ Fair   ☐ Poor

Item 2:
Indicate on a 1–10 scale your satisfaction with this system.

Item 3:
The new system is easier to use than the one it replaced.

☐ Strongly agree   ☐ Agree   ☐ No opinion   ☐ Disagree   ☐ Strongly disagree

Item 4:
How frequently have you used the new laboratory system?

☐ Most of the time   ☐ Some of the time   ☐ Never

Other Measurement Designs

We introduce briefly here two more complex measurement approaches that have appeared in the informatics literature. With one of these approaches, the "blinded mutual audit," the perceptions by the judges remain independent so an error rate for the measurement can be computed. The other, the "Delphi approach," uses a consensus-building approach whereby the responses of judges are deliberately shared, discussed, and then revised. Although this approach is appealing because it leads to an apparently settled consensus, from a methodological viewpoint it suffers by allowing no rigorous estimate of the error inherent in the result.

Mutual Audit

With the "blinded mutual audit" design, each judge reviews data from some fraction of the objects (usually test cases), giving his or her response. Data from each object are reviewed by at least two judges. Each opinion then is graded for correctness either by the same group of judges[22] or by a second group,[23] without knowing who originally provided it. This technique allows evaluators to calculate the inter- and intrajudge agreement (and thus error) rates and to ensure efficient use of the judges' time. Although we used a simplified version of it in the exercise in Chapter 5, the study of Hypercritic employed a variant of the mutual audit technique.

The mutual audit can be used in a pure measurement study; or, as shown in Figure 6.8, it can be employed in a hybrid measurement/demonstration study where a set of test cases is "reviewed" by a set of expert judges, an information resource, and the persons who provided the actual care on these cases.

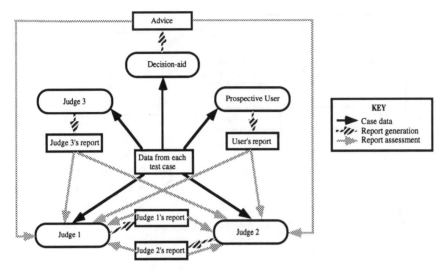

FIGURE 6.8. Possible design for blinded mutual audit.

Delphi Technique

The Delphi technique, as it applies to developing a consensus judgment of some attribute of a clinical case, is illustrated in Figure 6.9. Each judge reviews the data from all cases independently and records his or her opinion on a report form. The forms are passed to a moderator, who extracts the consensus opinion for each case and returns them and the case data to the judges for a second opinion, usually without informing them of their previous opinion. Judges continue to be asked for their opinions on each case until a convergence criterion is met. This technique is well established in a variety of fields[24] and is now being applied successfully in medicine.[25]

Answers to Self-Tests

Self-Test 6.1

1. Predicted reliability is 0.432, which is not usually acceptable.
2. The standard error of measurement is 0.34.
3. Content validity is somewhat built into the study through the choice of expert raters. It could be further ensured by asking the judges to write the rationale for their ratings for a subset of the patients and checking these rationales against published standards of care where possible. Criterion-related validity could be explored by selecting a subset of patients for whom the system's advice had been followed and comparing clinical outcomes seen in patients where the

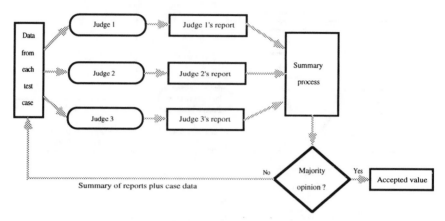

FIGURE 6.9. Dephi technique

advice had been highly rated in comparison with those patients where the advice was poorly rated. Construct validity might be assessed by examining some case properties with which the system's correctness might be hypothesized to be correlated. For example, cases that are more complex, as measured by the number of clinical variables they include, might be hypothesized to be truly more difficult and thus expected to generate lower scores from the raters. Cases with diagnoses that are more prevalent might be hypothesized to be less difficult and expected to generate higher scores.

Self-Test 6.2

1. More observations are needed to increase the reliability. The observations in the set are generally well behaved.
2. It appears that two attributes are being measured. Items 1–3 are measuring one attribute, and Items 4–6 are measuring the other.
3. Judge H displays the highest corrected part–whole correlation (0.55) and thus can be considered the "best" judge. Judge E is a close second with a part–whole correlation of 0.50. Judge C may be considered the worst judge, with a part–whole correlation of –0.27. Removing Judge C raises the reliability from 0.29 to 0.54 in this example. Such a large change in reliability is seen in part because the number of objects in this example is small. Judges B and D can in some sense be considered the worst, as they rendered the same result for every object and their part–whole correlations cannot be calculated.

Self-Test 6.3

The object class comprises patients who are to be admitted. In this case, "observers" (five levels), "times of day" (three levels), and "hospitals" (four levels) are facets of the measurement study.

Self-Test 6.4

The "observer" facet belongs to the "judges" category. The "times of day" and "hospitals" facets belong to the "logistical factors" category.

Self-Test 6.5

1. Each (of two) objects-by-observations matrixes would have 111 rows (for cases as objects) and three columns (for judges as observations). One matrix would be generated for actual care cases and the other for TraumAID's recommendations.
2. There is no compelling evidence for rater tendency errors. The mean ratings of the judges are roughly equal and near the middle of the scale. Central tendency effects can be ruled out because the standard deviations of the ratings are substantial.
3. From a reliability standpoint, the ratings are more than adequate. However, the validity of the ratings must be questioned because the judges are from the institution where TraumAID was developed.
4. The data seem to suggest that TraumAID's advice is accurate, as the judges preferred how TraumAID would have treated the patients over how the patients were actually treated. However, the concern about validity of the ratings would cast some doubt on this conclusion.

Self-Test 6.6

Item 1: Accuracy should be defined. The response categories should be replaced by alternatives that are more behavioral or observable.

Item 2: Ten response options is too many. The respondent needs to know whether 1 or 10 corresponds to a high level of satisfaction. The numerical response options have no verbal descriptors.

Item 3: "No opinion" does not belong on the response continuum. Having no opinion is different from having an opinion that happens to be midway between "strongly agree" and "strongly disagree."

Item 4: The logic of the response options does not match the stem. There are not enough response options, and they are not well spaced semantically.

References

1. Issac S, Michael WB: Handbook in Research and Evaluation. San Diego: EdITS Publishers, 1989.
2. Cureton EE, D'Agostino RB: Factor Analysis, an Applied Approach. Hillsdale, NJ: Lawrence Erlbaum, 1983.

3. Kim J, Mueller CW: Factor Analysis: Statistical Methods and Practical Issues. Beverly Hills, CA: Sage, 1978.

4. Brennan RL.: Elements of Generalizability Theory. Iowa City: American College Testing Program, 1983.

5. Anderson JG, Jay SJ, Schweer HM, et .al: Why doctors don't use computers: some empirical findings. J R Soc Med 1986;79:142–144.

6. Brown SH, Coney RD: Changes in computer anxiety and attitudes related to clinical information system use. J Am Med Inf Assoc 1994;1: 381–394.

7. Elstein AS, Shulman LS, Sprafka SA: Medical Problem Solving. Cambridge, MA: Harvard University Press, 1978.

8. Schmidt HG, Norman GR, Boshuizen HPA: A cognitive perspective on medical expertise: theory and implications. Acad Med 1990;65:611–621.

9. Stillman P, Swanson D, Regan MB, et al: Assessment of clinical skills of residents using standardized patients. Ann Intern Med 1991;114:393–401.

10. Swets JA: Measuring the accuracy of diagnostic systems. Science 1998; 240:1285–1293.

11. Jain R: The Art of Computer Systems Performance Analysis. New York: Wiley, 1991.

12. Friedman CP: Anatomy of the clinical simulation. Acad Med 1995;70: 205–208.

13. Berk RA (ed): Performance Assessment: Methods and Applications. Baltimore: Johns Hopkins Press, 1986.

14. Murphy KR, Cleveland JN: Understanding Performance Appraisal: Social, Organizational, and Goal-Based Perspectives. Thousand Oaks, CA: Sage, 1995.

15. Guilford JP: Psychometric Methods. New York: McGraw-Hill, 1954.

16. Thorndike RL, Hagen E: Measurement and Evaluation in Psychology and Education. New York, Wiley, 1977.

17. Wyatt J: A method for developing medical decision-aids applied to ACORN, a chest pain advisor. DM thesis, Oxford University, 1991.

18. Clarke JR, Webber BL, Gertner A, Rymon. KJ: On-line decision support for emergency trauma management. Proc Symp Comput Applications Med Care 1994;18:1028.

19. Landy FJ, Farr JL: Performance rating. Psychol Bull 1980;87:72–107.

20. Detmer WM, Friedman CP: Academic physicians' assessment of the effects of computers on health care. Proc Symp Comput Applications Med Care 1994;18:558–62.

21. Miller GA: The magical number seven, plus or minus two: some limits on our capacity for processing information. Psychol Rev 1956;63:46–49.

22. Quaglini S, Stefanelli M, Barosi G, Berzuini A: A performance evaluation of the expert system ANAEMIA. Comp Biomed Res 1987;21:307–323.

23. Yu VL, Fagan LM, Wraith SM, et al: Antimicrobial selection by computer: a blinded evaluation by infectious disease experts. JAMA 1979;242:1279–1282.

24. Delbecq AE: Group Techniques for Program Panning : A Guide to Nominal Group and Delphi Processes. New York: Scott, Foresman, 1975.

25. Kors JA, Sittig A, van Bemmel JH: The Delphi method used to validate diagnostic knowledge in a computerised ECG interpreter. Methods Inf Med 1990;29:44–50.

26. Shavelson RJ, Webb NM, Rowley GL: Generalizability theory. Am Psychol 1989;44:922–932.

Appendix A: Generalizability Theory

Using an approach known as generalizability theory,[4, 26] investigators can address many-facet measurement studies. They can analyze multiple potential sources of error and can model the relations among them. This additional power is of potential importance in medical informatics because it can mirror the complexity of all measurement problems addressed in the field. Generalizability theory (G-theory) allows computation of a "generalizability coefficient," which is analogous to a reliability coefficient in classical theory.

Although the specific computational aspects of G-theory are beyond this discussion, the theory has great value as a heuristic for measurement study design. If an informatics researcher can conceptualize and formulate a measurement problem in terms appropriate to study via G-theory, a psychometrician or statistician can handle the details. The basic idea is the same as in classical theory but with extension to multiple facets, whereas classical theory is limited to one facet. The basic strategy employed is portrayed in Figure 6.2. Analytical methods derived from the analysis of variance (ANOVA) are used to decompose the total variance of the measurement study, which is the total variability of the measurements made on the objects included in the study. The basics of ANOVA are discussed in Chapter 7. The total variability is decomposed into variability due to objects, variability due to the multiple facets and their statistical interactions, and variance due to other sources not explicitly modeled by the facets included by the investigator in the measurement study.

The generalizability coefficient is represented by:

$$\rho = \frac{V_{objects}}{V_{total}} = \frac{V_{objects}}{V_{objects} + V_{facets} + V_{other}}$$

Formally, the subscripted V's in the above formula are variance components, which can be computed using methods derivative from the ANOVA. V_{facets} and V_{other} are taken to represent sources of measurement error. Expressions for V_{facets} explicitly involve the number of levels of each facet, which makes it possible to use G-theory to model the effects on "reliability" of changing the number of levels of any of the facets that are part of the measurement process. For example, for the basic one-facet models that have been developed throughout this chapter, the formula for the generalizability coefficient is:

$$\rho = \frac{V_{objects}}{V_{objects} + (V_{objects \times observations} / N_{observations})}$$

This equation is exactly equivalent to the Spearman-Brown prophecy formula.

A major value of G-theory derives from its applicability to more complex measurement problems than classical theory allows. In addition to measurement studies with multiple facets, more complex designs can be considered, including nested designs of the type portrayed in Figure 6.5.

7

Design, Conduct, and Analysis of Demonstration Studies

Demonstration studies answer questions about an information resource, exploring such issues as the resource's value to a certain professional group or its impact on the processes and outcomes of health care.[1] Recall from Chapter 4 that measurement studies are required to test, refine and validate measurement processes before they can be used to answer questions about a resource or its impact. Chapters 5 and 6 explained these ideas and how to conduct measurement studies in more detail. In this chapter we assume that measurement methods are available and have been verified by appropriate measurement studies. To answer questions via a demonstration study, appropriate evaluation strategies and study designs must be formulated, the sample of subjects and tasks defined, any threats to validity identified and either eliminated or controlled for, and the results analyzed.[2, 3] These issues are discussed in this chapter.

In Chapter 3 we discussed the main attributes of information resources that can be measured, and we introduced eight kinds of studies that can be used to: verify the need for the resource; validate its design and structure; test its function in laboratory and field settings; study its impact on care providers in either laboratory or field settings; and study its impact on patient care and outcomes in field settings. These various studies may invoke different generic approaches to evaluation, as introduced in Chapter 2, and may entail different formal demonstration study designs, as introduced in Chapter 4. For example, validation of resource design and structure requires inspection of design documentation and the system components by a panel of judges. It invokes a subjectivist "professional review" approach to evaluation and has no formal demonstration study design. By contrast, studying the impact of the resource on care providers or patient care invokes a comparison-based approach using controlled, "experimental" demonstration studies. This chapter primarily addresses the more complex, controlled studies concerned with resource function and impact.

We discussed in Chapter 2 how different stakeholders in the evaluation process often have different questions they wish to answer and in Chapter 3 how the questions of interest tend to hinge on the resource's current stage in the developmental life cycle. In Chapter 4 we saw that demonstration study questions may be classed broadly as "pragmatic" (What is the impact of the information resource on working practices?) or "explanatory" (Why does the information resource change working practices?).[4] The needs of a pragmatic question may be well served by a relatively simple study design. Studies of an information resource at any early stage of development are usually designed to answer pragmatic questions. To answer an explanatory question about why an information resource changes working practices may require studies of resource function, its impact on care providers in both laboratory and field settings, and even its impact on patient care and broader health care activity.

Study Designs

In the following sections we start with a generic method for classifying study designs and describing their components before illustrating the studies that are possible. We use the running example of an antibiotic reminder system. A brief paragraph at the end of each study design section illustrates how the particular design can be described using the generic language developed in this first section. Expressing a study design using generic language can be useful when communicating with statisticians and other experimental scientists or methodologists; it also helps the evaluator to step back from the details of the study to see what is being planned.

Descriptive, Correlational, and Comparative Studies Revisited

Recall from Chapter 4 that objectivist demonstration studies can be divided into three kinds: descriptive, correlational, and comparative.

A *descriptive* design seeks only to estimate the value of a variable or set of variables in a selected sample of subjects. For example, to ascertain the "ease of use" of a nursing information system, a group of nurses could be given a rating form previously validated through a measurement study. The mean value of the "ease of use" variable would be the main result of this demonstration study. Descriptive studies can be tied to the "objectives-based" approach to evaluation described in Chapter 2: When an investigator seeks to determine if a resource has met a predetermined set of performance objectives, the logic and design of the resulting study are often descriptive.

Correlational studies explore the relations among a set of variables the researcher measures but does not manipulate in any way. Correlational studies can be seen as primarily linked to the "decision facilitation" approach to evaluation discussed in Chapter 2, as they are linked to pragmatic questions and cannot typically settle issues of cause and effect. For example, a correlational study may reveal a statistical relationship between clinical performance at some tasks and the extent of use of an information resource to accomplish those tasks.

In a *comparative* study, the investigator typically creates a contrasting set of conditions to compare the effects of one with another. Usually the motive is to correctly attribute cause and effect or to further explore questions raised by earlier studies. Extending the example from the previous paragraph, a comparative study can address whether use of the information resource *causes* improved performance. After identifying a sample of subjects for his or her study, the researcher assigns each subject, often randomly, to one or a set of conditions. Some variable of interest is then measured for each subject. The aggregated values of this variable are then compared across the conditions. Comparative studies are of course aligned with the "comparison-based" approach to evaluation introduced in Chapter 2.

Terminology for Demonstration Studies

In this section we develop a terminology and several ideas necessary to design studies of information resources. At this point, the reader may wish to refer to Chapter 4 where terminology for measurement and demonstration studies were first introduced. For the purposes of the immediate discussion, the terms of most importance are as follows.

Subjects: Subjects in a study are the entities about which data are collected. A specific study employs one sample of subjects, although this sample might be subdivided if, for example, subjects are assigned to conditions in a comparative design. It is key to emphasize that subjects are often people—care providers or care recipients—but subjects also may be information resources, groups of people, or organizations. Subjects in a demonstration study are analogous to objects in a measurement study.

Variables: Variables are specific characteristics of subjects that are purposefully measured by the investigator or are self-evident properties of the subjects that do not require measurement. Each variable in a study is associated with a level of measurement, as described in Chapter 5. In the simplest descriptive study, there may be only one variable. In comparative and correlational studies, there must be at least two variables, and there may be many more.

Levels of variables: A categorical (nominal or ordinal) variable can be said to have a discrete set of levels corresponding to each of the measured values the variable can have. For example, in a hospital setting, physician-members of a ward team can be classified as residents, fellows, or attending physicians. In this case, the "physician's level of qualification" variable is said to have three levels.

Dependent variables: The dependent variables are a subset of the variables in the study that capture the outcomes of interest to the investigator. For this reason, dependent variables are also called "outcome variables." A study may have one or more dependent variables. Studies with one dependent variable are referred to as "univariate," and studies with multiple dependent variables are referred to as "multivariate." In a typical study, the dependent variable is computed, for each subject, as an average over a number of tasks.

By definition, the subjects in a study are the entities on which the dependent variables are measured. This point is important in informatics because medical care is conducted in hierarchical settings with naturally occurring groups (a "doctor's patients"; "care providers in a ward team"). It raises often-challenging questions of exactly who are the subjects.

Independent variables: The independent variables are those included in a study to explain the measured values of the dependent variables. Note that a descriptive study has no independent variables, whereas comparative and correlational studies can have one or many independent variables.

Measurement challenges of the types discussed in Chapters 5 and 6 almost always arise during assessment of the outcome or dependent variable for a study. Often, for example, the dependent variable is some type of performance measure that invokes all of the concerns about reliability and validity of measurement. Depending on the study, the independent variables may also raise measurement challenges. When the independent variable is gender, for example, the measurement problems are relatively straightforward. However, if the independent variable is an attitude, level of experience, or extent of resource use, profound measurement challenges can arise.

Study Types Further Distinguished

Using our terminology, we can now sharpen the differences between descriptive, correlational, and comparative studies. Studies of all three types are, in a profound sense, designed by the investigator. In all three, the investigator chooses the subjects, the variables, and the measurement methods and logistics used to assign a value of each variable to each subject. In a descriptive study, however, there are no further decisions to be made. The defining characteristic of a descriptive study is the absence of independent variables. The state of a set of subjects is described by measuring one or more dependent variables. Although a descriptive study may report the relations among the dependent variables, there is no attempt to attribute variation in these variables to some cause.

In correlational studies, the investigator hypothesizes a set of relations among variables that, in the study, are measured but not manipulated for a group of subjects. The variability in these measures is that which occurs naturally in the sample of subjects included in the study. Correlational studies can be retrospective, involving analyses of archival data, or prospective, involving data collected according to a plan generated in advance of the study. Some researchers believe that assertions of cause and effect can occasionally be derived from the pattern of statistical relations observed in correlational studies, although this topic remains controversial.[5, 6] Measurement studies that explore the construct validity of a new measure, as discussed in Chapter 5, employ the logic of correlational studies.

The defining characteristic of a comparative study is the purposeful manipulation of the independent variables to enable sound inference of cause and effect from data. To this end, the investigator creates one or more new independent variables that define the study groups and typically take on values such as "intervention," "control," or "placebo." The investigator usually assigns subjects randomly to different levels of these independent variables. If all sources of variation in the dependent variables are controlled, either by statistical randomization or specific assignment to groups, cause-and-effect relations among the independent and dependent variables can be rigorously attributed. When the dependent variable is continuous (with interval or ratio properties), this can be achieved by employing methods such as analysis of variance (ANOVA) to demonstrate differences among the levels of the independent variables that are explicitly part of the design. When the dependent variable is discrete (binary or categorical), contingency table analysis and receiver operating characteristics (ROC) curves are customarily used. There is an extensive literature on designs of comparative studies,[7-9] and this chapter contains an exploration of some of the most important study designs.

The contrasts between descriptive, correlational, and comparative studies are summarized in Table 7.1. Readers are also referred to Figure 4.3.

Generic Issues in Demonstration Study Design

As we move into a more technical discussion of study design, we introduce three key issues that always arise: defining the intervention, choosing the subjects, and selecting the tasks for the subjects to undertake. When evaluating therapeutic technologies such as drugs, the subjects are usually patients. For evaluating interventions such as health education, a vaccination program, or information resources, the subjects can be care providers, departments, or even hospitals. [10, 11] In studies where the care providers are subjects, we usually consider the patients these care providers treat to be "tasks" and average the performance of each care provider over a set of tasks.

When studying an information resource, evaluators should be aware that its performance or impact may vary greatly among subjects (e.g., clinicians may vary greatly in the information they obtain from the clinical laboratory system, perhaps

Table 7.1. Summary of descriptive, correlational, and comparative studies

Parameter	Descriptive study	Correlational study	Comparative study
Goal of study	To describe a resource in terms of variables	To explore the relations between variables	To assign causality to the relation between variables
Independent variables	None	One or more as selected by investigator	One or more, with at least one created by the investigator
Dependent variables	One or more	One or more as selected by the investigator	One or more as selected by the investigator
Logic of data analysis	Descriptive statistics about dependent variables	Analysis of patterns of relationships among variables	Continuous variables: ANOVA. Discrete variables: contingency table, ROC analyses

because of differing experience) or between different kinds of tasks (e.g., the system may only improve the management of certain groups of patients, such as those in intensive care, irrespective of which clinician is looking after them). This means that evaluators should be aware of both the range of subjects and the range of tasks to be included in their study. In laboratory studies the investigator often can directly control both the subjects included in the study and the tasks with which they are challenged. In field studies, this level of control may not be possible, as the identity of care providers who work in clinical units and the patients who receive care in these units are often not manipulable. Even when the subjects and tasks are out of the investigator's direct control, she should carefully document the samples that were involved in the study, so others know how far the results can be generalized.

Defining the Intervention

One way of answering an explanatory question is to split the information resource up into its components and evaluate them separately. When we use the phrase "information resource" we have deliberately not defined precisely what the resource or system includes. However, particularly when trying to answer questions such as "How much difference is the resource likely to make in a new setting?" it is important to isolate the effects due to the information resource itself from effects due to other activities surrounding its development and implementation. For example, if a department were to implement a computer-based set of practice guidelines, a considerable amount of time might be spent on developing the guidelines before any implementation took place. Changes in clinical practice following the implementation of the information resource might be largely due to this guideline development process, not to the computer technology.[12] Transplanting the guideline system to a new hospital without repeating the guideline development process at the new site might yield results different from those seen at the development site. When evaluating new information resources it is often necessary to offer training, feedback, or other support to system users; they could also be considered part of the intervention.

A more specific example from the literature is the Leeds Abdominal Pain Decision Support System. Various components of this system were tested for their effects on the diagnostic accuracy of 126 junior doctors in a multicenter trial in 12 hospitals.[13] Table 7.2 shows the average percentage improvement due to each component of the "system." The data are extracted from a 2-year study of four groups of junior doctors working for 6 months in 12 emergency rooms, each group being exposed to a different level of implementation of decision support. The investigators measured diagnostic accuracy after the doctors had been in place for 1 and 6 months. The first row shows that there was minimal improvement when no information resource was in place. The second row shows the improvement in diagnoses due to what may be called a "checklist effect," described in more detail later in the chapter. Decision making improved when

TABLE 7.2. Effects due to components of an information resource

	Change in diagnostic accuracy from baseline (%)	
Intervention	End of month 1	End of month 6
None	0	+1
Data collection forms	+11	+14
Monthly feedback and data collection forms	+13	+27
Computer advice, feedback, and forms	+20	+28

Data from Adams et al.[13]

structured forms were used to assist clinical data collection. In the third group the doctors were given monthly feedback about their diagnostic performance as well as using the forms, and marked learning is seen. The fourth group received diagnostic probabilities calculated by a computer-based advisory system at the time of decision making as well as monthly feedback and using data collection forms.

The advice apparently aided diagnoses during the early months only, because in later months diagnostic accuracy in the third and fourth groups was similar. Also, the computer advice is contributing less to improving diagnostic accuracy than either the data collection forms or the individual feedback. If the information resource is defined as the computer advice alone, it is contributing only one-third of the 20% improvement in diagnostic accuracy seen at month 1, and one-thirtieth of the 28% improvement at month 6. (Of the 20% improvement seen at month 1, only the difference between row 3 and row 4, which is 7%, is attribute to the computer advice. Of the 28% improvement seen at month 6, only 1% appears due to the computer advice.)

Thus careful definition of the information resource and its components is necessary in demonstration studies to allow the evaluator to answer the explanatory question: "Which component of the information resource is responsible for the observed effects?" It is critical that the investigator define the resource before the study begins and use that definition consistently through the entire effort.

Selection of Subjects

The subjects selected for demonstration studies must resemble those to whom the study results will be applied. For example, when attempting to quantify the likely impact of an information resource on clinicians at large there is no point in studying its effects on the clinicians who helped develop it, or even built it, as they are likely to be technology enthusiasts and more familiar with the resource than average practitioners. Characteristics of subjects that typically need to be taken into account include age, experience, clinical role, attitude toward computerized information resources, and extent of their involvement in the development of the resource. These factors can be formalized as a set of selection criteria to include only a certain class of subjects in the study, or they can be made into explicit study variables if their effects are to be explored.

Volunteer Effect

A common bias in the selection of subjects is the use of volunteers. It has been established in many areas that people who volunteer as subjects, whether to complete questionnaires,[14] participate in psychology experiments, or test-drive new cars or other technologies are atypical of the population at large, being more intelligent, open to innovation, and extroverted. Although volunteers may make willing subjects for measurement studies or pilot demonstration studies, they should be avoided in definitive demonstration studies, as they considerably reduce the generality of findings. It is better to recruit a random sample of all the clinicians meeting the study selection criteria, following up invitation letters with telephone calls to achieve as near 100% recruitment of the sample as possible.

Number of Subjects Needed

The financial resources required for an evaluation study depend critically on the number of subjects needed. The required number in turn depends on the precision of the answer required from the study and the risk investigators are willing to take of failing to detect a significant effect by chance (discussed later). Statisticians can advise on this point and carry out sample size calculations to estimate the number of subjects required. Sometimes, in order to recruit the required number of subjects, some volunteer effect must be tolerated; often there is a trade-off between obtaining a sufficiently large sample and ensuring that the sample is representative.

Selection of Tasks

In the same way that subjects must be carefully selected to resemble the people likely to use the information resource, any tasks the subjects complete must also resemble those that will generally be encountered. Thus when evaluating a clinical order entry system intended for general use, it would be unwise to use only complex cases from, for example, a pediatric endocrinology practice. Although the order entry system might well be of considerable benefit in endocrine cases, it is inappropriate to generalize results from such a limited sample to the full range of cases seen in ambulatory care. For example, Van Way et al.[15] developed a scoring system for diagnosing appendicitis and studied the resource's accuracy using exclusively patients who had undergone surgery for suspected appendicitis. This method allowed the true cause of the abdominal pain to be obtained with near certainty. However, the symptoms were more severe and the incidence of appendicitis was five to ten times higher in these patients who had surgery for suspected appendicitis than for the typical patient in whom such a scoring system would be used. Thus the accuracy obtained with laparotomy patients would be a poor estimate of the system's accuracy in routine clinical use.

If the functions of an information resource are measured on a small number of hand-picked cases, the functions may appear spuriously complete. This is especially likely if these cases are similar to, or even identical with, the "training set" of cases used to develop or tune the information resource before the evaluation is carried out. When a statistical model is carefully adjusted to achieve maximal performance on training data, this adjustment may worsen its accuracy on a fresh set of data due to a phenomenon called overfitting.[16] Thus it is important to obtain a new set of cases and evaluate performance on this "test set."

Sometimes developers omit cases from a sample if they do not fall within the scope of the information resource, for example if the final diagnosis for a case is not represented in a diagnostic system's knowledge base. This practice violates the principle that a test set should be representative of all cases in which the information resource will be used and overestimates its effectiveness with unseen data. Some guidelines for the selection of test cases are given in Table 7.3.

Control Strategies for Comparative Studies

One of the most challenging aspects of demonstration study design is how to obtain "control" in comparative studies because we need some way to monitor all the other changes taking place that are not attributable to the information resource. In clinical medicine it is occasionally possible to predict patient outcome with good accuracy from a handful of initial clinical findings, for example the survival of patients in intensive care.[17] In these unusual circumstances where we have a close approximation to an "evaluation machine" (see Chapter 2) that can tell us what would have happened to patients if we had not intervened, we can compare what actually happens with what is predicted to draw tentative conclusions about the benefit of the information resource. Such accurate predictive models, however, are unusual in medicine,[16] so it is generally impossible to determine what health care workers would have done or the patient outcome had no information resource been available. Instead, we use various types of controls, defined as subjects and tasks that are not affected by the intervention of interest.

In the following sections we review a series of specific strategies, using as an anchor point the least controlled approach that is a purely descriptive study, and moving to increasingly more sophisticated approaches. We employ as a running example a reminder system that prompts doctors to order prophylactic antibiotics for orthopedic patients to prevent postoperative infections. In this example, the intervention is the installation and commissioning of the reminder system; the subjects are the physicians; and the tasks are the patients cared for by the physicians. The dependent variables include physicians' rate of ordering antibiotics (a process measure) and the rate of postoperative infection averaged across the patients cared for by each physician (an outcome measure). The independent variables in each example below are an inherent feature of the study design and derive from the specific control strategies employed. Although they are not explicitly discussed, measurement issues of the types addressed in Chapters 5 and 6 (e.g., determining whether each patient's infection can be accurately judged a "postoperative" infection) abound in this situation.

TABLE 7.3. Guidelines for selection of test cases

- Cases should be representative of those in which the information resource will be used; consecutive cases or a random sample are superior to volunteers or a hand-picked subset
- There should be a sufficient number and variety of cases to test most functions and pathways in the resource
- Case data should be recent and preferably from more than one, geographically distinct site
- Include cases abstracted by a variety of potential resource users
- Include a percentage of cases with incomplete, contradictory, or erroneous data
- Include a percentage of normal cases
- Include a percentage of difficult cases and some that are clearly outside the scope of the information resource
- Include some cases with minimal data and some with comprehensive data

Descriptive (Uncontrolled) Experiments

In the simplest possible design, a descriptive or "uncontrolled" study, we install the reminder system, allow a suitable period for training, then make our measurements. There is no independent variable. Suppose we discover that the overall postoperative infection rate is 5% and that physicians order prophylactic antibiotics in 60% of orthopedic cases. Although we have two measured dependent variables, it is difficult to interpret these figures without any comparison; it is even possible that there has been no change attributable to the system. This point is of course the weakness of the descriptive study. One way to understand the significance of these figures is to compare them with the same measurements made using the same methods in a comparison group, which transforms the study from a descriptive to a comparative one. Two types of comparison groups are possible: (1) historical controls, comprising the same patient care environment (doctors and their patients) before the system was installed; or (2) "simultaneous controls" comprising a similar patient care environment not provided with the reminder system.

Historically Controlled Experiments

As a first improvement to a descriptive study, let us consider a "historically controlled" experiment, sometimes called a "before–after" study. The investigator makes "baseline" measurements of antibiotic ordering and postoperative infection rates before the information resource is installed and then makes the same measurements after the information resource is in routine use. The independent variable is "time" and has two levels: before and after resource installation. Let us say that at baseline the postoperative infection rate was 10% and doctors ordered prophylactic antibiotics in only 40% of cases; the post-intervention figures are the same as before (Table 7.4).

The evaluators may claim that halving the infection rate can be safely ascribed to the information resource, especially because it was accompanied by a 20% increase in doctors' prophylactic antibiotic prescribing. Many other factors might

TABLE 7.4. Hypothetical results of a historically controlled study of an antibiotic reminder system

Time	Antibiotic prescribing rate (%)	Postoperative infection rate
Baseline (before installation)	40	10
After installation	60	5

have changed in the interim, however, to cause these results, especially if there was a long interval between the baseline and postintervention measurements. New staff could have taken over, the case-mix of patients could have altered, new pro-phylactic antibiotics might have been introduced, or clinical audit meetings might have highlighted the infection problem causing greater clinical awareness. Simply assuming that the reminder system alone caused the reduction in infection rates is naive. Other factors, known or unknown, could have changed meanwhile, making the assumption that our intervention is responsible for all of the observed effects untenable.

The weakness of crediting all benefit to the information resource in a histori-cally controlled study is highlighted by considering the likely response of medical informatics workers to a situation where measurements worsen after installing the information resource. Most workers, particularly if they had helped develop the resource, would search long and hard for other factors to explain the deterioration. However, there would be no such search if measurements improved, even though the experimental design is the same.

Evidence for the dubious value of before–after studies comes from a paper that compared the results of many historically controlled studies of antihypertensive drugs with the results of simultaneous randomized controlled trials carried out on the same drugs.[18] About 80% of the historically controlled studies suggested that the new drugs evaluated were effective, but this figure was confirmed in only 20% of the randomized studies that evaluated the same drugs. It appeared that in the before–after studies clinicians were unconsciously selecting those patients who were likely to obtain better control of their blood pressure to receive the new drug.

No assignment or manipulation of the subjects or their environment is involved with "before and after" studies, other than introduction of the information resource itself. For this reason, some label these studies correlational, not comparative.

Simultaneous Nonrandomized Controls

To address some of the problems with historical controls we might use simultane-ous controls, making our outcome measurements in doctors and patients not influ-enced by the prophylactic antibiotic reminder system but who are subject to the other changes taking place in the environment. If these measurements are made both before and after intervention, it strengthens the design because it gives an estimate of the changes due to the "nonspecific" factors taking place during the study period.

This study design is a parallel group comparative study with simultaneous controls. Table 7.5 gives some hypothetical results of such a study, focusing on postoperative infection rate as a single outcome measure or dependent variable. The independent variables are "time," as in the above example, and "group," which has the two levels of intervention and control. There is the same improvement in the group where reminders were available, but no improvement (indeed slight deterioration) where no reminders were available. This design provides suggestive evidence of an improvement that is most likely to be due to the reminder system. This inference is stronger if the control doctors worked in the same wards during the period the system was introduced, and if similar kinds of patients, subject to the same nonspecific influences, were being operated on during the whole time period.

Even though the controls in this example are now simultaneous, skeptics may still refute our argument by claiming that there is some systematic, unknown difference between the clinicians or patients in the reminder and control groups. For example, if the two groups comprised the patients and clinicians in two adjacent wards, the difference in the infection rates could be attributable to systematic or chance differences between the wards. Perhaps hospital staffing levels improved in some wards but not others, or there was cross infection by a multiply resistant organism but only among patients in the control ward. To overcome such criticisms, we could expand the study to include all wards in the hospital—or even other hospitals—but this measure would clearly take considerable resources. We could try to measure everything that happens to every patient in both wards and build complete psychological profiles of all staff to rule out systematic differences, but, we are still vulnerable to the accusation that something we did not measure—did not even know about—explains the difference between the two wards. A better strategy is to ensure that the controls are truly comparable by randomizing them.

Simultaneous Randomized Controls

The crucial problem in the previous example is that although the controls were simultaneous there may have been systematic, unmeasured differences between them and the subjects receiving the intervention. A simple, effective way to remove systematic differences, whether due to known or unknown factors, is to randomize the assignment of subjects to control or intervention groups. Thus we could randomly allocate half of the doctors on both wards to receive the antibiotic reminders, and the remaining doctors could work normally. We would then measure and compare postoperative infection rate in patients managed by doctors in the reminder and control groups. Providing that the doctors never look after each others' patients, any difference that is statistically significant can reliably be attributed to the reminders, as the only way other differences could have emerged is by chance.

Table 7.6 shows the hypothesized results of such a study. The baseline infection rates in the patients managed by the two groups of doctors are similar as

TABLE 7.5. Hypothetical results of a simultaneous nonrandomized controlled study of an antibiotic reminder system

Time	Postoperative infection rate (%)	
	Reminder group	Control group
Baseline	10	10
After intervention	5	11

TABLE 7.6. Results of a simultaneous randomized controlled study of an antibiotic reminder system

Time	Postoperative infection rate (%)	
	Reminder physicians	Control physicians
Baseline	11	10
After intervention	6	8

would be expected, because they were allocated to the groups by chance. There is a greater reduction in infection rate in patients of reminder physicians than those treated by the control physicians. The only systematic difference between the two groups of patients is receipt of reminders by their doctors. Provided that the sample size is large enough for these results to be statistically significant, we might conclude with some confidence that giving doctors reminders caused the reduction in infection rates. One lingering question is why there was also a small reduction, from baseline to postinstallation, in infection rates in control cases. Four explanations are possible: chance, the checklist effect, the Hawthorne effect, and contamination. These possibilities are discussed in detail in later sections.

When analyzing studies in which doctors or teams are randomized but measurements are made at the level of patients ("randomization by group"), data analysis methods must be adjusted accordingly. These corrections depend on the within- and between-doctor variance; further details and examples were suggested by Diwan et al.[11] and Cornfield.[19] In general, when randomizing doctors or hospitals, it is a mistake to analyze the results as if patients had been randomized—known as the "unit of analysis error." This problem and potential methods for addressing it are discussed in the section on hierarchical or nested designs (later in this chapter).

Externally Controlled Before–After Studies

An alternative approach to randomized simultaneous controls, lacking the rigor of the randomized study but that can occasionally be useful, is to use external controls in a before–after study. The logic here is that if we can argue, by measuring one or more appropriate external factors, that nothing else in a clinical environment is changing during the period of a before–after study, any change in the measurement of interest must be due to the information resource. Pursuing our antibiotic reminder system example, we need to identify actions by the same doctors and outcomes in the same patients that are not affected by the reminders but would be affected by any of the confounding, nonspecific changes that a skeptic alleges have occurred. An "external" clinical action that would reflect changes in prescribing is the prescribing rate of antibiotics for chest infections, and an external patient outcome that would reflect general postoperative care is the rate of postoperative deep venous thromboses (DVTs).[*] Any general improvements in clinical practice should be revealed by changes in these measures; however, providing reminders to doctors about prescribing prophylactic antibiotics to orthopedic patients should not affect either measure, at least not directly. Table 7.7 shows the hypothetical results from such a controlled before–after study.

The increase in prescribing for chest infections (5%) is much smaller than the increase for prophylaxis of wound infections (20%), and the postoperative DVT rate increased if anything. The evidence suggests that antibiotic prescribing in general has not changed much (using prescribing for chest infections as the external control), and that postoperative care in general (using DVT rate as the external control) is unchanged. Although less convincing than randomized simultaneous controls, the results rule out major confounding changes in prescribing or postoperative care during the study period, so the observed improvement in the target measure, postoperative infections, can be cautiously attributed to introduction of the reminder system. This argument is strengthened by the 20% increase in prophylactic antibiotic prescribing observed. Unfortunately, interpretation of the results of externally controlled before–after studies that are performed in the real world is often much more difficult than in this hypothetical example.

Crossover Studies

In crossover studies measurements are made on the same subjects with and without access to the information resource. Evaluators assume that the subject has not changed except for gaining (or losing) access to the information resource—that there is no "carryover." Thus in a crossover study of our antibiotic reminder system, evaluators must assume that the user's performance is not subject to learning, an assumption that usually needs to be tested. One way to conduct a randomized crossover design and measure any learning would be to randomize one-half of the doctors (group A) to use the information resource for the first half of the study and then withdraw access to it for the second study period; the other half (group B) would start with a control period followed by use of the information resource during the second period (Table 7.8). Learning from the decision support system is suggested by the lower postoperative infection rates in group A during their control period (which followed use of the reminder system) compared to group B during their control period.

---

[*] DVTs are blood clots in the leg or pelvic veins that cause serious lung problems if they become detached.

TABLE 7.7. Hypothetical results of an externally controlled before–after study of an antibiotic reminder system

Time	Antibiotic prescribed (%)		Postoperative infections	Postoperative DVT
	Prophylactic	Chest infections		
Baseline	40	40	10	5
After intervention	60	45	5	6

TABLE 7.8. Hypothetical results of a randomized crossover study of an antibiotic reminder system

Period	Postoperative infection rate (%)	
	Group A	Group B
First	5 (reminders)	10 (control)
Second	7 (control)	5 (reminders)

So long as there is no carryover, the crossover design overcomes the imperfections of historically controlled studies by arranging that there are simultaneous randomized controls during all phases of the experiment. Making the subjects act alternately as intervention and control also gives greater statistical power than a simple parallel group study and avoids the difficulty of matching control and information resource subjects or institutions. However, the crossover study can be used only with interventions that achieve a temporary improvement in the attribute being measured, so this approach cannot be employed to evaluate information resources that have significant carryover or educational effects. Showing that the intervention causes no carryover can require more subjects and tasks than conducting a more convincing randomized parallel groups study. Because withdrawing the information resource from subjects who have previously had free access to it may antagonize them if they believe it is beneficial, the crossover may have to be synchronized with staff changeover. To be valid, it requires the assumption that the next group of staff closely resembles the previous group. On the other hand, for studies where it may be unacceptable for subjects to be denied access to the information resource altogether—as often happens in education settings—the crossover may be the only feasible randomized design.

Matched Controls as an Alternative to Randomization

The principle of controls is that they should sensitively reflect all the nonspecific influences and biases present in the study population, while being isolated in some way from the effects of the information resource. As argued earlier, it is only by random assignment of controls that perfect matching, for all known and unknown factors, can be guaranteed. Careful matching of controls may occasionally be used instead if for some reason randomization is not feasible. In this case, controls should be matched to intervention cases or subjects for all the features likely to be relevant to the measurements being made. Usually, a pilot correlational study is needed to identify which factors are most important.

Summary

To summarize this section on controls and study designs, although evaluators may be tempted to use either no controls or historical controls in demonstration studies, we have illustrated, using a running example, why such studies are seldom convincing. If the goal of a demonstration study is to show cause and effect, simultaneous (preferably randomized) controls are required.[20] Otherwise there is no way of quieting those who inevitably and appropriately point out that confounding factors, known or unknown, could account for all of the improvements the investigator might attribute to the information resource.

Self-Test 7.1

For each of the scenarios given below: (a) name the independent variables and the number of levels of each; (b) identify the dependent variables and the measurement strategy used to assess them; (c) identify the subjects; and (d) indicate the control strategy employed by the study designers.

1. An new admission/discharge/transfer system is purchased by a major medical center. Evaluators administer a 30-item general attitude survey about information technology to staff members in selected departments 6 months before the resource is installed, 1 week before the resource is installed, and 1 and 6 months after it is installed.
2. A diagnostic decision support system in an early stage of development is employed to offer advice on a set of test cases. A definitive diagnosis for each test case had previously been established. The investigators measure the accuracy of the resource as the proportion of time the computer-generated diagnoses agree with the previously established diagnosis.
3. At each of two metropolitan hospitals, 18 physicians are randomized to receive computer-generated advice on drug therapy. At each hospital, one group receives advice automatically for all clinic patients; the second receives this advice only when they request it; the third receives no advice at all. Total charges related to drug therapy are measured by averaging across all relevant patients for each physician during the study period, where relevance is defined as patients whose conditions pertained to the domains covered by the resource's knowledge base.
4. A new reminder system is installed in a hospital that has twelve internal medicine services. During a 1-month period, care providers on six of the services, selected randomly, receive reminders from the system. On the other six ser-

vices the reminders are generated by the system but not issued to the care providers. An audit of clinical care on all services is conducted to determine the extent to which the actions recommended by the reminders were in fact taken.

5. A new computer-based educational tool is introduced in a medical school course. The tool covers pathophysiology of the cardiovascular (CV) system and gastrointestinal (GI) system. The class is divided randomly into two groups. The first group learns CV pathophysiology using the computer and GI pathophysiology by the usual lecture approach. The second group learns GI pathophysiology by the computer and CV pathophysiology by the lecture approach. Both groups are given a knowledge test, covering both body systems, after the course. [Example drawn from Lyon et al.[21]]

Formal Representation of Study Designs

In the previous section we introduced strategies for experimental control pragmatically using a running example. In this section, we discuss a more formal representation of designs of comparative studies. The designs introduced here cover most of the examples discussed in the previous section. These representational tools help researchers describe their designs to others and enable them to step back from the study details to adapt the design to meet specific needs or features of the environment in which they are conducted. This discussion assumes that all independent variables in a study are either nominal or ordinal, so each independent variable has discrete levels. We also assume that the dependent variables have ratio or interval properties.

Complete Factorial Designs

A complete factorial study is one of the designs that can be used to explore the effects of one or more independent variables on the dependent variable. "Factorial" means that a unique group of subjects is exposed to a unique set of conditions where each condition is a specified combination of the levels of each independent variable. "Complete" means that all possible conditions (combinations of each level of each independent variable) are included in the design. Consider our example of a randomized controlled trial of the effects of an antibiotic reminder system (Table 7.6) with doctors as the subjects. Let us assume that there are junior and senior doctors on the wards, and we wish to study (1) if reminders work at all and (2) the effects of seniority on the response to reminders. The dependent variable is postoperative infection rate, and the independent variables are exposure to antibiotic reminders (two levels: yes or no) and the experience of the doctor (two levels: junior or senior). No doctor is studied both with and without reminders. To run the complete factorial design, physicians at both levels of experience must be randomized to a "reminders" group or a "no reminders" group, so a unique group of

TABLE 7.9. Notation of a complete factorial design

| Physician experience level | Intervention in four subject groups (G1 – G4) | |
	Reminders	Control
Junior	G1	G2
Senior	G3	G4

physicians is exposed to each condition. This design can be represented as in Table 7.9. Note that the table expresses the plan for the study, not the results. The four unique groups of subjects are denoted G1 through G4.

When data are collected for factorial designs, the logic of the analysis is to compare the means of the groups, or cells, of the study. In the example in Table 7.9, the mean and standard deviation of infection rates for each of the four groups would be computed. Using the ANOVA technique, discussed later in the chapter, it is possible to test statistically for two so-called main effects: (1) if there is a difference in infection rate attributable to the reminders; and (2) if there is difference in infection rates attributable to the grade of doctor. It is also possible to test for an "interaction" between the grade of doctor and availability of decision support, which tests whether the effect of decision support on infection rates depends on the seniority of the doctor.

Thus a complete factorial design may be thought of as a matrix with each cell occupied by a unique group of subjects. Each dimension of the matrix corresponds to one independent variable. If there are N independent variables, the matrix is N-dimensional.

Nested (Hierarchical) Designs

Factorial designs tend to work well in laboratory settings, but investigators conducting field studies may find factorial designs unsuited to their needs because the real world presents situations where the independent variables are hierarchically related. This situation typically occurs when subjects in a study are part of groups inherent to the setting in which the study is conducted and thus cannot be disaggregated. Recall that in the earlier discussion of the antibiotic reminder system we assumed that physicians do not look after each others' patients. More typically, clinicians are part of ward teams that work closely together in patient care. If we wanted to retain clinicians as the subjects in a study conducted in this setting, a factorial design would not be acceptable, as individual clinicians within a team could not be randomly assigned to receive reminders because they work so tightly in groups. If we did randomize some team members to receive reminders and others to the control group, the differential effects attributable to the reminder system would be diluted through interactions among team members. In this setting, ran-

TABLE 7.10. A nested or hierarchical
design to study the effects of reminders

	Intervention	
Ward team	Reminders	Control
A	G1	
B	G2	
C	G3	
D		G4
E		G5
F		G6

domization must occur at the level of the ward team even though the dependent variable is measured for individual clinicians.

This situation calls for a "nested" (or hierarchical) design, as shown in Table 7.10. There are two independent variables: ward team (with six levels) and intervention (with two levels). Each subject belongs to one of six ward teams, and all subjects in each team are exposed to only one level of the independent variable by random allocation of the teams. The experimental groups (G1 through G6) are not created by the experimenter. They exist as part of the natural environment of the study. G1 is ward team A. The well-known study of reminder systems by McDonald et al.[22] used a nested design similar to this example. In general, nested designs can be used when naturally occurring *groups* of subjects (those on whom the dependent variables is measured) are the units of randomization.

In such a nested design, it is possible to test for a main effect for each independent variable. In the example in Table 7.10 it would be possible to determine if there is a difference attributable to the availability of reminders and if there is a difference attributable to ward teams. It is not possible, however, to explore a possible statistical interaction between reminders and ward team, which could potentially tell us if some ward teams benefited more from the intervention than others. In general, factorial designs are preferable to nested designs,[9] but investigators in informatics often are presented situations where the nested design is the only rigorous option.

Repeated Measures Designs

In the complete factorial design and the nested design, each subject is exposed to only one combination of the independent variables and thus appears only once in a table representing the design. By contrast, in repeated measures designs, each subject appears in two or more cells in the table and is, in effect, reused during the study. Thus in a repeated measures design, subjects are said to be employed as their own controls. The hypothetical study discussed above, under Simultaneous Randomized Controls, provides a perfect example of a repeated measures design.

Each subject, a physician, is randomly assigned to one of two groups (G1 or G2), and all the postoperative infection rates of their patients are measured before and after any antibiotic reminders are issued. Using our design notation, this study is illustrated in Table 7.11.

Note that each group, and thus each subject in each group, appears twice in this design. In the terminology of experimental design, time is a "within subject" variable because the same subjects appear at multiple levels of that variable: before and after installation. Reminder delivery method is a "between subject" variable because each subject appears in only one level of that variable: reminder or control. The crossover design, discussed above, is another example of a repeated-measures design.

Self-Test 7.2

Using the notation developed in the previous section, diagram the studies described in Scenarios 1, 3, 4, and 5 of Self-Test 7.1. Scenario 4, as worded, can be interpreted two ways. For purposes of this exercise, treat it as a nested design with care providers as the subjects and clinical services as the unit of randomization.

Threats to Inference and Validity

Internal and External Validity

We all want our demonstration studies to be valid.[*] There are two aspects to validity: internal and external. If a study is internally valid, it means that we can be confident in the conclusions drawn from the specific circumstances of the experiment: the population of subjects studied, measurements made, and interventions provided. Are we justified in concluding that the differences observed are due to the attributed causes? There are many potential threats to internal validity, called "confounders," which we discuss later. Even if all these threats to internal validity are overcome to our satisfaction, we also want the study to have external validity. This means that the conclusions can be generalized from the specific setting, subjects, and intervention studied to the broader range of settings others encounter. Thus even if we demonstrate convincingly that our antibiotic reminder system reduces postoperative infection rates in our own hospital, it is of little interest to others unless we can convince them that the results can safely be generalized to other reminder systems in other hospitals. Threats to external validity are also discussed below.

---

[*] Here we see another difference in the terminology of measurement and demonstration studies. Validity of a demonstration study design, discussed here, is different from validity of measurement, discussed in Chapter 5.

TABLE 7.11. Repeated measures design

Time	Intervention	
	Reminders	Control
Baseline	G1	G2
After installation	G1	G2

Inference and Error

When we conduct a demonstration study, there are four possible outcomes. We illustrate these outcomes in the context of a demonstration study exploring the "effectiveness" of an information resource using an appropriate comparative design. Four possible outcomes are:

1. The information resource was effective, and our study shows it.
2. The information resource was ineffective, and our study shows it.
3. The information resource was effective, but for some reason our study mistakenly failed to show it—a "type II" error.
4. The information resource was ineffective, but for some reason our study mistakenly suggested it was effective—a "type I" error.

Outcomes 1 and 2 are salutary from a methodological viewpoint; the results of the study mirror reality. Outcome 3 is a false negative result, or type II error. (In the language of inferential statistics, we mistakenly accept the null hypothesis.) Type II errors can arise because the size of the information resource's effect on the measure of interest is small, and too few subjects have been included in the study to detect it[23]; or we may have failed to measure the outcome variable on which the resource is having an impact. In outcome 4 we have concluded that the resource is valuable when in reality it is not: a false-positive result, or type I error. (We have mistakenly rejected the null hypothesis.) The risk of a type I error is built into every study. When we accept, for example, the value of $p < 0.05$ as a criterion for statistical significance, we are consciously accepting a 5% risk of making a type I error as a consequence of using randomization as a mechanism of experimental control.

Study Power

Every demonstration study has a probability of detecting a difference of particular size between the groups. This probability is known as the statistical power of the design. By increasing the number of subjects, the power can be increased. Study power is an important consideration in study design. A study with insufficient subjects, which is unlikely to detect the minimum worthwhile difference between the groups, will make poor use of the subjects' time and the investigators' resources. While a detailed discussion of statistical power is beyond the scope of this volume, a clear and comprehensive discussion is found in the text by Cohen.[24] In general, the formulas used to compute statistical power include the target difference between the means of the dependent variables—the amount of difference between the groups the study is designed to detect—as well as the anticipated standard deviations of the group means. For simple two-group studies with equal numbers of subjects allocated to each group, nomograms are a convenient way of determining the required sample size (e.g., p. 456 in Altman[7]). When studies are designed to demonstrate equivalance (as opposed to differences), to measure the time till an event occurs, or when there are more than two groups or one outcome variable, investigators are advised to consult a statistician for advice.

Validity and Confounding in Demonstration Studies

The motive for conducting demonstration studies is to provide reliable conclusions that are of interest to those making decisions. Usually, we want to inform decisions not only about the particular information resource in the context in which it was studied but also about similar resources in other possible contexts in which they may be installed. We want our results to be reliable and free from any threat to internal validity, or bias.

Threats to Internal Validity: Biases and How to Avoid Them

Assessment Bias

It is important to ensure that no one involved in a demonstration study can allow his or her own feelings and beliefs about an information resource, whether positive or negative, to bias the results. Simply asking study participants to ignore their feelings so as to avoid consciously biasing the study is unrealistic; we must ensure that they cannot affect the results consciously or unconsciously. The people who could bias a study include those designing it, those recruiting subjects, those using the information resource, those collecting follow-up data, and those who participate as judges in making measurements of dependent or independent variables.

Consider a study in which the users of an antibiotic reminder system also collect data needed for determining whether the advice generated by the system was correct. If they were computer skeptics they might collect additional data to prove themselves right and the reminder system wrong. Thus they might record that a patient was suffering from chest symptoms to justify an antibiotic prescription that the reminder system had not advised, or collect bacteriological specimens from a wound infection in such a way that the laboratory was unable to culture any pathogens in a patient in whom the system reminded them to prescribe an antibiotic but they had ignored its advice. Thus if the users collect important data or even provide "gold standard" judgments as part of the measurement process, evaluators are completely reliant on their impartiality about the information resource.

Alternatively, if the judges of the "gold standard" for each case used in a study know in which cases the information resource was used, they might be prejudiced in their judgment about whether the users' decisions or actions were correct, particularly if they participated in the development of the information resource, or if the criteria used for judging the correctness of decisions or outcome are poorly formulated.

To eliminate these biases, everyone involved in the collection of case data and the judgments about cases should be blinded to whether the information resource was used in each case. If follow-up data about a case are necessary to establish a final diagnosis, for example, the follow-up data should ideally be obtained by a second group of clinicians after an independent person removes any evidence of information resource use from the notes. Blind determination of "gold standards" means that external independent observers make these determinations from data provided by the study team without revealing if it is an intervention or control case.[25, 26] If outcomes could be classified without need to resort to human judgments, it would alleviate the problem; unfortunately, such measures are rarely available in medicine.

Allocation and Recruitment Bias

Early studies of information resources often take place in the environment in which they were developed and frequently arouse strong positive (or negative) feelings among study subjects. In a study where patients are randomized and the clinicians have strong beliefs about the information resource, two biases may arise. Clinicians may cheat the randomization method and systematically allocate easier (or more difficult) cases to the information resource group (allocation bias), or they may avoid recruiting easy (or difficult) cases to the study if they know in advance (by obtaining a copy of the randomization list or holding randomization envelopes up to a light) that the next patient will be allocated to the control group (recruitment bias).[27] These biases would either over- or underestimate the information resource's value. In a study where care providers or departments are randomized, bias can arise if the care providers' enthusiasm for the information resource is inversely correlated with their level of experience or competence. Thus inexperienced care providers might drop out of a study less often if they are in the information resource group, confounding the benefit of the information resource with the care providers' inexperience and reducing the information resource's apparent benefit.

The solution to these problems is to define the population of patients and subjects eligible as subjects for the trial, screen them strictly for eligibility, randomize patients as late as possible before the information resource is used, and conceal the allocation of patients to intervention or control groups until they have been irrevocably recruited to the study.[27] It is wise to check whether subjects can cheat the randomization method (e.g., check if randomization envelopes are translucent), quantify the number of patients or care providers who are *not* recruited, and analyze the study according to the principle of *"intention to provide information,"* as discussed in a later section.

The Hawthorne Effect

The Hawthorne effect—the tendency for humans to improve their performance if they know it is being studied—was discovered by psychologists measuring the effect of ambient lighting on workers' productivity at the Hawthorne factory in Chicago.[28] Productivity increased as the room illumination level was raised, but when the illumination level was accidentally reduced, productivity increased again, suggesting that it was the study itself, rather than changes in illumination, that caused the increase. During a study of a medical information resource, the Hawthorne effect can lead to an improvement in the performance of all subjects in all study groups. This "global" Hawthorne effect is particularly likely to occur when care providers' performance is low because they lack some simple knowledge or insight that is easy for them to correct.[25] The net result is to increase performance in both control and information resource groups, potentially causing the benefit of the information resource to be underestimated. To quantify a global Hawthorne effect requires a preliminary low-profile study of the performance of care providers before any large-scale study. Disguising the true intention of this "baseline" study may take some ingenuity, but is a necessary evil if the Hawthorne effect is not to bias this study too.

A better approach is to ensure that the Hawthorne effect acts only on some of the subjects' activities by using a distracting task in what is known as a balanced incomplete block design. Here investigators introduce two similar interventions and allocate each subject randomly to one of them without telling any subjects what is happening to other subjects. The investigators make two sets of measurements: One set measures the effects of the first intervention on the first group of subjects and uses the second group as control; the other measurements assess the effects of the second intervention on the second group, using the first group as the controls. Subjects are randomized to the two groups, so there is no systematic difference between groups. Because both groups of subjects experience what appears to be an important experimental intervention, the Hawthorne effect is equal, and each group can safely act as a control for the other. The two interventions should be made similar, for example providing anesthetists with reminders about prophylactic antibiotics for preoperative orthopedic patients or for preoperative cardiac patients (Table 7.12). The postoperative infection rates in orthopedic patients whose doctors received orthopedic reminders was half that of patients whose doctors received reminders about cardiac patients. Both groups of doctors were receiving reminders about some of their patients, so the Hawthorne effect is not responsible. Equally, the postoperative infection rates in cardiac patients whose doctors received cardiac reminders was nearly half that of patients whose doctors received reminders about orthopedic patients, suggesting that the cardiac reminders were also effective.

Data Collection Biases

Checklist Effect

The checklist effect is the improvement observed in decision-making due to more complete and better-structured data collection when paper- or computer-based

TABLE 7.12. Hypothetical results of a balanced incomplete block design of two antibiotic reminder systems

| | Postoperative infection rate (%) | |
Patients	Orthopedic reminders	Cardiac reminders
Orthopedic	5	10
Cardiac	18	11

forms are used to collect patient data. As shown earlier (Table 7.1), the impact of forms on decision-making can equal that of computer-generated advice,[13] so it must either be controlled for or quantified. It is most likely to occur when inexperienced care providers collect complex data under critical time pressures, as with trauma care. To control for the checklist effect, the same data should be collected in the same way in control and information resource cases, even though the information resource's output is only available for the latter group.[25] To quantify the magnitude of this effect, a randomly selected "data collection only" group of patients can be recruited.[13]

Data Completeness Effect

In some studies the information resource itself may collect the data used to assess a dependent variable. Thus more data are available in intervention cases than in controls. It may cut both ways. For example, consider a field study of an intensive care unit (ICU) information system where the aim is to compare recovery rates from adverse events, such as transient hypotension, between patients monitored by the information system with those allocated to traditional manual data recording. Because the information system logs episodes that may not be recorded by the manual system, the recovery rate may apparently *fall* in this group of cases, as more adverse events are being detected. To detect this bias, the completeness and accuracy of data collected in the control and information resource groups should be compared against some third method of data collection, perhaps in a short pilot study, or all events should be logged by computer but with the computer record made available only to care providers in the computer group. When analyzing the study, all data from control patients are reviewed for evidence of hypotensive episodes, whether logged by hand or computer.

Feedback Effect

As mentioned in the earlier discussion, one interesting result of the 1986 study of the Leeds Abdominal Pain System[13] was that the diagnostic accuracy of the control house officers spending 6-months in a training level failed to improve over the period, whereas the performance of the doctors given both data collection forms and monthly feedback did improve: starting at 13% above control levels at month 1 and rising to 27% above control levels at month 6 (Table 7.1). Thus providing the doctors with the opportunity to capture their diagnoses on a form and encouraging them to audit their performance monthly did improve their performance. Many information resources provide a similar opportunity for easy audit and feedback of personal performance. To ensure that the effects of any decision support or advice can be distinguished from the effects of such feedback, either controls should be provided with the same audit and feedback or the study should include a third "audit and feedback group" to quantify the size of the improvement caused by this factor alone, as was done in the Leeds study.[13] Those who doubt the importance of this effect should read a discussion about how much of the original Hawthorne effect may have been due to enhanced feedback and opportunities for operant conditioning and increased piecework income offered to workers by the counting equipment installed in the relay assembly test room.[29]

Carryover Effect

The carryover effect is a contamination of the management of the "control" condition by care providers who also have, or have previously had, access to the information resource. It is most likely to occur with information resources that have an educational effect, such as decision support systems. A carryover effect will reduce the measured difference in performance between information resource and control care providers. To eliminate the carryover effect, it is probably best to randomize at the level of the care provider instead of the patient[22, 30] or department instead of care provider.[13] This creates a nested design as discussed earlier. The procedure has implications for the method of statistical analysis.[19] To quantify the carryover effect, investigators can conduct a study with alternating information resource and control periods[31] as discussed under crossover studies that allows carryover after the information resource is withdrawn to be quantified, so long as all time-related trends can be safely attributed to the information resource.

Placebo Effect

In some drug trials simply giving patients an inactive tablet, or "placebo," causes them to recover. This "placebo effect" may be more powerful than the drug effect itself and may even obscure a complete absence of therapeutic benefit. In a medical information resource study, if some patients watch their doctors consult an impressive workstation while others have no such experience, it can unbalance the groups and overestimate the value of the information resource. It is also possible that some patients believe that a care provider who needs a computer workstation is less competent. The problem is most likely to arise when the attributes being measured are attitudes or beliefs (e.g., the patients' satisfaction with therapy) or when the computer is used in front of the patient. Possible remedies are for all care providers to leave the patient for the same brief period (when some would use the information resource) or for all care providers to use computers but the system output would available only be to intervention care providers. Measuring features of the patients' condition that are less dependent on the patients' perceptions makes the study more immune to the placebo effect.

"Second-Look" Bias

When conducting a laboratory impact study of the effects of an information resource on clinical decision-making using written case scenarios, the usual procedure is to ask clinicians to read the test scenario and state their initial decision. They are then allowed to use the information resource (e.g., a decision support system) and are asked again for their decision.[32] Any improvements in decision-making are credited to the decision support system. However, there is a potential bias here: The subjects are being given a second opportunity to review the same case scenario, which allows them more time and further opportunities for reflection, which can itself improve decision-making. This "second-look bias" can be reduced or eliminated by increasing the interval between the two exposures to the stimulus material to some weeks or months[33] or by providing a different set of case data, matched for difficulty with the first, for the second task.[34] Alternatively, the size of the effect can be quantified by testing subjects on a subset of the test data a second time without providing them access to the information resource.

External Validity Issues

Even if we believe that the study findings are internally consistent and the conclusions are correct, evaluators and recipients of evaluation reports (see Chapter 2) must be able to generalize from the specific details of the study to a range of other, similar settings. It requires the study to demonstrate external validity. Possible threats to external validity are discussed below.

Generalizing from the Sample

We have already mentioned the risks of using homogeneous sets of selected cases and subjects when conducting demonstration studies, such as patients with abdominal pain severe enough to require laparotomy.[15] Unless the evaluators have sampled cases and subjects that reflect the variability to be expected everywhere,[35] the results of the study apply to narrow circumstances only and fail attempts at replication.[16] A classic example is a prognostic model to predict relapse from asthma that performed very well in the center where it was developed but had near-zero discriminatory power in a second, similar center.[36]

Risks of Resource Developers also Evaluating the Resource

If the developers of an information resource also attempt to evaluate it, and human judgment is required to decide whether the resource is "correct" or agrees with the gold standard, there may be bias in favor of the resource. This event is a special problem during laboratory studies of resource function (see Chapter 3) when test cases are input and the information resource's output may be recorded by a member of the development team, or when the gold standard diagnosis or treatment for a particular test case is unclear. If data items for a test case are missing or ambiguous, the developer may know how to persuade the information resource to produce the "right" output. The problem also arises if there is an incomplete or ambiguous mapping between the information resource's output and the scoring scheme, for example if a decision support system advises on the presence or absence of ischemic heart disease but the only diagnosis available for each case is whether they have suffered a myocardial infarction. The developers and their associated clinicians know how to use the information resource to best effect; others outside the center of development do not, so the study results may not apply elsewhere.

Also, medical information resources seldom encompass every aspect of medicine, even in a subarea, so it is common for a given information resource to be confronted with novel combinations of case data when tested on a new set of cases. Developers sometimes suspend the tests while the information resource is modified to cater for the novel case and then quote its accuracy on the whole series, forgetting that the modifications may now cause the information resource to fail on some of the previous cases. If the tests are performed by impartial evaluators, they can only report the resource's performance on the whole case series, without modification.

Selection of Tasks: Representative Versus Homogeneous

There is an inevitable compromise when selecting subjects or tasks for a demonstration study: whether to choose a homogeneous group with selected characteristics or a random or comprehensive sample that encompasses all the variation seen in care providers and cases at large. The study is easier to conduct with the former but suffers from lack of generality or external validity because of the selection of subjects and cases. Evaluators must decide where to set the trade-off: completing the study with limited resources and maximum attention to internal validity by controlling potential sources of bias, or emphasizing external validity, requiring attention to identifying representative cases, subjects, and judges and potentially needing larger resources for a multicenter study.

Evaluation Paradox

In a demonstration study, users are understandably reluctant to act on the output of an information resource until its value has been established. However, to establish the information resource's value, its output must be acted on. This "evaluation paradox" applies especially to so-called black box information resources, which provide little if any insight into the reasons for their output[37] and would cause care providers to ignore the information resource's output and thus lead to its benefits being underestimated. Although one solution might be to deliberately exaggerate the benefits of following system output, we prefer to give care providers an honest account of the information resource's scope and performance in laboratory tests, the differences between its reasoning method and the input data it processes compared to those used by care providers, and examples of cases when people's decisions were superior to that of the information resource and vice versa. This method encourages care providers to treat the information resource as an aid, not as a black-box dictator. There is little reason to instruct care providers to always follow the information resource's output during a demonstration study, as it is certainly not the case when the resource is released for general use.

Analysis by "Intention to Provide Information"

In a demonstration study, there are many instances when the information resource is not used as intended[25, 38] or when its output is ignored. When analyzing the results of the study, it may be tempting to exclude such cases, thereby increasing the difference between control and information resource groups. There is a close analogy when analyzing the results of drug trials: To which group should one assign subjects who were randomized to a drug but failed to take it or who took it but were found not to absorb it? If one excludes from analysis all the patients who did not take the drug, the *average* benefit of giving the drug to patients described by the study entry criteria is overestimated, as we know that in real life a certain percentage of patients are noncompliant. Thus when analyzing drug trials, subjects are included in the group to which they were originally randomized. This method is called analysis by the principle of *"intention to treat."*

The same argument applies to medical information resources: The aim of demonstration studies is usually to measure the *average* impact of the information resource on care providers and patients to whom it is made available, not its *maximum* potential for benefit when everyone is forced to use it or nonusers are excluded. Indeed, this is the motivation for conducting demonstration studies. Thus we must analyze the study according to the principle of *"intention to provide information."* There are three possible scenarios.

Scenario 1: A control patient or control care provider when the information resource was illicitly accessed by the care provider.

If the care provider was sufficiently uncertain about the patient's care to consult the information resource, he or she might have sought information from elsewhere had the information resource not been available. The analogy here is self-medication by patients. Verdict: *retain case in the control group.*

Scenario 2: A control patient or control care provider where the care provider consulted someone else to obtain the same information that could have been obtained from the information resource.

If the care provider was sufficiently uncertain to consult someone else, this would probably have happened regardless of whether there was a study in progress. Again, the analogy is self-medication. Verdict: *retain case in the control group.*

Scenario 3: A case in which the care provider was supposed to use the information resource but failed to use it, used it incorrectly, or ignored its output or advice.

If the care provider was unwilling to use the information resource, failed to use it correctly, or ignored its output under the conditions of a trial when their performance was under scrutiny, they would probably not have used it in a real setting. The analogy is patient non-

compliance or failure to absorb the drug. Verdict: *retain case in the information resource group.*

Self-Test 7.3

For each of the following short study scenarios, try to identify any of the potential biases or threats to validity discussed in this chapter. Each scenario may contain more than one bias or threat to validity. Then consider how you might alter the system implementation or evaluation plans to reduce or quantify the problem.

1. As part of its initiative to improve patient flow and teamwork, a family practice intends to install an electronic patient scheduling system when it moves to new premises in 3 month's time. Evaluators propose a 1-month baseline study of patient waiting times and phone calls between clinicians, starting at 2 months and conducted prior to the move, to be repeated immediately after starting to use the new system in 3 months.
2. A bacteriology laboratory is being overwhelmed with requests for obscure tests with few relevant clinical data on the paper request forms. It asks the hospital information system director to arrange for electronic requesting and drafts a comprehensive three-screen list of questions clinicians must answer before submitting the request. The plan is to evaluate the effects of electronic test ordering on appropriateness of requests by randomizing patients to "paper request forms" or "electronic requests" for the next year. They intend to present their work at a bacteriology conference.
3. A renowned chief cardiologist in a tertiary referral center on the West coast is concerned about the investigation of some types of congenital heart disease in patients in her unit. A medical informatics expert suggests that her expertise could be represented as reminders about test ordering for the junior staff looking after these patients. She agrees, announces her plans at the next departmental meeting, and arranges system implementation and training. Each patient is managed by only one junior staff member; there are enough staff to allow them to be randomized. After the trial the appropriateness of test ordering for each patient is judged by the chief cardiologist from the entire medical record. It is markedly improved in patients managed by the doctors who received reminders. Based on these results, the hospital chief executive agrees to fund a start-up company to disseminate the reminder system to all U.S. cardiology units.

Analysis of Demonstration Study Results

When the time comes to analyze the data collected during a study, one of the most important factors determining the approach taken is the levels of measurement of the dependent (outcome) variable and independent variables. For the sake of simplicity, we dichotomize each of these as either discrete (nominal/ordinal) or continuous (interval/ratio). Table 7.13 suggests some of the possible methods of

TABLE 7.13. Methods of data analysis for the four main combinations of experimental variables

Dependent variable	Independent variables	
	Discrete	Continuous
Discrete	Contingency table methods, chi square	Discriminant analysis, logistic regression
Continuous	ANOVA, t-test	Pearson correlation, multiple regression

analysis for the various resulting combinations. For example, ANOVA can be used when the independent variables of a study are discrete and the outcome variable is continuous.

We discuss in the following sections two common situations that arise in informatics demonstration studies: discrete independent variables coupled with either discrete or continuous dependent variables. This section by no means covers all the possible analytical challenges, but it does address the analytical schemes employed in many studies in the literature and raises most of the generic issues.

Analyzing Studies with a Discrete Dependent (Outcome) Variable

Many descriptive and comparative studies employ discrete dependent (outcome) variables, such as whether elements of stored data are accurate, whether a computer-generated reminder caused an action, or whether the advice given corresponded with the advice accpted as a gold standard for the case. Such data can be analyzed using the contingency, or two by two (2 × 2) table approach.

Using Contingency (2 × 2) Tables

In many evaluations of information resource function the only measurement made is the percentage of agreements between the information resource and a gold standard for a set of test cases. Citing this "crude accuracy" alone can cause a number of problems. First, it gives the reader no idea of what accuracy could have been obtained by chance. For example, consider a diagnostic aid designed to detect a disease **D**, where the prevalence (prior probability) of disease **D** in the test cases is 80%. If a decision support system always suggests disease **D** no matter which case data are input, the measured accuracy over a large number of cases is 80%. If it was slightly more subtle, still ignoring all input data but advising diagnoses solely according to their prevalence, it would still achieve an accuracy of around 64% by chance because it would diagnose disease **D** on 80% of occasions, and on 80% of occasions disease **D** would be present.

The major problem with citing accuracy alone is that it ignores differences between types of errors. If a decision support system erroneously diagnoses disease **D** in a healthy patient, this false positive error may be less serious than if it pronounces that the patient is suffering from disease **E**, or that a patient suffering from disease **D** is healthy, a false negative error. More complex errors can occur if more than one disease is present, or if the decision support system issues its output as a list of diagnoses ranked by probability. In this case, including the correct diagnosis toward the end of the list is less serious than omitting it altogether but is considerably less useful than if the correct diagnosis is ranked among the top three.[39]

The disadvantages of citing agreement rates alone can be largely overcome by using a contingency table to compare the output given by the information resource against the gold standard, which (as discussed in Chapters 4 and 5) is the accepted value of the "truth," and by calculating a number of derived measures, Table 7.14.[40] This method allows the difference between false positive and false negative errors to be made explicit.

Errors can be classified as false positive (*FP* in the table) or false negative (*FN* in the table); these rates and other measures such as the specificity can be calculated. In a field study where an information resource is being used, care providers typically know the output and want to know how often it is correct; or they suspect a disease and want to know how often the information resource correctly detects it. In this situation, some care providers find the predictive value positive and the "detection rate,"[41] also known as sensitivity, intuitively more useful than the false-positive and false-negative rates. The positive predictive value has the disadvantage that it is highly dependent on disease prevalence, which may differ significantly between the test cases used in a study and the clinical environment in which an information resource is deployed. Sensitivity and positive predictive value are particularly useful, however, with information resources that issue alarms, as the accuracy, specificity, and false-positive rates may not be obtainable. This is because, in an alarm system that continually monitors the value of one or

TABLE 7.14. Example of a contingency table

Decision-aid's advice	Gold standard		Totals
	Attribute present	Attribute absent	
Attribute present	TP	FP	TP + FP
Attribute absent	FN	TN	FN + TN
Total	TP + FN	FP + TN	N

TP, true positive; FP, false positive; FN, false negative; TN, true negative. Accuracy: (TP + TN)/N; false-negative rate: FN/(TP + FN); false-positive rate: FP/(FP + TN); positive predictive value: TP/(TP + FP); negative predictive value: TN/(FN + TN); detection rate (sensitivity): TP/(TP + FN); specificity: TN/(FP + TN).

more physiological parameters, there is no way to count discrete true negative events.

Chi-Square Test and Cohen's Kappa

The basic test of statistical significance for 2 × 2 tables is performed by computing the chi-square statistic, which in its general form is:

$$\chi^2 = \Sigma_i \frac{(O_i - E_i)^2}{E_i}$$

where the summation is performed over all i cells of the table, O_i is the observed value of cell i and E_i is the value of cell i expected by chance alone. The expected values are computed by multiplying the row and column totals for each cell and dividing this number by the total number of observations in the table. For example, the Table 7.15 gives the results of a hypothetical laboratory study of an information resource based on 90 test cases. The columns give the "gold standard" verdict of a panel as to whether each patient had the disease of interest, and the rows indicate whether the patient was predicted by the system to have the disease of interest. Observed results are in boldface type; expected frequencies for each cell, given these observed results, are in parentheses.[*]

The value of chi-square for Table 7.15 is 9.8. A 2 × 2 contingency table is associated with one statistical degree of freedom. With reference to a standard statistical table, we note that this relation is signficant at about the 0.001 level, which means that we accept a 1 in 1000 chance of making a type I error if we conclude that there is a relation between the system's predictions and the verdict of the panel, which is the accepted "gold standard." As with any statistical test, there are cautions and limitations applying to its use. Chi-square should not be used (or should be "corrected for continuity") if the count in any of the table's cells is less than five.

Chi-square can tell us the probability of committing type I errors, but this statistic does not give a useful indication of the strength of association between the two variables represented in a contingency table. A useful index of agreement is given by Cohen's kappa (κ), which compares the agreement against that which might be expected by chance.[7, 42] The formula for calculating κ is:

$$\kappa = \frac{O_{Ag} - E_{Ag}}{1 - E_{Ag}}$$

where O_{Ag} is the observed fraction of agreements (the sum of the diagonal cells

---

[*] The reader should confirm the calculations of expected values. For example, the expected value for the "disease–disease" cell is obtained by multiplying the relevant row total (41) by the relevant column total (43) and dividing the product by the total number of subjects (90).

TABLE 7.15. Hypothetical study results as a contingency table

System's prediction	Panel verdict, observed results (no.)		Total
	Disease	No disease	
Disease	**27** (19.6)	**14** (21.4)	41
No disease	**16** (23.4)	**33** (25.6)	49
Total	43	47	90

Numbers in parentheses are the expected results.

divided by the total number of observations) and E_{Ag} is the expected fraction of agreements (the sum of the expected values of the diagonal cells, divided by the total number of observations). In our example above, $O_{Ag} = 0.67$ [(27 + 33)/90] and $E_{Ag} = 0.50$ [(19.6 + 25.6)/90], which makes the value of $\kappa = 0.33$.

Kappa can be thought of as the *chance-corrected proportional agreement,*[7] and possible values range from +1 (perfect agreement) via 0 (no agreement above that expected by chance) to –1 (complete disagreement). Some authorities consider a κ above 0.4 as evidence of useful agreement, but this threshold obviously depends on the clinical application.[43]

Cost Matrices

The measures derived from contingency tables can be converted to a total score or cost by combining the frequencies with a separate "cost matrix" (see example in Table 7.16). Here a correct classification of disease D has been assigned a score of +10 points, correct exclusion of D +2 points, a false-positive diagnosis –2 and false-negative diagnosis –10 points. These points are assigned by a panel of representative users of the information resource and attempt to take into account the utility of a correct classification and the dysutility of the two kinds of error. Such methods are especially useful when the information resource produces a list of alternatives or when it modifies its output with an expression of certainty.

Each case is then classified according to the cell of the cost matrix in which it falls. Thus if one decision-support system states that a certain patient in a test set has disease D and the gold standard states that disease D is absent, 2 points are subtracted from that decision aid's score. If a different system or the doctors managing the patient say that disease D is absent in that patient, 2 points are added to their score, and so on for all the cases in the test set. The system with the highest score is judged the best using this cost matrix. Note, however, that such a ranking is highly dependent on the specific costs in the cost matrix, as well as the prevalence of disease D in the test set.

The weighted κ is a similar statistic to Cohen's κ (discussed above) but incorporates different weights for each kind of disagreement, as in the cost matrix. Further discussion of the use of κ may be found in Altman[7] and Hilden et al.[44]

Table 7.16. Example of a cost matrix for a diagnostic decision support system

| | Gold standard | |
Decision aid's advice	Disease **D** present	Disease **D** absent
Disease **D** present	+10	−2
Disease **D** absent	−10	+2

ROC Analysis

Some information resources incorporate qualitative or quantitative thresholds as a criterion for rendering a binary (yes/no) decision. For example, in an antibiotic reminder system that reasons using probabilities, the probability of a postoperative infection may have to exceed 0.5 before an alert is issued. In these resources, the value fixed for the threshold may be a key determinant of its ability to provide accurate advice. If the incorrect threshold is chosen, the information resource's accuracy may appear lower than it can actually attain.

To assess variation in the accuracy of advice as an internal threshold is adjusted, it is valuable to plot a receiver operating characteristic (ROC) curve.[45] This curve plots the true-positive rate against the false-positive rate for varying threshold levels (Figure 7.1). If an information resource provides random advice, its ROC curve lies on the diagonal, whereas an ideal information resource would have a "knee" close to the upper left hand corner. The area under the ROC curve can be used as a measure of the discriminatory power of the information resource.[46] In other cases, an ROC curve can be plotted from results obtained as the number of input data items is varied or the number of facts in a decision support system's knowledge base are changed.[47] For a discussion of calibration, please see the Appendix to this chapter.

Choice of Metrics: Absolute Change, Relative Change, Number Needed to Treat

When we conduct demonstration studies, the goal is to inform and enhance decisions about information resources. We should not try to exaggerate the effects we have observed any more than we would deliberately ignore known biases or threats to generality. Thus it is important to describe the results of the study in terms that accurately convey their meaning. Consider the study results in Table 7.17. We can summarise these results in three main ways.

1. By citing the absolute difference (after intervention versus baseline) in the percentage infection rates due to the reminders (row 3 of Table 7.17). It may appear to be 5%, but a more conservative estimate is 3%. The 5% change in the reminder group should be corrected by the 2% change due to nonspecific factors in the control cases.

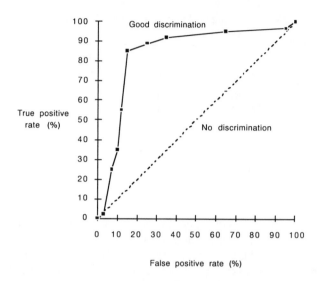

FIGURE 7.1. Sample receiver operating characteristic (ROC) curve.

2. By citing the relative difference in the percentage infection rates due to the reminders. It is a 46% fall, though again the more conservative estimate would be 26%: the 46% fall in the reminder group minus the 20% fall due to nonspecific factors in the control cases.

3. By citing the "number needed to treat" (NNT). This figure gives us an idea about how many patients would need to be "treated" by the intervention to produce the effect of interest in one patient. The NNT is the reciprocal of the absolute difference in rates (3%, or 0.03) and is 33 for these results. To put it another way, reminders would need to be issued for an average of 33 patients before one postoperative infection would be prevented.

$$NNT = \frac{1}{rate_1 - rate_2}$$

where: $rate_1$ = absolute rate of the event in group 1
         $rate_2$ = absolute event rate in group 2.

Several studies have shown that clinicians make much more sensible decisions about prescribing when the results of drug trials are cited as NNT rather than absolute or relative percentage differences.[48] As can be seen, in many ways the NNT is the most helpful way to visualize the effects of implementing an information resource and should be reported whenever possible.

TABLE 7.17. Hypothetical results of a simultaneous randomized controlled study of an antibiotic reminder system

Time	Postoperative infection rate (%)	
	Reminder cases	Control cases
Baseline	11	10
After intervention	6	8
Absolute difference	5	2
Relative difference	−46	−20

Analyzing Studies with Continuous Outcomes

Logic of Analysis of Variance (ANOVA)

Many comparative study designs employ one or more independent variables that have discrete values (at the nominal or ordinal level of measurement) and a dependent variable with continuous values (at the interval or ratio level of measurement). In the most basic true experiment, the intervention and control groups comprise two levels of a nominal independent variable. Statistical methods using analysis of variance (ANOVA), discussed briefly here, exist specifically to address these situations. If the outcome measure, the dependent variable, lends itself naturally to measurement at the interval or ratio level, there is no need to categorize it artificially. For example, if systolic blood pressure is the outcome measure, its measured value can and should be used for purposes of statistical analysis. Categorizing measured blood pressure values as "low," "normal," and "high" neglects potentially useful information and makes the results dependent on what might be arbitrary decisions regarding the thresholds.

Experimental design and ANOVA are the topics of major parts of entire textbooks.[9] We seek here to establish the basic principles using the results of an actual study as an example. Our example is based on preliminary and somewhat simplified results of a biomedical information retrieval study under way at the University of North Carolina.[49] The study explores whether Boolean or Hypertext access to a database results in more effective retrieval of information to solve biomedical problems. With the Boolean access mode, subjects framed their queries as combinations of key words joined by logical *and* or *or* statements. With the Hypertext mode, subjects could branch from one database node to another via a large number of preconstructed links. The biomedical data available to subjects were in the domain of bacteriology and infectious disease and were identical across the two access modes. The results to be discussed here are based on data collected from 42 medical students randomized to the Boolean or Hypertext access mode. Subjects were also randomized to one of two sets of clinical case problems, each set comprising eight clinical infectious disease scenarios. Students were given two passes through their eight assigned problems. On the first pass they were asked to generate diagnostic hypotheses using only their personal knowledge. Immediately thereafter, on the second pass, they were asked to generate another set of diagnostic hypotheses for the same set of problems but this time with aid from the database.

First we examine the basic structure of this study and note that it has two independent variables, each measured at the nominal level.

- The first independent variable is access mode: Boolean or Hypertext.
- The second independent variable is the particular set of eight case problems to which students were assigned, arbitrarily labeled set A and set B.

Because each of the two independent variables has two levels and is fully randomized, the study design is that of a complete factorial experiment (as discussed earlier in the chapter) with four groups as shown in Table 7.18. The table also shows the number of subjects in each group. The dependent variable is the improvement in the diagnostic hypotheses from the first pass to the second—the differences between the aided and unaided scores—summed over the eight assigned cases. This variable was chosen because it estimates the effect attributable to the information retrieved from the database, controlling for each subject's prior knowledge of bacteriology and infectious disease.

Interpreting ANOVA results

The logic of analyzing data from such an experiment is to compare the mean values of the dependent variable across the groups. Table 7.19 shows the mean and standard deviations of the improvement scores for each of the groups. For all subjects, the mean improvement score is 16.4 with a standard deviation of 7.3.

Take a minute to examine Table 7.19. It should be fairly clear that there are differences of potential interest between the groups. Across problem sets, the improvement scores are higher for the Hypertext access mode than the Boolean mode. Across access modes, the improvement scores are greater for problem set B than for problem set A. Are these differences statistically significant?

The methods of ANOVA allow us to determine if differences in the group means can be attributed statistically to each of the independent variables or to combinations of the independent variables. The former are called *main effects;* the latter are called *interactions.* The number of main effects is equal to the number of independent variables; the number of possible interactions increases geometrically with the number of independent variables. With two independent variables there is one interaction; with three independent variables there are four; with four independent variables there are eleven.[*]

In our example with two independent variables, we need to test for two main effects and one interaction. Table 7.20 shows the results of ANOVA for these

---

[*] With three independent variables (A,B,C), there are three two-way interactions (AB,AC,BC) and one three-way interaction (ABC). With four indcpendent variables (A,B,C,D), there are six two-way interactions (AB,AC,AD,BC,BD,CD), four three-way interactions (ABC,ABD,ACD,BCD), and one four-way interaction (ABCD).

TABLE 7.18. Structure of the example information retrieval study

Access mode	Structure, by assigned problem set	
	A	B
Boolean	G1	G2
	$(n = 11)$	$(n = 11)$
Hypertext	G3	G4
	$(n = 10)$	$(n = 10)$

TABLE 7.19. Results of the example information retrieval study

Access mode	Results, by assigned problem set (mean ± SD)	
	A	B
Boolean	11.2 ± 5.7	17.5 ± 7.3
	$(n = 11)$	$(n = 11)$
Hypertext	15.7 ± 7.2	21.8 ± 5.2
	$(n = 10)$	$(n = 10)$

TABLE 7.20. Analysis of variance results for the information retrieval example

Source	Sum of squares	df	Mean square	F ratio	p
Main effects					
Problem set	400.935	1	400.935	9.716	0.003
Access mode	210.005	1	210.005	5.089	0.030
Interaction					
Problem set by					
access mode	0.078	1	0.078	0.002	0.966
Error	1568.155	38	41.267		

data. Again, a full understanding of this table requires reference to a basic statistical text. For purposes of this discussion, note the following:

1. The *sum-of-squares* is an estimate of the amount of variability in the dependent variable attributable to each main effect or interaction. All other things being equal, the greater the sum-of-squares, the more likely is the effect to be statistically significant.

2. A number of statistical *degrees of freedom* (*df*) is associated with each source of statistical variance. For each main effect, *df* is one less than the number of levels of the relevant independent variable. Because each independent variable in our example has two levels, *df* = 1 for both. For each interaction, the *df* is the product of the *df*s for the interacting variables. In this example, *df* for the inter-

action is 1, as each interacting variable has a *df* of 1. Total *df* in a study is one
less than the total number of subjects.

3. The *mean-square* is the sum-of-squares divided by the *df*. It is analogous to a
measure of variance.

4. The inferential statistic of interest is the F ratio, which is the ratio of the mean-
square of each main effect or interaction to the mean-square for error. The
mean-square for error is the amount of variability that is unaccounted for statistically by the independent variables and the interactions among them. The *df*
for error is the total *df* minus the *df* for all main effects and interactions.

5. Finally, with reference to standard statistical tables, a p value may be associated with each value of the F ratio and the values of *df* in the ANOVA table. A
p value of less than 0.05 is typically used as a criterion for statistical significance. In Table 7.20, the p value of the effect for problem set depends of the
value of the F ratio ($F = 9.716$), the *df* for problem set ($df = 1$), and the *df* for
error ($df = 38$).

In our example, we see that both main effects are statistically significant, but
the interaction between the dependent variables is not. Note that the ANOVA
summary (Table 7.20) does not tell us anything about the directionality or substantive implications of these differences. Only by inspecting the mean values for
the groups, shown in Table 7.19, can we conclude that the Hypertext access mode
is associated with higher improvement scores and that the case problems in set B
are more amenable to solution with aid from the database than the problems in set
A. Because there is no statistical interaction, this superiority of Hypertext access
is consistent across problem sets.

A statistical interaction would be in evidence if, for example, the Hypertext
group outperformed the Boolean group on set A, but the Boolean group outperformed the Hypertext group on set B. To see what a statistical interaction means,
it is frequently useful to make a plot of the group means, as shown in Figure 7.2,
which depicts the study results represented in Table 7.19. Departure from paral-
lelism of the lines is the indicator of a statistical interaction. In this case, the lines
are nearly parallel.

Special Issues

In this section it was possible only to scratch the surface of analysis of experimental data. To close this section of the chapter, we point to three special issues.

1. In the special case where a study has one independent variable with two levels,
we have the familiar situation where the *t*-test applies. Applying ANOVA to
this case yields the same results as the *t*-test, with $F = t^2$.

2. The analysis example discussed above pertains only to a completely randomized factorial design. The methods employed for other designs, including
nested and repeated measures designs, are variants on this example.

3. Appropriate use of ANOVA requires that the dependent variables are well
behaved in particular ways. If the distributions fail to meet the assumptions,
corrective actions such as transformations of the data may be required.

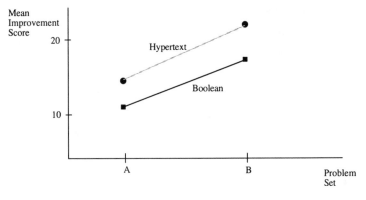

FIGURE 7.2. Graphing results as a way to visualize statistical interactions.

Self-Test 7.4

1. Given below are the data from the Hypercritic study discussed in Chapter 5. For these data, compute: (a) Hypercritic's accuracy, sensitivity, and specificity; (b) the value of chi-square; and (c) the value of Cohen's κ.

	Pooled rating by judges		
Hypercritic	Comment valid (≥ 5 judges)	Comment not valid (< 5 judges)	Total
Comment generated	145	24	169
Comment not generated	55	74	129
Total	200	98	298

2. Review scenario 3 in Self-Test 7.1. Hypothetical results of that study are summarized in the two tables below. Interpret these results. The first table gives means and standard deviations of the outcome measure, charges per patient, for each cell of the experiment. Note that $n = 6$ for each cell.

	Advice mode		
Hospital	Advice always provided	Advice when requested	No advice
A	58.8 ± 7.9	54.8 ± 5.8	67.3 ± 5.6
B	55.2 ± 7.4	56.0 ± 4.7	66.0 ± 7.5

The second table gives the ANOVA results.

Source	Sum-of-squares	df	Mean square	F ratio	p value
Main effects					
Hospital	12.250	1	12.250	0.279	0.601
Advice mode	901.056	2	450.528	10.266	< 0.000
Interaction					
Hospital					
by group	30.500	2	15.250	0.348	0.709
Error	1316.500	30	43.883		

Interpret these results.

3. Consider an alternative, hypothetical outcome of the information retrieval study as shown below. Make a plot of these results analogous to that in Figure 7.2. What would you conclude with regard to a possible statistical interaction?

	Mean ± SD, by assigned problem set	
Access mode	A	B
Boolean	19.3 ± 5.0 ($n = 11$)	12.4 ± 4.9 ($n = 11$)
Hypertext	15.7 ± 5.7 ($n = 10$)	21.8 ± 5.2 ($n = 10$)

Answers to Self-Tests

Self-Test 7.1

1. a. Independent variable(s): time with four levels.
   b. Dependent variable(s): attitude (presumably toward the new system); the measurement strategy is a questionnaire consisting of multiple items as the independent observations.
   c. Subjects are the hospital staff members.
   d. Control strategy is historical, before–after.
2. a. Independent variable(s): none, as this study is a descriptive one conducted in the laboratory.
   b. Dependent variable(s): agreement with definitive diagnosis, measured as yes–no for each case. The primary measurement strategy was completed earlier when the definitive diagnosis was established for each case, but also note that a further measurement challenge in this study may exist. It may not be clear in all cases whether the diagnosis offered by the system agrees with the definitive diagnosis, as the diagnostic categories built into the resource and those used to establish the definitive diagnosis may have been different.

In that situation, it may be necessary to create a panel to determine if the resource's diagnosis and the definitive diagnosis are in fact the same.

    c. Subjects in this particular study are the test cases themselves.

    d. There is no control strategy.

3. a. Independent variable(s): hospital (two levels) and mode of receiving advice (three levels).

    b. Dependent variable(s): charges related to drug therapy, averaged over all patients seen ("tasks") during the study period.

    c. Subjects are the physicians.

    d. Control strategy is simultaneous and nonrandomized, as physicians are not randomly assigned to hospitals.

4. a. Independent variable(s): whether care providers receive the reminders (two levels).

    b. Dependent variable(s): compliance by care providers with the action recommended by the reminders. The measurement strategy is a retrospective audit of patient care, with patients treated by care providers as the "tasks." For each patient it is necessary to determine whether the actions recommended by the reminders were followed.

    c. Subjects, in the most orthodox sense, are the clinical services because those are the units of randomization. The comparison of dependent variables would occur at the level of the clinical service, with $n = 6$ in each of the two study groups. (We have seen that it is also possible to consider care providers as subjects if we treat this design as hierarchical or nested.)

    d. Control strategy is simultaneous, randomized.

5. a. Independent variable(s): There are two independent variables: body system (GI or CV: two levels) and instructional mode (computer or lecture: two levels).

    b. Dependent variable(s): scores on knowledge tests. The measurement strategy is a written test consisting of several items.

    c. Subjects are the students.

    d. Control strategy is randomized with crossover.

Self-Test 7.2

Scenario 1: G1 (group 1): 6 months before, 1 week before, 1 month after, 6 months after.

Scenario 3:

Hospital	Mode of receiving advice		
	All patients	By request	None
A	G1	G2	G3
B	G4	G5	G6

Scenario 4:

	Intervention	
Services	Reminders	Control
A	G1	
B	G2	
C	G3	
D	G4	
E	G5	
F	G6	
G		G7
H		G8
I		G9
J		G10
K		G11
L		G12

Scenario 5:

	Studied by	
Body system	Computer	Lecture
CV	G1	G2
GI	G2	G1

Self-Test 7.3

1. Introduction of the new patient scheduling system is confounded with the move to new premises, which may be responsible for all the improvements in patient flow and teamwork. The baseline data are collected during the last month of working on the old site: Some staff may have left, others are helping to plan the move, so the data are atypical of current working patterns. The second 1-month data collection period starts too early: Staff are still adapting to the new scheduling system and patients will be adapting to the new premises. Also, any improvements observed may be due to unknown and unmeasured changes, such as a new organizational structure, new head of the clinic, or even the coming of Spring.

    Solution: Delay introduction of the patient scheduling system until 3 months after the move to new premises (which may prove organizationally beneficial too). Start the baseline study 1 month after the move, and delay the second data collection period until 2 months after introducing the new system to allow all staff to be trained with the system. In a before–after study such as this, it is impossible to exclude some unknown confounder. Measuring some aspect of patients the information system should not affect but any other changes might, such as patient satisfaction, may be helpful. This then becomes a before–after design with external controls.

2. The electronic request forms are more detailed than the paper forms, so some of the improvement in test orders are due not to the fact that orders are electronic but to the checklist effect (clinicians must fill out a more detailed form, so their decisions improve). Also, randomizing patients leads to carryover (contamination). Each doctor uses both electronic requests and paper requests, causing test ordering for paper-request patients to improve.

   Solution: To eliminate the checklist effect and quantify the benefit of electronic ordering per se, the control should be a paper version of the electronic request form; or the new electronic form could be a clone of the original paper form. To reduce carryover, doctors or even teams of doctors should be randomized.

3. This is a markedly atypical setting: Both the patients and the clinicians are unusual, so it is difficult to believe that the results will generalize to other hospitals. Also, the chief cardiologists' opinions about test ordering may not be shared elsewhere. Second, knowing that the chief of cardiology wrote the reminders and that their performance is being measured, junior staff improve their patient management anyway—the Hawthorne effect. Third, the chief cardiologist is judging the quality of test ordering "open"—knowing which doctors managed which patients from their record—so can easily infer for which patients the reminders were available, leading to an assessment bias.

   Solution: To improve generality, patients, doctors, and experts in test ordering from other centers should be involved in developing and evaluating the system. To reduce Hawthorne effects, two kinds of reminder could be made available to the junior doctors (e.g., test ordering to one group of doctors and prescribing to the another). The Hawthorne effect then influences both groups equally, and each can act as a control for the other. To eliminate assessment bias, the appropriateness of test (or drug) ordering must be judged blind to the reminders the doctor received. This means extracting enough data to make the judgment from each patient's notes or otherwise obscuring the identity of the doctor managing the patient and if any reminders were received.

Self-Test 7.4

1. (a) Accuracy $= (145 + 74)/298 = 0.73$; sensitivity $= 145/200 = 0.72$; specificity $= 74/98 = 0.75$. (b) chi-square $= 61.8$ (highly significant with $df = 1$). (c) $\kappa = 0.44$.
2. By inspection of the ANOVA table, the only significant effect is the main effect for the advice mode. There is no interaction between hospital and group, and there is no difference, across groups, in mean charges for the two hospitals. Examining the table of means and standard deviations, we see how the means are consistent across the two hospitals. The mean for all subjects in hospital A is 60.3 and the mean for all subjects in hospital B is 59.1. This small difference is indicative of the lack of a main effect for hospitals. Also note that, even though the means for groups vary, the pattern of this variation is the same

across the two hospitals. The main effect for the groups is seen in the differences in the means for each group. It appears that the difference occurs between the "no advice" group and the other two groups. Although the F test used in ANOVA can tell us only if a global difference exists across the three groups, methods exist to test differences between levels of the dependent variables.

3. Nonparallelism of lines is clearly suggestive of an interaction. A test using ANOVA is required to confirm that the interaction is statistically significant.

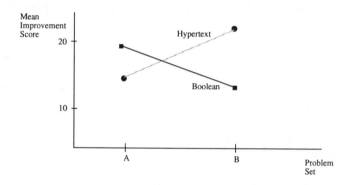

References

1. Donabedian A: 1966. Evaluating the quality of medical care. Millbank Mem Q 1966; 44:166–206.
2. Wasson JH, Sox HC, Neff RK, Goldman L: Clinical prediction rules: applications and methodological standards. N Engl J Med 1985;313:793–799.
3. Wyatt J, Spiegelhalter D: Evaluating medical expert systems: what to test and how? Med Inf (Lond) 1990;15:205–217.
4. Schwartz D, Lellouch J: Explanatory and pragmatic attitudes in therapeutic trials. J Chron Dis 1967;20:637–648.
5. Anderson C: Measuring what works in health care. Science 1994;263:1080–1081.
6. Byar DP: Why data bases should not replace randomised controlled clinical trials. Biometrics 1980;36:337–342.
7. Altman D: Practical Statistics for Medical Research. London: Chapman & Hall, 1991.
8. Cochran WG, Cox GM: Experimental Designs. New York: Wiley, 1957.
9. Winer BJ: Statistical Principles in Experimental Design. New York: McGraw Hill, 1991.
10. Buck C, Donner A: The design of controlled experiments in the evaluation of non-therapeutic interventions. J Chronic Dis 1982;35:531–538.
11. Diwan VK, Eriksson B, Sterky G, Tomson G: Randomization by group in studying the effect of drug information in primary care. Int J Epidemiol 1992;21:124–130.
12. Grimshaw JM, Russell IT: Effect of clinical guidelines on medical practice: a systematic review of rigorous evaluations. Lancet 1993;342:1317–1322.

13. Adams ID, Chan M, Clifford PC, et al: Computer aided diagnosis of acute abdominal pain: a multicentre study. BMJ 1986;293:800–804.
14. Myers DH, Leahy A, Shoeb H, Ryder J: The patient's view of life in a psychiatric hospital: a questionnaire study and associated methodological considerations. Brit J Psychiatry 1990;156:853–860.
15. Van Way CW, Murphy JR, Dunn EL, Elerding SC: A feasibility study of computer-aided diagnosis in appendicitis. Surg Gynecol Obstet 1982;155:685–688.
16. Wyatt JC, Altman DG: Prognostic models: clinically useful, or quickly forgotten? BMJ 1995;311:1539–1541.
17. Knaus W, Wagner D, Lynn J: Short term mortality predictions for critically ill hospitalised patients: science and ethics. Science 1991;254:389–394.
18. Sacks H, Chalmers TC, Smith H: Randomised vs. historical controls for clinical trials. Am J Med 1982;72:233–240.
19. Cornfield J: Randomisation by group: a formal analysis. Am J Epidemiol 1978; 108:100–102.
20. Tierney WM, Overhage JM, McDonald CJ: A plea for controlled trials in medical informatics. J Am Med Inf Assoc 1994;1:353–355.
21. Lyon HC Jr, Healy JC, Bell JR, et al: PlanAlyzer, an interactive computer-assisted program to teach clinical problem solving in diagnosing anemia and coronary artery disease. Acad Med 1992;67:821–828.
22. McDonald CJ, Hui SL, Smith DM, et al: Reminders to physicians from an introspective computer medical record. A two-year randomized trial. Ann Intern Med 1984; 100:130–138.
23. Freiman JA, Chalmers TC, Smith H, Kuebler RR: The importance of beta, the Type II error and sample size in the design and interpretation of the randomised controlled trial. N Engl J Med 1978;299:690–694.
24. Cohen J: Statistical Power Analysis for the Behavioral Sciences. Hillsdale, NJ: Lawrence Erlbaum, 1988.
25. Wyatt J: Lessons learned from the field trial of ACORN, an expert system to advise on chest pain. In: Barber B, Cao D, Qin D (eds) Proceedings of the Sixth World Conference on Medical Informatics, Singapore. Amsterdam: North Holland 1989:111–115.
26. Yu VL, Fagan LM, Wraith SM, et al: Antimicrobial selection by computer: a blinded evaluation by infectious disease experts. JAMA 1979;242:1279–1282.
27. Schultz KF, Chalmers I, Hayes RJ, Altman DG: Dimensions of methodological quality associated with estimates of treatment effects in controlled trials. JAMA 1995; 273:408–412.
28. Roethligsburger FJ, Dickson WJ: Management and the Worker. Cambridge, MA: Harvard University Press, 1939.
29. Parsons HM: What happened at Hawthorne ? Science 1974;183:922–932.
30. Pozen MW, d'Agostino RB, Selker HP Sytkowski PA, Hood WB: A predictive instrument to improve coronary care unit admission in acute ischaemic heart disease. N Eng J Med 1984;310:1273–1278.
31. Murray GD, Murray LS, Barlow P, et al: Assessing the performance and clinical impact of a computerized prognostic system in severe head injury. Stat Med 1986; 5:403–410.
32. deBliek R, Friedman CP, Wildemuth BM. Martz JM, Twarog RG, File D: Information retieval from a database and the augmentation of personal knowledge. J Am Med Inf Assoc 1994;1:328–338.
33. Cartmill RSV, Thornton JG: Effect of presentation of partogram information on obstetric decision-making. Lancet 1992;339:1520–1522.

34. Suermondt HJ, Cooper GF: An evaluation of explanations of probabilistic inference. Comput Biomed Res 1993;26:242–254.
35. Horrocks JC, Lambert DE, McAdam WAF, et al: Transfer of computer-aided diagnosis of dyspepsia from one geographical area to another. Gut 1976;17:640–644.
36. Centor RM, Yarbrough B, Wood JP: Inability to predict relapse in acute asthma. New Eng J Med 1984;310:577–580.
37. Hart A, Wyatt J: Evaluating black boxes as medical decision-aids: issues arising from a study of neural networks. Med Inf (Lond) 1990;15:229–236.
38. Wellwood J, Spiegelhalter DJ, Johannessen S: How does computer-aided diagnosis improve the management of acute abdominal pain ? Ann R Coll Surg Engl 1992;74:140–146.
39. Indurkhya N, Weiss SM: Models for measuring performance of medical expert systems. AI Med 1989;1:61–70.
40. Titterington DM, Murray GD, Murray LS, et al: Comparison of discriminant techniques applied to a complex data set of head injured patients (with discussion). J R Stat Soc A 1981;144:145–175.
41. Wald N: Rational use of investigations in clinical practice. In: Hopkins A (ed) Appropriate Investigation and Treatment in Medical Practice. London: Royal College of Physicians, 1990:7–20.
42. Cohen J: Weighted kappa: nominal scale agreement with provision for scaled disagreement or partial credit. Psychol Bull 1968;70:213–220.
43. Fleiss JL. Measuring agreement between two judges on the presence or absence of a trait. Biometrics 1975;31:357–370.
44. Hilden J, Habbema DF: Evaluation of clinical decision-aids: more to think about. Med Inf (Lond) 1990;15:275–284.
45. Hanley JA, McNeil BJ: The meaning and use of the area under a receiver operating characteristic (ROC) curve. Radiology 1982;143:29–36.
46. Swets JA: Measuring the accuracy of diagnostic systems. Science 1988;240:1285–1293.
47. O'Neil M, Glowinski A: Evaluating and validating very large knowledge-based systems. Med Inf 1990;15:237–252.
48. Bobbio et al: Completeness of reporting trial results: effect on physicians' willingness to prescribe. Lancet 1994;343:1209–1211.
49. Friedman CP, Wildemuth BM, Gant SP, Muriuki M, File DD: A comparison of Boolean and Hypertext access to a basic science database. Presented to the Annual Conference on Research in Medical Education, November 1995 [abstract].
50. Habbema JDF, Hilden J, Bjerregaard B: The measurement of performance in probabilistic diagnosis; general recommendations. Meth Inf Med 1981;20:97–100.
51. Murphy AH, Winkler RL: Probability forecasting in meteorology. J Amer Statist Assoc 1984;79:489–500.

Appendix A: Further Indices Derived from Contingency Table Analysis, Including Calibration

As well as issuing output, some decision support systems also estimate the probability that their output is true or use a qualitative term corresponding to a probability range. For example, the system may state "Diagnosis **D** is likely" when the calculated probability of **D** lies between 0.7 and 0.9. If the information resource's probability estimate is overoptimistic or pessimistic, it may mislead the user just as much as if the wrong diagnosis was given.

It is important to measure the accuracy of the probability estimate, or its "calibration." To measure calibration, evaluators should divide the test cases up into ten "bins" according to which probability band they were assigned by the information resource: 0.01–0.10, 0.11–0.20, and so on. The number of test cases in each probability band from $p(D) = m$ to $p(D) = n$ in which the information resource's output was correct should then be divided by the total number of cases allocated to that band, to give $p(\text{correct})_{m\text{-}n}$:

$$p(\text{correct}) = \frac{[N(\text{output correct} \cap (m \leq p(D) < n)]}{N(m \leq p(D) < n)}$$

where $N(...)$ indicates the number of cases satisfying the condition.

If the probability estimate is accurate, $p(\text{correct})_{m\text{-}n}$ should equal $(m + n)/2$. If this equality holds throughout the range of probability estimates, the information resource's output is said to be well calibrated. Although it is possible to derive a single measure for calibration,[50] a useful method to explore calibration is to plot $P(\text{correct})_{m\text{-}n}$ against $p(D)$. A sample of such a curve, showing the excellent calibration that can be achieved, is given in Figure 7.3. There are a number of other methods for summarizing the calibration and precision of predictions, such as the Brier score[51] and proper scoring rules, which penalize predictive errors in proportion to their direction and size.

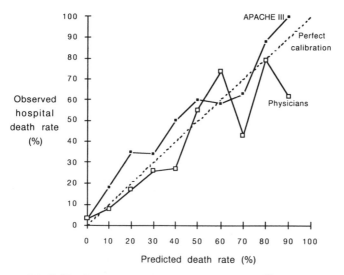

FIGURE 7.3. Calibration curve. (Redrawn from Knaus et al.,[17] with permission.)

8

Subjectivist Approaches to Evaluation

As usual, the most significant results of the project are not measurable with a t-*test.*

(M. Musen, summarizing his experience with a 5-year project, personal communication, 1996)

With this chapter we turn a corner. The previous four chapters have dealt almost exclusively with objectivist approaches to evaluation. These approaches are useful for answering some, but by no means all, of the interesting and important questions that challenge investigators in medical informatics. The subjectivist approaches, introduced here and in Chapter 9, address the problem of evaluation from a different set of premises as first discussed in Chapter 2. These premises derive from philosophical views that may be unfamiliar and perhaps even discomforting to some readers. They challenge some fundamental beliefs about scientific method and the validity of our understanding of the world that develops from objectivist research. They argue that, particularly within the realm of evaluation of information resources, the kind of "knowing" that develops from subjectivist studies may be as useful as that which derives from objectivist studies. While reading what follows, it may be tempting to dismiss subjectivist methods as informal, imprecise, or "subjective." When carried out well, however, these studies are none of the above. They are equally objective, but in a different way. Professionals in informatics, even those who choose not to conduct subjectivist studies, can come to appreciate the rigor, validity, and value of this work.

Chapter 2 introduced four subjectivist approaches to evaluation: connoisseurship, quasi-legal, professional review, and illuminative/responsive. Chapters 8 and 9 focus on what we have called the illuminative/responsive approach to evaluation. This approach is rooted in the disciplinary traditions of ethnography and social anthropology, which in turn have been extensively applied to the general problem of evaluating social programs, educational programs, and information technology. Our emphasis on this approach derives from the applicability it has found in evaluation and from the extensive methodological literature that has developed for it over the past three decades. Appendix A lists several books that describe the methodology in more detail than we can provide here.

The major goals of this chapter are to establish the scientific legitimacy of subjectivist methods and a general framework for understanding how studies using these methods are conducted. Chapter 9 provides a much more detailed tour through the methods of illuminative/responsive evaluation and seeks to provide insight into how the thought processes of those who conduct these studies must differ from those who do objectivist work.

Motivation for Subjectivist Studies: What People Really Want to Know

In Chapter 2 we presented some prototypical evaluation questions.

- Is the information resource working as intended?
- How can it be improved?
- Does it make any difference?
- Are the differences it makes beneficial?
- Are the observed effects those envisioned by the developers or are they different?

We also noted that we could append "why or why not?" to each of these questions listed above. The reader should take a moment to examine these questions carefully and begin to think about how we might go about answering them. When subjected to such further scrutiny, the questions quickly become more ornate and intricate.

- Is the resource working as intended?

  As who intended? Were the intentions set realistically? Did these intentions shift over time? What is it really like to use this resource as part of everyday professional activity?

- How can it be improved?

  How does one distinguish important from idiosyncratic suggestions for improvement? Which suggestions should be addressed?

- Does it make any difference?

  Was it needed in the first place? What features are making the difference?

- Are the differences it makes beneficial?

  To whom? From whose point of view? Are all the pertinent views represented?

- Are the observed effects those envisioned by the developers or are they different?

  How do you detect what you do not anticipate?

The more specific, more explanatory, and more probing questions, shown in italics, are often what those who commission evaluation studies—and others who have interest in an information resource—want to know. Some of these deeper questions are difficult to answer using objectivist approaches to evaluation. It may be that these questions are never discussed, or are deferred as interesting but "sub-jective" issues, during discussions of what should be the foci of an evaluation study. These questions may never be asked in a formal or official sense because of a perception that the methods do not exist to answer them in a credible way. This chapter and Chapter 9 beg the reader to suspend his or her own tendencies to this belief.

Many of these deeper questions derive their importance from life in a pluralistic world. As discussed in Chapters 1 and 2, information resources are typically introduced into complex organizations where there exist competing value systems: different beliefs about what is "good" and what is "right," which translate into different beliefs about what changes induced by information resources would constitute benefits. These beliefs are real to the people who hold them and difficult to change. Indeed, there are many actors playing many roles in any real-world setting where an information resource is introduced. Each actor, as an individual and a member of multiple groups, brings a unique viewpoint to questions about fuzzy constructs such as need, quality, and benefit. If these constructs are explored in an evaluation study, perhaps the actors should not be expected to agree about what these constructs mean and how to measure them. Perhaps need, quality, and benefit do not inhere in an information resource. Perhaps they are dependent on the observer as well as the observed. Perhaps evaluation studies should be conducted in ways that document how these various individuals and groups "see" the resource, and not in ways that assume there is a consensus when there is no reason to believe one exists. Perhaps there are many "truths" about an information resource, not just one.

Definition of the Responsive/Illuminative Approach

The responsive/illuminative approach to evaluation is designed to address the deeper questions: the detailed "whys" and "according to whoms" in addition to the aggregate "whethers" and "whats." As defined in Chapter 2, the responsive/ illuminative approach seeks to represent the viewpoints of those who are users of the resource or otherwise significant participants in the clinical environment where the resource operates. The goal is "illumination" rather than judgment. The investigators seek to build an argument that promotes deeper understanding of the information resource or environment of which it is a part. The methods used derive largely from ethnography. The investigators immerse themselves physically in the environment where the information resource is or will be operational and collect data primarily through observations, interviews, and reviews of documents. The designs—the data collection plans—of these studies are not rigidly predetermined and do not unfold in a fixed sequence. They develop dynamically and nonlinearly as the investigators' experience accumulates. The study team begins with a minimal set of orienting questions; the deeper questions that receive more thorough study evolve from initial investigation. Investigators keep records of all data collected and the methods used to collect and analyze them. Reports of reponsive/illuminative studies tend to be written narratives. Such studies can be conducted before, during, or after the introduction of an information resource.

Support for Subjectivist Approaches

It is not surprising that endorsements for subjectivist approaches come from those who routinely undertake such studies. A more compelling endorsement may come from designers of information resources themselves who believe that subjectivist methods can provide a deeper understanding of their own work and thus more useful information to guide their future efforts. As suggested by the quotation which began this chapter, the results of a study, when reduced to tables and tests of statistical significance, may no longer capture what the developers see as most important. To the extent that a study is "for" the developers, this can be a serious shortcoming.

Although subjectivist approaches may run counter to most readers' notions of how one conducts empirical investigations, these methods and their conceptual underpinnings are not at all foreign to the worlds of information and computer science. The pluralistic, nonlinear thinking that underlies subjectivist investigation shares many features with modern conceptualizations of the information resource design process. Consider the following statements from two highly regarded works addressing issues central to design. Winograd and Flores[1] argued that:

In designing computer-based devices, we are not in the position of creating a formal 'system' that covers the functioning of the organization and the people within it. When this is attempted, the resulting system (and the space of potential action for people within it) is inflexible and unable to cope with new breakdowns or potentials. Instead we design additions and changes to the network of equipment (some of it computer based) within which people work. The computer is like a tool, in that is brought up for use by people engaged in some domain of action. The use of the tool shapes the potential for what those actions are and how they are conducted....Its power does not lie in having a single purpose...but in its connection to the larger network of communication (electronic, telephone, paper-based) in which organizations operate [p. 170].

Norman[2] added:

Tools affect more than the ease with which we do things; they can dramatically affect our view of ourselves, society, and the world [p. 209].

These thoughts from the work of system design alert us to the multiple forces that shape the "effects" of introducing an information resource, the unpredictable character of these forces, and the many viewpoints on these effects that exist. These sentiments are highly consonant with the premises underlying the subjectivist evaluation approaches.

Another connection is to the methodology of formal systems analysis, generally accepted as an essential component of information resource development. Systems analysis uses many methods that resemble closely the subjectivist methods for evaluation that we introduce here. It is recognized that systems analysis requires a process of information gathering about the present system before a design for an improved future system can be inferred. Systems analysis requires a process of information gathering, heavily reliant on interviews with those who use the existing system in various ways. Information gathering for systems analysis is typically portrayed as a cyclical, iterative process rather than a linear process.[3] In the literature of systems analysis we find admonitions, analogous to those made by proponents of subjectivist evaluation, about an approach that is too highly structured. An overly structured approach can misportray the capabilities of workers in the system's environment, misportray the role of informal communication in the work accomplished, underestimate the prevalence of exceptions, and fail to account for political forces within every organization that shape much of what happens.[4] Within the field of systems analysis, then, there has developed an appreciation of some of the shortcomings of objectivist methods and the potential value of subjectivist methods drawn from ethnography that we discuss here.[5]

Also worthy of note is the high regard in which studies using subjectivist methods are held when these studies are well conducted. In medicine, one prominent example is Becker's classic *Boys in White*.[6] Another is Bosk's superb work, *Forgive and Remember: Managing Medical Failure*.[7] Several valuable studies in informatics are introduced in the following section.

When Are Subjectivist Studies Useful in Informatics?

It is possible to argue that subjectivist approaches are applicable at all stages of development of an information resource, but they are most clearly applicable at two points in this continuum. First, as part of the design process, a subjectivist study can document the need for the resource and clarify its potential niche within a given work environment.[8, 9] Indeed, it is possible for system developers to misread or misinterpret the needs and beliefs of potential users of an information resource[10, 11] in ways that could lead to failure of an entire project. Formal subjectivist methods, if applied appropriately, can clarify these issues and direct resource development toward a more valid understanding of user needs. There is already a substantial literature and sense of general support for use of subjectivist methods at the design stage of a resource.[8–12] At this point, the relation between subjectivist evaluation and the methods of formal systems analysis is most evident.

Second, after an information resource is mature and has been tested in laboratory studies, further study using subjectivist approaches can describe the impact of the resource on the work environments in which it is installed.[13–15] At this developmental stage the insights that can derive from objectivist and subjectivist studies are different and potentially complementary.[16] Objectivist methodology, and specifically the comparison-based approach, has dominated the literature on the impact of information resources. The randomized clinical trial has been put forward as the standard against which such studies should be measured.[17] Although the randomized trial can estimate the magnitude of an "effect of interest" for an information resource, this method cannot elucidate the meaning of this effect for users of the resource and other interested parties and typically sheds little light on whether the "effect of interest" was the effect of most importance. Whether the impact of a resource is better established by objectivist methods derived from the clinical-trials tradition or by subjectivist methods derived from the ethnographic tradition is and should be a matter of ongoing discussion. Overall, subjectivist study of deployed information resources remains an unexploited opportunity in medical informatics.

Rigorous, But Different, Methodology

The subjectivist approaches to evaluation, like their objectivist counterparts, are empirical methods. Although it is easy to focus only on their differences, these two broad classes of evaluation approaches share many features. In all empirical studies, for example, evidence is collected with great care; the investigator is always aware of what he or she is doing and why. The evidence is then compiled, interpreted, and ultimately reported. Investigators keep records of their procedures, and these records are open to audit by the investigators themselves or by individuals outside the study team. The principal investigator or evaluation team leader is under an almost sacred scientific obligation to report the methods in detail, ideally in enough detail to enable another investigator to replicate the study. Failure to do that invalidates a study. The two approaches also share a dependence on theories that guide investigators toward explanations of the phenomena they observe as well as a dependence on the pertinent empirical literature: published studies that address similar phenomena or similar settings. With both classes of approaches there are rules of good practice that are generally accepted. It is therefore possible to distinguish a good study from a bad one. Finally, a neophyte can learn both types of research, initially by reading textbooks and other methodological literature (see Appendix A) and ultimately by conducting studies under the guidance of experienced mentors.

There are, however, many fundamental differences between objectivist and subjectivist approaches. First and foremost, subjectivist studies are "emergent" in design. Objectivist studies typically begin with a set of hypotheses or specific questions and a plan for addressing each member of this set. There is also an assumption by the investigator that, barring major unforeseen developments, the plan will be followed exactly. (When objectivist researchers deviate from their plan, they do so apologetically.) To do otherwise, in fact, might introduce bias, as the investigator who sees negative results emerging from the exploration of a particular question or use of a particular measurement instrument might change strategies in the hope of obtaining more positive findings. By contrast, subjectivist studies typically begin with some general "orienting issues" that stimulate the early stages of investigation. Through these initial investigations, the important questions for further study begin to emerge. The subjectivist investigator is willing, at virtually any point, to adjust future aspects of the study in light of the most recent information obtained. Subjectivist investigators are incrementalists; they live from day to day and have a high tolerance for ambiguity and uncertainty. (In this respect, they are much like good software developers.) Also like software developers, skilled subjectivist investigators must develop the ability to recognize when a project is finished: when further benefit can be obtained only at great cost in time and effort.

A second feature of subjectivist studies is a "naturalistic" orientation: a reluctance to manipulate the setting of the study, which in most cases is the environment into which the information resource is introduced. To do otherwise might alter the environment in order to study it. Control groups, placebos, purposefully altering information resources to create contrasting interventions, and other techniques central to the construction of objectivist studies are typically not used. Subjectivist studies do employ quantitative data for descriptive purposes and may additionally offer quantitative comparisons when the research setting offers up a natural experiment where such comparisons can be made without altering the setting under direct study. Subjectivist researchers are opportunists where pertinent information is concerned; they use what they see as the best information available to illuminate a question under investigation.

A third important distinguishing feature of subjectivist studies is that they result in reports written in narrative prose. Although these reports can be lengthy and may require a more significant time investment on the part of the reader, no technical understanding of quantitative research methodology or statistics is required to comprehend them. Results of subjectivist studies are therefore accessible—and even entertaining—to a broad community in a way that results of objectivist studies are not. Reports of subjectivist studies seek to engage their audience.

Subjectivist Arguments and Their Philosophical Premises

Subjectivist studies do not seek to prove or demonstrate. They strive for insightful description—what has been called "thick description"[18]—leading to deeper understanding of the phenomenon under study. They offer an argument; they seek to persuade rather than demonstrate.[19]*

It has been emphasized that the purpose of evaluation is to be useful to various "stakeholders": those with a need to know. These needs vary from study to study, and within a given study the needs vary across the different stakeholder groups and over time. A major feature of subjectivist approaches is their responsiveness[20] to these needs. The foci of a study are formulated though a process of negotiation, to ensure their relevance from the outset. These foci can be changed in light of accumulating evidence to guarantee their continuing relevance. Subjectivist methods are therefore concordant with the basic tenets of evaluation as a process that, in order to be successful, must be useful in addition to truthful.

As our discussion of subjectivist methods unfolds, it becomes clear that there are numerous features working to ensure that well-executed studies meet the dual criteria of utility and veracity. At this point, we might ask whether a method that is so open-ended and responsive can also generate confidence in the veracity of the findings. We come immediately to the issue of what makes evidence credible.

---

* At this point, the reader is encouraged to refer to the Evaluation Mindset section of Chapter 2 to see the concordance between subjectivist methods and the broad purposes of evaluation as described earlier.

Objectivist studies rely on methods of quantitative measurement, discussed in great detail earlier in this book, which in turn are based on the principle of inter-subjectivity, what might also be called *quantitative objectivity*.[21] Simply stated, this principle holds that the more independent observers who agree with an observation, the more likely it is to be correct. (Recall that in Chapter 5 we developed a specific methodology for implementing this principle.) Indeed, within the objectivist mindset, unless we can show that several observers agree to an acceptable extent, their observations are prima facie not credible. One observer is not to be trusted. By contrast, the principle of *qualitative objectivity* is central to subjectivist work. It holds that an experienced, unbiased observer is capable of making fundamentally truthful observations and may in fact be superior to a panel of observers who agree but are all wrong because of some bias they share. Subjectivist approaches can be seen to be as objective (i.e., truthful) as objectivist studies. They rely, however, on a different definition of objectivity.

We can also contrast objectivist and subjectivist approaches on the ways they address issues of cause and effect. How can cause-and-effect relations be established without the experimental control customary to randomized trials? In subjectivist research a case for cause and effect can be made in much the same way that a detective determines the perpetrator of a crime or a forensic pathologist infers cause of death.[22] Through detailed examination of evidence, the investigator recreates the pertinent story, often depicting in great detail a number of critical events or incidents. Via this portrayal, the investigator crafts a logical, compelling case for cause and effect. In the end, such a portrayal can be as compelling as the result of a controlled experiment that is subject to the manifold biases described in Chapter 7.

Natural History of a Subjectivist Study

As a first step in describing the methodology of subjectivist evaluation, Figure 8.1 illustrates the stages or natural history of a study. These stages comprise a general sequence; but, as mentioned earlier, the subjectivist investigator must always be prepared to revise his or her thinking and possibly return to earlier stages in light of new evidence. Backtracking is a legitimate aspect of this model.

1. *Negotiation of the "ground rules" of the study:* During any empirical research, and particularly for evaluation studies, it is important to negotiate an understanding between the study team and those commissioning the study. This understanding should embrace the general aims of the study; the kinds of methods to be used; access to various sources of information including health care providers, patients, and documents; and the format for interim and final reports. The aims of the study might be formlulated in a set of initial "orienting questions." Ideally, this understanding is expressed in a memorandum of understanding, analogous to a contract, signed by all interested parties. By analogy to a contract, these ground rules can be changed during a study with the consent of all parties. (Although essential to a subjectivist study, a memo of understanding or evaluation contract is recommended for all studies, irrespective of methodology employed.)

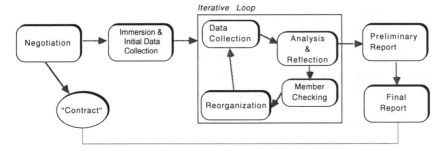

FIGURE 8.1. Natural history of a subjectivist study.

2a. *Immersion into the environment:* At this stage the investigators begin spending time in the work environment. The activities range from formal introductions to informal conversations and the silent presence of the investigators at meetings and other events. Investigators use the generic term "field" to refer to the setting, which may be multiple physical locations, where the work under study is carried out. Trust and openness between the investigators and those in the field are essential elements of subjectivist studies. If a subjectivist study is in fact to generate insights with minimal alteration of the envrionment under study, those in the field must feel sufficiently comfortable with the presence of the investigators to go about their work in the customary way. Therefore, time invested in building such a relationship pays compound interest in the future.

2b. *Initial data collection to focus the questions:* Even as immersion is taking place, the investigator is already collecting data to sharpen the initial questions or issues guiding the study. The early discussions with those in field and other activities primarily targeted toward immersion inevitably begin to shape the investigators' views. Immersion and initial data collection are labeled "2a" and "2b" to convey their close interaction. Almost from the outset, the investigator is typically addressing several aspects of the study simultaneously.

3. *Iterative loop:* At this point the procedural structure of the study becomes akin to an iterative loop as the investigator engages in cycles of data collection, analysis and reflection, and reorganization. Data collection involves interview, observation, document analysis, and other methods. Data are collected on planned occasions as well as serendipidously or spontaneously. The data are carefully recorded and interpreted in the context of what is already known. Reflection entails the contemplation of the new findings during each cycle of the loop. Reorganization results in a revised agenda for data collection in the next cycle of the loop.

Although each cycle within the iterative loop is depicted as linear, even this is somewhat misleading. The net progress through the loop is clockwise, as shown in Figure 8.1, but backward steps are natural and inevitable. They are not reflective of mistakes or errors. An investigator may, after conducting a series of interviews and studying what participants have said, decide to speak again with one or two participants to clarify their positions on a particular issue.

An important element of the iterative loop, which can be considered part of the reflection process, is sharing of the investigator's own thoughts and beliefs with the participants themselves. (This step is called "member checking" and is discussed in more detail in Chapter 9.) With objectivist research, member checking would "unblind" the study and introduce catastrophic bias. With subjectivist research, the views of informed participants on the investigators' evolving conclusions are considered a key resource.

4. *Preliminary report:* The first draft of the final report should itself be viewed as a research instrument. By sharing this report with a variety of individuals, a major check on the validity of the findings can be obtained. Typically, reactions to the preliminary report generate useful clarifications and a general sharpening of the study findings. Sometimes (but rarely if previous stages of the study have been carried out with care), reactions to the preliminary report generate major needs for further data to be collected. Because the report is usually a narrative, it is vitally important that it be well written, in language understood by all intended audiences. Circulation of the report in draft can ensure that the final document communicates as intended. Liberal use of anonymous quotations from interviews and documents makes a report highly vivid and meaningful to readers.

5. *Final report:* The final report, once completed, should be distributed as negotiated in the original memo of understanding. In subjectivist evaluation studies, distribution of the report is often accompanied by "meet the investigator" sessions that allow interested persons to explore the study findings interactively and in greater depth.

As shown in Figure 8.2, the natural history of a subjectivist study results in the progressive focusing of issues. The process was well described by Parlett and Hamilton.[23]

The transition from stage to stage, as the investigation unfolds, occurs as problem areas become progressively clarified and re-defined. The course of the study cannot be charted in advance. Beginning with an extensive data base, the researchers systematically reduce the breadth of their enquiry to give more concentrated attention to the emerging issues. This "progressive focusing" permits unique and unpredicted phenomena to be given due weight. It reduces the problem of data overload and prevents the accumulation of a mass of unanalyzed material [p. 18].

Data Collection Methods

What data collection strategies are in the subjectivist researcher's black bag? There are several, and they are typically used in combination. We discuss each one assuming a typical setting for a subjectivist study in medical informatics: the introduction of an information resource into patient care activities in a hospital.

1. *Observation:* Investigators typically immerse themselves in the setting under study. It is done in two ways. The investigator may act purely as a detached observer, becoming a trusted, unobtrusive feature of the environment but not a participant in the day-to-day work and thus reliant on multiple "informants" as

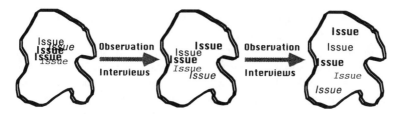

FIGURE 8.2. Process of progressive focusing.

sources of information. True to the naturalistic feature of this kind of study, great care is taken during the investigator's immersion into the environment. This diminishes the possibility that the presence of the observer will skew the work activities that occur, or that the observer will be rejected outright by the ward team. An alternative approach is participant-observation where the investigator becomes a member of the work team. Participant-observation is more difficult to engineer, as it may require the investigator to have training in some aspect of health care. It is also much more time-consuming but can give the investigator a more vivid impression of life in the work environment. During both kinds of observation, data accrue continuously. These data are qualitative and may be of several varieties: statements by health care providers and patients, gestures and other nonverbal expressions of these same individuals, and characteristics of the physical setting that seem to affect the delivery of health care.

2. *Interviews:* Subjectivist studies rely heavily on interviews. Formal interviews are occasions where both the investigator and interviewee are aware that the answers to questions are being recorded (on paper or tape) for direct contribution to the evaluation study. Formal interviews vary in their degree of structure. At one extreme is the unstructured interview where there are no predetermined questions. Between the extremes is the semistructured interview where the investigator specifies in advance a set of topics he or she would like to address but is flexible as to the order in which these topics are addressed and open to discussion of topics not on the prespecified list. At the other extreme is the structured interview with a schedule of questions that are always presented in the same words and in the same order. In general, the unstructured and semistructured interviews are preferred for subjectivist research. Informal interviews, spontaneous discussions between the investigators and members of a ward team as occur during routine observation, are also part of the data collection process. Informal interviews are invariably considered a source of important data.

3. *Document/artifact analysis:* Every project produces a trail of papers and other artifacts: patient charts, various versions of a computer program and its documentation, memos prepared by the project team. Unlike the day-to-day events of patient care, these artifacts do not change once created or introduced. They can be examined retrospectively and referred to repeatedly as necessary over the course of a study. Also included under this heading are so-called unobtrusive measures, which are records accrued as part of the routine use of the information resource.

They include, for example, user log files of an information resource. Data from these measures are often quantifiable.

4. *Anything else that seems useful:* Subjectivist investigators are supreme opportunists. As questions of importance to a study emerge, the investigator collects the best information he or she perceives to bear on these questions. This does not preclude clinical chart reviews, questionnaires, tests, simulated patients and other methods more commonly associated with the objectivist approaches. Rarely, however, does a subjectivist study deliberately manipulate the work setting, as is common to objectivist experiments, for the purpose of collecting data.

Qualitative Data Recording and Analysis

As mentioned earlier, subjectivist researchers keep careful records of their procedures and are extremely diligent in their handling of qualitative data. Data gathered from observations, interviews, and document analysis are recorded and usually reviewed within 24 hours of the initial recording. In the case of interviews and other discussions with participants in the work setting, this review is particularly important if there is no permanent record of the discussion on tape and the only documentation that exists is the investigator's own notes ("trigger notes") rapidly jotted during the conversation. Even when the interview has been tape recorded, listening to the tape soon after the interview was conducted can stimulate thoughts that might not occur to the investigator later. During this review the investigator should annotate the notes, being careful to maintain the distinction between what was recorded during the interview itself and what is subsequent annotation or interpretation. Some investigators do this by writing their annotations in a different color than the original notes; others use a two column format where original notes appear on the left, annotations on the right. A careful investigator must also distinguish between verbatim quotations and different degrees of paraphrase of what an interviewee said.

There are many procedures for analyzing qualitative data. The important thing to note is that the analysis is conducted systematically. In general terms, the investigator looks for themes or trends emerging from several sources. Thus it is important to be able to collate individual statements and observations by theme as well as by source. Some investigators transfer these observations to file cards so they can be sorted and resorted in a variety of ways. Others use software especially designed to facilitate analysis of qualitative data.[24] At the present level of technology, the investigator must key in all his or her handwritten notes, but the flexibility afforded by the software often justifies the effort. Pen-based computers may eventually change the way subjectivist research is carried out.

The analysis process is fluid, with analytical goals shifting as the study becomes more mature. At an early stage the goal is primarily to focus the questions that are to be the targets of further data elicitation. At the later stages of study, the primary goal is to collate data that address these questions. The investigator must recognize that the data often raise new questions in addition to answering pre-existing ones. Sometimes new data do not alter the basic conclusions of a study but reveal to the investigator a significant reorganization of the results that lends greater clarity to their exposition. (This situation is analogous to a linear transformation in mathematics; the same information is contained in the set but is expressed relative to a different and more useful set of axes.)

It should be clear that subjectivist study requires a different frame of mind on the part of the investigator. The agenda is never closed. The investigator must always be alert to new information that may require a systemic reorganization of everything he or she has done so far. For these reasons, many heuristic strategies and safeguards are built into the process. Just as there are well-documented procedures for collecting data while conducting subjectivist studies, there is also a set of strategies used by investigators to validate results and insights. A few are noted here and are discussed in more detail in Chapter 9.

Triangulation is a strong check on the veracity of study findings. The subjectivist researcher looks across different types of information (observation of work events, interviews of individuals from a variety of roles, analysis of documents) to determine if a consistent picture emerges for any given theme of the results. This is the subjectivist analogy to the objectivist strategy of using multiple, independent measures to estimate the quantitative error in a measurement process.

Of course, it is possible that the study is generating accurate answers to the questions it explored, but one cannot tell if the right questions were explored. Here the related principles of *closure, saturation,* and *convergence* come into play. If the investigators remain properly open-ended throughout their approaches to participants and no longer hear anything substantially new, it is likely that they have exhausted the views available on this particular issue. These principles will be examined in greater detail in Chapter 9.

Verification by individuals external to the study and by participants themselves is another important check on the veracity of the findings. When people familiar with the setting of a study read a report or a preliminary document, the message should be meaningful or insightful to them. They should say, perhaps with enthusiasm, "Yes, that's right. You've portrayed it correctly." External verification might occur by asking an experienced investigator not associated with this particular study to conduct an audit to review the data and the derived conclusions for logical consistency. What is sought here is not necessarily agreement with the conclusions themselves but, rather, an affirmation that the conclusions were reached in a scientifically competent and responsible manner and that the conclusions are consistent with the data on which they are based. Members of a study team routinely audit each other, but the addition of external reviewers reduces the possibility that some perspective affecting the entire team will skew the results.

Comparing Objectivist and Subjectivist Studies: Importance of a Level Playing Field

When all is said and done, how do we know that the findings of a subjectivist study are "correct?" How do we know if the findings carry any truth? What makes a study of this type more than one person's opinion or the opinion of a research team that may share a certain perspective on the resource under study? To explore this question fairly, subjectivist studies should be seen, along with objectivist studies, as part of the larger family of methods for empirical investigation. Neither approach should be placed on the defensive and required to prove itself against a set of standards produced by proponents of the other. When seen in this light, the credibility of both objectivist and subjectivist approaches derives from five sources.

- Belief in the philosophical basis of the approach
- Existence of rules of good practice
- Investigators' adherence to these rules
- Accessibility of the data
- Value of the resulting studies to their respective audiences

We discussed these factors as they apply to objectivist studies earlier in the book, and we have discussed them as they apply to subjectivist studies to some extent in this chapter. A more thorough discussion is found in Chapter 9.

Ultimately, each reader must make a personal judgment about the credibility of any evaluation approach. None of the approaches is beyond challenge. We caution the reader making such an appraisal against establishing the objectivist approaches, particularly the randomized clinical trial, as a standard and then comparing subjectivist approaches to the specific characteristics of this standard. This would inequitably frame the comparison using the logic, definitions, and assumptions of only one of the entities being compared. For example, can subjectivist approaches establish causality as well as objectivist approaches? If cause and effect is defined as objectivists define it, of course the answer is no. If cause and effect is defined more generically, however, both objectivist and subjectivist approaches can address such issues. They just do it differently.

It is human nature to compare anything relatively new to an idealization of what is familiar. Because objectivist studies may be more familiar, it is tempting to base a comparison of subjectivist methods on the perfect objectivist study, which is never realized in practice. Every objectivist study has limitations that are usually articulated at the end of a study report. Many such reports end with a lengthy list of limitations and cautions and a statement that further research is needed. For these reasons, rarely has any one study, objectivist or subjectivist, ended a controversy over an issue of scientific or social importance.

Two Example Abstracts

To convey both the substance and some of the style of subjectivist work in informatics, we include below abstracts of two published studies. The first is Forsythe's 1992 work,[10] which had substantial impact on a project at the design stage. The second is Aydin's 1989 work,[13] which addressed the impact of a deployed information resource.

The problem of user acceptance of knowledge-based systems is a current concern in medical informatics. User acceptance should increase when system-builders understand both the needs of potential users and the context in which a system will be used. Ethnography is one source of such understanding. This paper describes the contribution of ethnography (and an anthropological perspective) during the first year of a 3-year interdisciplinary project to build a patient education system on migraine. Systematic fieldwork is producing extensive data on the information needs of migraineurs. These data call into question some of the assumptions on which our project was based. Although it is not easy to rethink our assumptions and their implications for design, using ethnography has enabled us to undertake this process relatively early in the project at a time when redesign costs are low. It should greatly improve our chances of building a system that meets the needs of real users, thus avoiding the troublesome problem of user acceptance [Forsythe's study].

This paper explores the effects of computerized medical information systems on the occupational communities of health care professionals in hospitals. Interviews were conducted with informants from the pharmacy and nursing departments at two hospitals currently using medical information systems for communicating physicians' medication orders from the nursing station to the pharmacy. Results showed changes in tasks for both pharmacy and nursing, resulting in increased interdependence between the two departments. This interdependence was accompanied by improved communication and cooperation, providing an opportunity [to] encourage better working relationships between departments. The use and maintenance of the common computerized data base became a superordinate goal for the two groups, with the computer system itself as the topic of communication [Aydin's study].

Food for Thought

1. Return to Self-Test 2.2. After rereading the case study presented there, consider the following questions.
   a. What specific evaluation issues in this case are better addressed by objectivist methods and which are better addressed by subjectivist methods?
   b. If you were conducting a subjectivist study of the T-HELPER project, consider the various data collection modalities you might employ. Whom would you interview? What events would you observe? What artifacts would you examine?
   c. How would you immerse yourself into the environment of this project?
2. Consider the following about subjectivist studies:
   a. Are they/can they be credible in the world of biomedicine?
   b. What personal attributes must a subjectivist researcher have?
   c. Which of these attributes do you personally have?
   d. Should medical informatics professionals themselves perform these studies, or should they be "farmed out" to anthropologists or other social scientists?

References

1. Winograd T, Flores F: Understanding Computers and Cognition: A New Foundation for Design. Reading, MA: Addison-Wesley, 1987.
2. Norman DA: The Psychology of Everyday Things. New York: Basic Books, 1988.
3. Davis WS: Business Systems Design and Analysis. Belmont, CA: Wadsworth, 1994.
4. Bansler JP, Bødker K: A reappraisal of structured analysis: design in an organizational context. ACM Transact Inf Syst 1993;11:165–193.
5. Zachary WW, Strong GW, Zaklad A: Information systems ethnography: integrating anthropological methods into system design to insure organizational acceptance. In: Hendrick HW, Brown O (eds) Human Factors in Organizational Design and Management. Amsterdam: North Holland, 1984:223–227.
6. Becker H: Boys in White: Student Culture in Medical School. Chicago: University of Chicago Press, 1963.
7. Bosk CL: Forgive and Remember: Managing Medical Failure. Chicago: University of Chicago Press, 1979.
8. Fafchamps D, Young CY, Tang PC: Modelling work practices: input to the design of the physician's workstation. Symp Comput Applications Med Care 1991;15:788–792.
9. Forsythe DE, Buchanan BG: Broadening our approach to evaluating medical information systems. Symp Comput Applications Med Care 1991;15:8–12.
10. Forsythe DE: Using ethnography to build a working system: rethinking basic design assumptions. Symp Comput Applications Med Care 1992;16:505–509.
11. Forsythe DE: Using ethnography in the design of an explanation system. Expert Applications 1995;8:403–417.
12. Osheroff JA, Forsythe DE, Buchanan BG, Bankowitz RA, Blumenfeld BH, Miller R: Analysis of clinical information needs using questions posed in a teaching hospital. Ann Intern Med 1991;14:576–581.
13. Aydin CE: Occupational adaptation to computerized medical information systems. J Health Soc Behav 1989;30:163–179.
14. Kaplan B: Initial impact of a clinical laboratory computer system. J Med Syst 1987; 11:137–147.
15. Wilson SR, Starr-Schneidkraut N, Cooper MD: Use of the Critical Incident Technique to Evaluate the Impact of MEDLINE. Palo Alto, CA: American Institutes of Research, 1989. Final Report to the National Library of Medicine under contract N01-LM-8-3529.
16. Kaplan B, Duchon D: Combining qualitative and quantitative methods in information systems research: a case study. MIS Quarterly 1988;12:571–586.
17. Johnston ME, Langton KB, Haynes RB, Matthieu D: A critical appraisal of research on the effects of computer-based decision support systems on clinician performance and patient outcomes. Ann Intern Med 1994;120:135–142.
18. Geertz C: The Interpretation of Cultures. New York: Basic Books, 1973.
19. House ER: Evaluating with Validity. Beverly Hills: Sage, 1980.
20. Stake RE: Evaluating the Arts in Education: A Responsive Approach. Columbus, OH: Merrill, 1975.
21. Scriven M: Objectivity and subjectivity in educational research. In: Thomas LG (ed) Philosophical Redirection of Educational Research. National Society for the Study of Education. Chicago: University of Chicago Press1972.
22. Scriven M: Maximizing the power of causal investigations: the modus operandi method. In: Popham WJ (ed) Evaluation in Education. Berkeley, CA: McCutchan, 1974.

23. Parlett M, Hamilton D: Evaluation as illumination. In: Parlett M, Dearden G (eds) Introduction to Illuminative Evaluation. Cardiff-by-the-Sea, CA: Pacific Soundings, 1977.
24. Fielding NG, Lee RM: Using Computers in Qualitative Research. Newbury Park, CA: Sage, 1991.

Appendix A: Additional Readings

This chapter was designed to develop an appreciation and respect for subjectivist methods, and some sense of their applicability to medical informatics. If this reading has developed a further curiosity about these methods, it has served its purpose. To satisfy this curiosity, several readings are recommended.

The duo of Egon Guba and Yvonna Lincoln have written several outstanding texts. Their first is *Effective Evaluation* (Jossey-Bass, 1981). These were followed by *Naturalistic Inquiry* (Sage Publications, 1985) and *Fourth Generation Evaluation* (Sage Publications, 1989).

A classic work in this area is by Hamilton et al (eds). *Beyond the Numbers Game: A Reader in Educational Evaluation* (McCutchan, 1977). This book contains, as part of its introduction, the seminal paper "Evaluation as illumination" by Parlett and Hamilton.

Elliot Eisner is a leading proponent of the connoisseurship or art criticism approach to evaluation. His most recent book, *The Enlightened Eye* (Macmillan, 1991), is a treasure.

Another popular and important work is *Qualitative Evaluation Methods* by Michael Q. Patton (Sage Publications, 1980).

9

Design and Conduct of Subjectivist Studies

ALLEN C. SMITH III

This chapter extends our discussion of the use of qualitative or subjectivist approaches in research and evaluation in informatics. With a combination of theoretical and practical points, it provides direction to the reader who chooses to answer questions that are difficult if not impossible to study with more traditional, objectivist approaches. Four introductory issues must be explored before we begin to outline a realistic model for qualitative inquiry.

First, qualitative inquiry is intended to offer a two level answer to research and evaluation questions. The conclusion that emerges from a study must offer a "thick, rich description" of the events in question.[1] It must also provide an explanation of those events. Subjectivist approaches have the potential to build durable arguments that assert a relationship between theory and data. To achieve the potential, research and evaluation questions must be answered with confidence based on objective data, methodological rigor, and theoretical clarity. If a research conclusion is to have utility, it must go beyond a simple record of what the data "look like." If an evaluation conclusion is to offer a useful indication of the value inherent in a program, it must do more than present the apparent facts. Qualitative inquiry, like all other serious inquiry, must combine description with explanation.

Throughout this chapter, the term "theory" refers to three interactive levels of thinking about the way events or variables are related to each other. First, an individual investigator develops personal, informal schemes to provide some order in the rush of specific data. It is presumptuous to call this first line thinking "theory," but it is the first step in theoretical thinking. A second level of theory is drawn from the work of others who have studied situations comparable to the problem that defines the current study. The earlier research offers an abstract argument that explained the data encountered there. The third level of relatively formal theory offers explanation beyond the specific kinds of events evident in a current study. At this level the theorist is arguing for a deeper relationship between events and theory that would be evident in a wide variety of situations.

Personal theory, ranging from an initial hunch to a confident argument, is obviously related to the investigator's professional training and background. "Previous studies" theory, which was originally tied to the authors' personal theories, claims increasing legitimacy as it survives professional review and proves useful to others. The more often this theory is cited and supported, the more substantial it is assumed to be. "Formal theory," certainly the most abstract of the three levels, is often framed in relation to specific events but is tested against data drawn from a range of situations.

A simple example can illustrate. After preliminary study of the use of a new computerized patient record system in a clinic, an investigator begins to believe (a personal theory) that most physicians do not make use of the information resource unless they can find at least one other person to join them in learning. Reviewing the literature on new informatics programs, the investigator finds that innovations are more effective when they are introduced into small organizational units so individuals can support each other (theory from previous studies). On talking with a colleague in education, the investigator encounters social learning theory (a formal theory), which argues that the social risk involved in attempting a new technology is enough to inhibit most individuals unless they can enlist support. In this case the three levels of theory are aligned and provide a basis for forming an argument about events in the new clinic situation.

The second introductory issue is based on the sequence of intellectual events within a study. With objectivist studies, the familiar sequence progresses along a linear path from the research problem, through a literature review, the development of a research design, the collection and analysis of data, and finally a statement of conclusions. Each of these steps is included in qualitative work, but the sequence is neither linear nor predictable. To use a familiar term, qualitative work is inductive, flowing from data toward an argument that explains the data.[2] Objectivist work is deductive, flowing from a theoretical premise toward analysis that tests the theory against objective data. Subjectivist work asks "What is happening here and why?" Objectivist work asks "Is X happening here as theory predicts?" Qualitative work is meant to develop theory. Quantitative work is meant to test theory. The classic sequence of pure deductive analysis is an ideal in objectivist work. It is deliberately changed in subjectivist work.

Furthermore, there is no single sequence characteristic of qualitative work. In fact, we might argue that the several kinds of thinking implied in the inductive sequence are conducted simultaneously, mutually interacting with each other. As discussed in Chapter 8, the inductive path implies that every element of a study— the questions, relevant literature, research design, and interpretive argument—are continually refined throughout the life of the study. Work proceeds continuously through the iterative loop with constant adjustments as the data and theory are gradually combined into explanation. We can define a starting place for a study, where a decision is made to invest significant resources into a question, though the work to answer the question inevitably began before the decision. We can also define a stopping place, where a decision is made that an argument has been assembled that adequately captures and explains the significant data, though the work can always continue and lead into another cycle of questions. The process between beginning and end is inherently flexible, and the degree of flexibility varies across legitimate qualitative studies.

Third, in qualitative work the natural context surrounding specific events is taken as part of the study. Ultimately, events cannot be understood except in relation to their social, physical, organizational, and cultural context so an argument attempting to explain the events must capture salient features of the context as well as the narrowly defined events themselves.[3, 4] A clinician's success in mastering a new computerized patient record system, for example, depends in part on whether the system is consistent with other forces (e.g., colleagues and staff routines) in the clinic. Apart from the intellectual adjustments the physician must make to the language and structure of the software, a qualitative study examines a range of forces that shape the clinician's work. Changes in practice are not trivial. The significance of context means that there is an important problem in defining the boundaries of a study—clarifying which aspects of the events and their context will be studied. It is also important that the study comes to draw on a potentially wider variety of theory than the focused objectivist study, which focuses more precisely on the events and controls contextual factors.

Case Example

The rest of this chapter proceeds in the context of an example. We return to it repeatedly, adding to our hypothetical "case" with new points to illustrate new concepts. You could easily add to the illustration based on your own situation and experience. We hope you will. Note that the way we frame the illustration at the beginning is important, leading us toward an exploratory, qualitative approach.

The Up-To-Date Clinic has recently installed a computer-based patient record system in one of its community practices. After a year of exploration and consultation, management determined that it had found the most effective system and has now decided that after a 3-month transition all patient records will be prepared and maintained using the new system. Anticipating some adjustment problems, they have asked a consultant to evaluate the new system and the transition, expecting the report to provide the basis for smoothing out the rough spots in the system and the training they provide to staff. Their working assumption is that the clinical staff will grumble during the transition but will respect the system after they proceed through a short period of learning.

From this point on the evaluation project could develop in any number of ways. Any consultant would have any number of questions before officially starting to work. No one approach to the project would be the single right way, but each would require careful thought and professional attention to method.

All of the points in this introduction point toward one strategic tip. The investigator should consider finding colleagues to help in all phases of a subjectivist study. Furthermore, thought should be given to finding colleagues who can bring new theory and perspective to the study. Recruiting an organizational psychologist, for example, can enrich the effort to understand the organizational context surrounding the events to be studied. A sociologist with training in subjectivist approaches can add depth to the study of the norms and authority issues among the subjects. A team including members from different disciplines can become intellectually complex. It can take time to be sure that the team members are using a common vocabulary despite the differences in their theories and disciplines. It can be awkward to establish a balance of theory and practicality in the team, as the members have different norms based on their different training. The complex team can enrich the project in important ways, however, most notably in the depth of the explanatory argument they achieve.

The balance of this chapter is presented in four sections, each written to provide a mixture of practical tips and theoretical issues: (1) five kinds of subjectivist thinking; (2) safeguards to protect the integrity of the work; (3) special issues involved in subjectivist evaluations; and (4) special problems in reporting on subjectivist work. We return often to our example the Up-To-Date Clinic.

Five Kinds of Subjectivist Thinking

The heart of this chapter is organized on the premise that the initial questions and the work done over the life of a project fall generally into five categories, each requiring a different kind of thinking. All five must be thoughtfully developed, recorded, and eventually completed, albeit in an unpredictable sequence. Each has its own implications and its own kinds of rigor. After a brief overview, we discuss the five kinds of thinking in detail. The order of our discussion here was chosen to make explanation simpler. The sequence suggests nothing about the nonlinear sequence in which they are involved in a project.

1. *Sensing the data:* This step entails searching for, recognizing, finding, collecting, and recording objective data according to the emergent design of the study. All of the senses can be involved. Innumerable facts can become important. The process is inevitably shaped by theory and assumptions that evolve with the study but rests ultimately on the five human senses.

2. *Reflecting on subjective experience:* This phase concerns developing awareness of the investigator's personal memories, feelings, and values as they become active while working on site with the data and in the library with theory. These subjective reactions can distort the investigator's vision and interpretation, and they can provide powerful suggestions about what the situation is like for the subjects of the study.

3. *Building the argument:* This intellectual process is conserned with building an argument that captures and explains the events. It involves analytical acuity, creativity, and intuition as the data and useful theory are progressively brought together, from the initial hunches to the final argument. Data illustrate the theory, and theory explains the data. The argument represents the intellectual achievement of the work—an integrated, persuasive statement of what the investigator believes as a result of the study.

4. *Reviewing available theory:* Subjectivist investigators use the work of others for help in understanding and explaining the data they collect. Reviewing theory can involve libraries and consultants, sometimes from fields that seem far afield at first. The theory may come from other studies of comparable events or from more abstract frameworks developed in other situations.

5. *Planning next steps:* Throughout the emergent study the investigator must make frequent decisions about what happens next. Each next step might be understood as an action statement within the four other kinds of thinking. Depending on the degree of "chaos" that develops in the project, however, planning can best be seen as a fifth kind of thinking in which next steps are seen across the other domains and recorded systematically to improve the likelihood that the steps are taken in a deliberate way and to provide a chronicle for subsequent review.

Sensing the Data

The first major step in sensing the data is to enter the field, the site where the events occur and where the subjects work. The first steps are typically taken informally and privately, but as the study becomes a project we establish ourselves in the setting with a legitimate role. This step involves negotiating with some key players and providing at least a minimal explanation to others. There is no standard formula for making the initial introductions, clarifying the project, explaining the process, clarifying the subjects' rights, or answering the subjects' initial questions. In fact, the process of "entering the field" defines a stage in the project, not an event.[5]

The natural circumstances within which the project continues make the subjects relax after an initial time of curiosity and concern. It allows us a candid look at the people and events, but it also implies that we should occasionally remind the subjects of our roles and promises, and that we accept a continuing responsibility not to exploit the candor we solicit. Obviously, if we have a participant's role in the situation as well as that of an investigator, we can move smoothly in the field. But there is a real ethical problem involved in concealing the investigator behind the participant.[6] The subjects need to know both of our roles, and we should sometimes take pains to remind them.

Once in the field, including those first informal visits, we collect data for qualitative studies in three basic ways: observing events and situations, talking with people, and reviewing written messages and other artifacts.[2] There are numerous variations of each basic strategy. Data collection might occur on the primary site of the project or anywhere else the issues and the people involved take us. Returning to the Up-To-Date Clinic, a consultant might plan a simple set of initial strategies, depending in part on her initial beliefs and expectations.

She might observe at the computer stations, at the nurses' station, in the hallways and examining rooms, or in offices, laboratories, and staff meetings. She might notice the people who make use of the records and the system, the kinds of paper records and notes they produce, the gestures they make, the clutter they leave behind. She might talk with some physicians and nurses casually and then ask a selection of them to give her more than just casual comments, moving into a range of scheduled interviews. She might read the data summaries the system produces and follow their use in staff meetings. She might review the minutes of formal committees. She might ask a nurse to keep a journal. Throughout the process, she might choose to be "unobtrusive," using a participant role to justify her presence and interest, or to become an obvious observer with a known role as evaluator.

There is no single right way to gather the data for this or any other study. The evaluation project would have to take shape on the basis of the questions that need answers and the opportunities available.

The data collection methods in a given project vary, and overlap. Observation includes a range of talk with the subjects of the study, much of which can be understood as interview data. Interviews can be understood only in a context that must be examined through observation. Documents range from official reports, to personal calendars, to informal statements on bulletin boards and elevator walls. The specific types of data-gathering strategy vary between and within qualitative studies. It is both useful and necessary to think about and plan for the various kinds of data collection, but it is ultimately artificial to separate the strategies into three distinct categories. It is almost as certain that the data would be collected using a mixture of strategies because each kind of data has its own advantages and limitations.

Whatever the data collection method, it is important to enter the situation each time with a set of focal, orienting questions in mind. They may be broad and open-ended, or they may be narrow and specific, depending on whether the purpose at that time is to explore or confirm some aspect of the emergent argument. It is also important to keep track of priorities. Which questions, if any, are critical now, given that there may not be another chance to talk with this person? Working to articulate the questions and hunches before a specific session of data collection provides a perspective from which to observe and listen. It also clarifies the unspoken ideas, which would have influenced perceptions anyway.

Exploration–Confirmation Cycle

The data to be collected at any given time are determined in relation to a continuing cycle of exploration and confirmation.[7] There are cycles of data collection in which the deliberate effort is to explore—to find data that suggest something new. This means maintaining a simple openness to events and details, an almost child-like freedom to notice, to be curious about what and why, to wonder.

There are other times when the purpose is to seek data that either confirm or conflict with the emergent argument. Confirmatory data work includes the effort to ensure that the findings from one field experience are cross-checked against other times and places in a sampling process. It also includes a search for other kinds of data that should be evident or absent if current thinking is accurate. "If my hunch in right, X should be evident at the end of their staff meetings." At times, confirmation takes imagination as the search for new kinds of data continues. At other times, it takes courage as conflicting data become evident.

The switch between confirmation and exploration can be described with a simple photographic metaphor. With a confirmatory filter, we scan for details that relate directly to the interpretation of the facts we are gradually building (see below). Sometimes the data confirm our ideas. Sometimes they conflict. With an exploratory filter, we scan the same scene for details that might lead to new ideas or new questions, some of which become central elements of the study. The challenge is in the discipline required to watch through two filters while a single situation unfolds.

Once in the field, in the situation with the people who are the subjects in the study, the first practical task is to observe and listen. Neither is as simple as it appears. In most circumstances people routinely devote most of their time to internal thinking in response to the events around them. When someone offers a comment, the listener stops listening after a few seconds and begins to assemble a response or to remember something or someone else. The natural interplay between external events and internal response is an essential aspect of qualitative inquiry, but the process must be slowed. With practice, the investigator can put the internal thinking "on pause" while noticing and recording more of the external details. The important job in collecting data is to hear what is said and see what happens. There is time for interpretation later.

Recording the Data

While gathering data the paramount mechanical task is to record what the senses detect. The significance of this step is the simple fact that the resulting pages become the data set on which the remainder of the research or evaluation must be based. Most of the data are recorded using two kinds of notes, which make the process both reasonable and durable.[8] First are "trigger notes," simple, abbreviated notes taken at the moment or immediately after and adequate as a reminder of details some hours later when preparing the complete "field notes," which capture the events in as much detail as possible.

Trigger notes are prepared in the field, sometimes during contact with the events, sometimes during short breaks. These notes could be taken using a small notebook, perhaps a dictaphone, and sometimes a small computer. However they are recorded, these notes are rough and brief, including just enough words and phrases to provide a reminder later. With experience, the investigator develops his own shorthand with symbols and words that represent whole comments. At times he captures a complete quote, though it is difficult. At times he uses a code to refer to an idea or a question. A "2A" for example, might mean that he asked the question noted as 2A on the interview guide (discussed below.) A "Q resist" might mean that he asked a question about how the subjects resist the change discussed in a meeting. Trigger notes must also include a quick header with the date and a simple reminder of the scene itself (e.g., "staff meet, 3/15–4:30").

Trigger notes also include inserts representing the four other kinds of thinking. These inserts arise from the private thinking that is inevitably part of the process. Noting these thoughts briefly in the trigger notes allows the investigator to return more quickly to the data. The investigator might include, inside brackets for example, a brief note standing for her own sense of surprise at the events. Some investigators make this comment with "I surpr" to emphasize that "I" am feeling something, or "RN" for reflective notes (see below). A quick thought that the scene is a good example of an idea already included in the code words from earlier observations might be inserted with a large A (for Argument) in large parentheses, (A.code word), to note where the data might be used in the emerging argument. To return to our example of the Up-To-Date Clinic, the insert might read "A.lang" to refer to a cluster that covers the ways physicians modify their language to fit into the automated record system. Other inserts might connect to the review of formal theory, planning, or future data collection. Instead of fighting off these private thoughts while gathering data, the investigator records them briefly. That makes them available for review later and frees her to return to more spontaneous observation and listening, with confidence that the thought is recorded.

Trigger notes are sometimes taken during the events, on the scene. At other times they are recorded during short breaks. Plan to show these notes to some of the subjects of the study to respond to their curiosity and suspicion about the process. The notes are typically illegible, but we can explain them, indirectly answering questions about the kinds of things we are capturing. It also provides an opportunity for our subjects to correct something we may have misunderstood (see below under Safeguards, Member Checking). In general, the tactic of sharing notes, ideas, and code words with subjects depend on how well we have explained the project and our roles to the people on the scene.

Particularly during planned interviews, data are often recorded on audiotape. It is a convenient tactic that allows detailed review of an exact record later. This can be reassuring when accurate quotes are important and when the analytical focus is on the subject's exact language. However, there are important limitations. First, the process of transcribing audiotapes can become expensive, particularly when there are more than two voices involved. It can take 4 hours or more to transcribe the results of a 1-hour, one-person interview. Furthermore, it takes considerable time to review the transcripts. More important, the investigator can be lulled into complacency if she relies too heavily on the transcripts, losing some of the important interview data that cannot be captured on tape.

One strategy with audio recordings is to use the tapes to regain full details of a segment of the interview that the investigator's trigger and field notes mark as important. Often without transcripts, the tapes can be reviewed to provide details that were not recalled when preparing field notes. This approach forces the investigator to maintain concentration on the interview and to maintain good trigger notes.

It is also possible to record interview and observation data using video technology. Again, this technique provides detailed review, though at some expense in time. Again there are limitations. Depending on the camera system used, the data do not in fact provide an accurate image of the scene as the investigator observed it. There are inevitable distortions based on the camera's perspective and the quality of the lens and microphone. Certain facts are recorded faithfully. Many other facts are changed. As with audiotapes, it is essential that the investigator maintain good trigger notes without relying too heavily on the video recordings.

Within a day after recording trigger notes, the investigator should prepare full field notes, an expanded effort to capture the details of the events in as much detail as our trigger notes, memory, and time allow. The extent of the details in the field notes depends on the argument we are building and the time we have to record them. In some studies, it takes 2 days of work to prepare field notes after a single day of observation and interviews. At another point in the project cycle or in another study it might be possible to cover a day's events within 2 to 3 hours of writing the field notes. The time taken also depends on the quality of the trigger notes written on site. At this point it becomes clear that qualitative work can be surprisingly time consuming. Clearing our calendar for a half-day to observe in a clinic, for example, could mean clearing an additional day to make sure the field notes, the data for the study, are complete and useful.

Basic word processing software is an immense support at this stage, independent of the more complex programs used to help with analysis of the data. Practically, it is useful to prepare field notes using different fonts for the different kinds of thinking involved. Alternatively, indent the private thoughts prompted by the scene and capture the data statements on a wider format. This method facilitates quick identification of different thoughts later on. Similarly, when we print field notes, and we all but certainly will, we should double space and provide a 3-inch left margin for making interpretive notes and adding handwritten "code words." Many programs include features that provide for prearranged formats to facilitate this process. Be careful when devising a system for naming files and directories to make it possible to review them easily later. Selection of software for data entry should be compatible with any other programs we plan to use for data analysis later.

Throughout the data collection process, it is important to understand that sensing data cannot be a purely objective process. The process of selecting which data to sense and record and then arraying those data in a descriptive statement involves important intellectual and personal acts. If we were asked to describe a clinical situation, perhaps the Up-To-Date Clinic, we could not proceed without reference to the theoretical schemes we possessed at the time, primitive or well developed. Description is itself an important step toward interpretation. It is difficult to separate them when describing even a simple object. It is impossible to separate them when the subject is a human situation in its natural context. In this sense, gathering data is inseparable from the other four kinds of thinking inherent in qualitative inquiry.

Sensing data includes careful attention to what is evident to the several senses and a deliberate effort to note what is not evident. It is one thing to notice and establish that the people in the field are talking about some pattern of issues. It takes a different kind of attention to note that they are not discussing something else. That silence may be important, indicating that the unspoken issue is extraneous to them or perhaps taboo. Similarly, data can reveal patterns of stability and change over time. The fact that the data are not the same in two situations does not mean that either set of data is faulty. It simply means that the situations were different. The difference can become a significant element of the analysis.

During data collection we often need to pause, sometimes to jot down notes, sometimes to capture a thought, sometimes simply to rest or to call the mechanic about the car. The pause might last 10 seconds, while our mind wanders away from the observation or interview; or it might last 15 minutes while we catch up on notes. It might last a week or more as we "come home" from the field to get away from the people and the project or to catch up on something else. It is always important to sense the timing of these pauses, acknowledge the need, and plan the shifts in our attention.

Finally, some data are collected deliberately and officially. In an ongoing project, however, rich data are often encountered accidentally and informally. In the same way, although some data are collected in the present, we almost certainly possess data that we encountered before the study began—perhaps long before. New and old, deliberate and accidental—they can all be useful data. It is wrong to treat all data uniformly, but it would also be wrong to ignore it just because we did not have our official research hats on when we encountered them.

Reflecting on Subjective Experience

Our personal or subjective experience during a project exists at two connected levels. First, personal psychology, individual philosophy, and professional training all shape the way we perceive and interpret the events around us. Many elements of these personal traits can become active during a qualitative study, often in unpredictable ways.[9] In the Up-To-Date case study, for example, we may begin to take sides with some players in an unspoken power struggle with others, based in part on our own political values. The physicians, the patients, or the staff might claim our attention more than the others, in part because of our own sense of the human and political values involved in health care reform. Another investigator might see the same situation differently.

At another level, subjectivity exists in momentary memories, impulses, and feelings. Memories and feelings stimulated by on-site experience can be understood as flags indicating that some events are personally significant. Quiet reflection can reveal the significant events and lead to new ideas and questions. If we were surprised or disappointed by something in the situation, for example, it would indicate that we expected something to happen that did not. What was the expectation? It may become clear that the expectation was a purely personal thing, essentially extraneous to the study and relatively safe in terms of its power to distort your thinking once it is acknowledged. In fact, surprise about your personal beliefs might lead you to realize that people in the same situation have a different understanding of the events and therefore different expectations. The difference could be significant for your study.

At Up-To-Date, the consultant might feel a sense of surprise on noticing a physician smile when the business manager reminds her that diagnostic labels should be drawn from the codes prespecified on the system. On reflection, he recognizes that he expected the physician to feel angry. When he later asks about the situation, the physician responds that she had helped to create the codes herself and realized that she had been a little lazy when completing that record. The consultant moves from his original sense of surprise to a new curiosity about how the physicians came to accept elements of the computerized system as "their own." Without recognizing the surprise, the new questions would not have emerged.

This example could be reframed with many other feeling words describing the consultant's embarrassment, sadness, anger, boredom, fatigue, or conflict. The reflective process begins with the investigator identifying his feeling, memory, or impulse and connecting it to or separating it from events in the situation. The process continues with a consideration of the situation as the subjects understand it.

There are other important indicators of subjective experience. For example, you are often tempted to tell some stories of the events you are studying when you are away from the study and among friends. Which stories are tempting? (Note that you should generally not tell them at all, depending on your agreements about confidentiality.) Why are these stories particularly fascinating to you? What issues about the project do the stories highlight? The same is true for the dilemmas you face during the project (e.g., ethical decisions), for your tendency to prefer some people and avoid others, and for your sense of clumsiness in handling certain situations.

Our subjective responses to events in the field are important factors in two ways. As evident in objectivist research and evaluation, subjectivity is a threat to the integrity of a study across the entire process. Objectivist designs have controls, such as "blinding," built in to contain this threat, promising that the data are truly detached from the people collecting them. The same dangers exist in subjectivist approaches. It is also recognized that subjectivity can be a powerful ally as well as a dangerous enemy, providing useful guides to important questions which can add significant depth to the project. For both reasons, reflecting on personal subjectivity is a routine part of the qualitative research process, offering protection from distorted analysis and suggestions for new dimensions of inquiry.

Unfortunately, through both cultural and professional socialization, most investigators have learned some dysfunctional lessons about handling subjectivity. Feelings in particular are understood as part of private life, markers of a failure in our professional lives if they occur vividly or if we express them openly. Viewing our subjectivity as a regrettable part of our professional lives and setting it aside as unworthy of serious attention, let alone public expression, leaves the feelings in place to influence our work outside of our own awareness and control.

The simplest practical steps involved in awareness and reflection were mentioned above when discussing trigger notes and field notes. As the notes are prepared, we simply insert notes describing our subjective response to the events using a simple code to mark them as our personal reactions, distinct from the "objective" events. This practice, however, presumes that we can freely and quickly label our reactions, and we often cannot. The code in our notes may simply indicate that we were "pleased" or "upset" with something. Continued reflection later helps clarify the response.

Given the personal nature of our subjectivity, it is often wise to find a trusted colleague with whom we can discuss our experience relatively openly. It is important to negotiate clearly about such confidences, agreeing to confidentiality and ensuring that the colleague understands the positive approach to subjectivity. The colleague can then become a useful support for clarifying the issues and asking questions about how you can use the directions your responses provide while working to guard your subsequent interpretations from unreasonable distortion.

Building the Argument

An investigator conducts a qualitative research or evaluation project in order to understand something better, to answer some questions with confidence. Throughout the process and certainly during the final stages, she will be gradually building an argument that describes and explains the situation and answers the questions in a way she and others can respect. At the end, she can argue that an explanatory relationship exists between the data and theory. The argument is the intellectual work of the project, the progressive effort to find and clarify the elements of a new understanding and to assemble them into a coherent whole.

Despite its inductive approach, qualitative work assumes that there is some intellectual starting place at the beginning of a project based on the investigator's professional training and personal biography. Often there is a tendency at the beginning to impose a "theoretical" scheme onto a problem that provides the basis for the first questions and concerns. What are the first things someone would want to know about Up-To-Date Clinic? What does she (perhaps secretly) hope to find? Assuming that she acknowledges this vague "theoretical" starting place (see above under Reflecting on Personal Experience), the process of building an explanatory argument proceeds from that point.

Over time, the argument progresses from small, tentative possibilities to a coherent, confident whole. At the beginning, and at many stages, the work focuses on "hunches," tentative ideas about the events and how they can be understood. These ideas bring small segments of data into clusters that can be described and labeled. The labels, often called "code words," are terms that begin to give the clusters more general meaning and then to connect the clusters into a wider scheme with intellectual links and bridges. Gradually, each piece can be seen as part of a broader issue or concept. It is likely that the investigator has some simple, often implicit theory in mind about the data as she selects these labels or code words. It is vital to begin the process by working with small pieces of data, avoiding for some time the effort to find a theoretical scheme broad enough to include all of the pieces.

In the Up-To-Date project, we may have begun with a sense that the largest potential problem exists in the staff's ability to learn the new system and to make small adjustments in their work to use it routinely. Accordingly, the consultant may begin to find clusters of data from early observations and interviews that fit into an explanatory theory focusing on learning. The first code words might be "frustration," "support," and "practice." At the same time, however, she might begin to note that some staff are expressing anger. In a conversation/interview, she might learn that one senior physician is upset because management did not consult with her about the new system or its installation. One of the nurses also shows concern about the system but quietly begins to keep small written notes on his patients. These observations lead to new code words as hunches develop.

Because our example is an evaluation study, it is urgent to note that management, the client of the study, provided the opening premise. During every evaluation it is critical to keep track of whose questions and hunches are guiding the study.

Each of the ideas in the hypothetical summary above would be expanded and explored gradually. Each would lead to another round of data collection to expand the "sample" and probe for the meaning of observed behavior. The list of code words would expand. As the interpretive process continues, there is a continual transition back and forth between building the argument and sensing the data. At times the effort is to find data that provoke new ideas, to explore the situation with an open mind. At other times the purpose is to confirm some part of the emergent argument. In the ongoing cycle of exploration and confirmation we introduced above, the emergent argument is gradually extended and tested against the data.

A practical step in building the argument is to accep the hunches that emerge and work to give them a chance to survive. Many are discarded, but some survive; it is difficult to distinguish the useful from the useless until they are developed through an initial process. It is often useful simply to jot down an idea, writing about it without trying to be sophisticated or precise. It might involve three or four paragraphs, or a sketch. It involves wondering and guessing—intellectual play while the idea takes some shape.

A complementary approach involves describing the situation metaphorically. With reference to the example of the new electronic patient record, we might compare the staff physician's first attempts to use the computer-based record with a child's first attempts to ride a bike. The youngster may find the two wheeler intimidating. He or she may have painful accidents while learning to ride. Friends may succeed more quickly and laugh at the slow learner. Success may come only after it becomes clear that the bicycle can serve a useful purpose, providing rapid, pleasant transportation and a new social activity. This metaphor, which presumes that learning to use the computer is both beneficial and possible, suggests a variety of questions that may be involved in the process of adopting the new patient record system. All metaphors, however, have obvious limits. In the present example, we might allow children to choose their own time to learn to ride, whereas we know that the clinic requires the physician to learn the new record system promptly.

As the interpretive process continues, it becomes important to develop a separate list of the code words in use. As the set of code words evolves, dated lists can gradually become an outline of the emerging argument. What are the terms, and how do they relate to one another? Feel free to adjust the specific vocabulary of the code words, noting that the changes produce related adjustments in the argument itself. Sometimes the language colors the meanings of the argument in subtle ways that should be noticed and controlled. Sometimes the changes make relations among the ideas much more obvious.

Another interpretive tool is the matrix. Classically, it involves arraying ideas on one dimension and data sources on the other, allowing cross-checks and comparisons. This subject is expanded below under Triangulation. Another approach is the relationship diagram in which we connect the numerous elements of our argument through a series of arrows that suggest cause or sequence. Miles and Huberman have provided a rich source of variations on these basic ideas.[10] The mechanics can become overpowering, but the ideas are useful.

As code words are refined and an interpretive outline is developed, it becomes possible to connect the terms to the data they represent. The process is simultaneously vital and difficult. In order to use the data that reside in the field notes, they must be edited to include the code words. This means that we must go back to the hard copy of the notes and insert the code words clearly into the paragraphs of the field notes where they fit. We also mark the code words as our own thoughts about the data. This step is initially done in the margins of a printed copy of the field notes, discussed above under Sensing the Data.

As some of the field notes are reviewed and coded in writing (keeping a clean copy of the raw notes available), we strengthen the conceptual outline by sensing the variety of data that exist within the category labeled with each code word. In the Up-To-Data project, we might find several sentiments and behaviors clustered under the heading "frustration." The differences might give the cluster a richer meaning, or they might suggest that the cluster should be subdivided or given a new label. This step leads to a deeper outline based on better code words and the variation evident in the data. Each code word stands for a complex idea, not a single statement. Note that an outline that interrelates the code words is in fact an outline of the emerging argument.

At a later stage, when we are more confident about our code words and outline, we enter the code words into the computer files, using special symbols to set them off from the data. (The symbols, e.g., brackets, depend in part on the software we are using.) This maneuver makes it possible to automate the process of shuffling the data into piles defined by the code words. We can combine into one file all of the paragraphs in our field note that include the label "frustration." Once shuffled into the outline of code words, the material is semiorganized as the basis for a rough draft. Word processing software sharply reduces the time it takes, as the process previously required photocopying the field notes, writing on them, making copies, and then cutting and sorting the notes into conceptual piles.

The process of inserting code words and sorting the data leads to further revisions in our overall outline, sometimes to changes in the code words and sometimes to another stage of inserting code words and sorting the paragraphs. The cyclic pattern explains why we do not insert the code words throughout the data set on the first attempt. At the end, the interpretive clusters are refined, and the result is a rough draft of our report, complete with quotes and descriptions from the raw data. This process may seem lengthy and time-consuming, but computer software has made the progressive revisions much more efficient and has therefore allowed us to produce much stronger arguments.

The array of computer programs designed to assist in the interpretive process within qualitative inquiry is expanding rapidly. Weitzman and Miles have provided a useful overview of the current market.[11] In general, after we have taken the critical steps to clarify the conceptual language of our argument and then insert it into the data, software can serve a variety of purposes for interpretation. Briefly, programs can count the occurrences of our terms (or of select natural language terms in the raw data.) More important, software can find all of the paragraphs to which we have attached certain codes and then create new files including all of these paragraphs. (Ideally, the paragraphs copied into these new files include specifications of their original location in the raw data.) Because most paragraphs have multiple code words attached, we must edit these files to extract the specific data that fit with the associated term. Depending on the overall size of the data set, we edit all or some of these paragraphs.

When turning to the newer software supports, it is critical to understand one principle. The computer cannot take the interpretive step involved in specifying the code words and conceptual labels. That step is our responsibility, and it represents the essential intellectual moment, the delicate human achievement. Software helps but cannot accept responsibility for the interpretive step between data and explanation.

Eventually, it is in the interpretive mode that we complete the process of building an argument that fits the data and that works when explaining the events. The first draft of the overall report represents only a first step, albeit a long step, toward understanding. It requires polishing, and the polishing reveals significant changes, additions, and improvements. The second draft and the third each present a stronger argument. The rewrites involve yet more cycles through the five kinds of thinking, but each cycle usually becomes smoother.

One word of warning. You cannot achieve an argument that adequately explains all of the significant events. There are always some data that conflict with your argument. The fit between data and theory is never perfect. You will have to refine your work repeatedly to achieve an argument that fits the data and works theoretically,[12] but you must stop the interpretive process before it is perfect. One step that often requires some help from the outside is deciding when to stop the process.

Using Existing Theory

The purpose of a subjectivist study is to create an argument that combines data and theory, description, and explanation. Whereas the objectivist investigator draws together the relevant literature at the beginning of his work to help frame the research question and methods, the subjectivist investigator turns to the literature often throughout the project. New literature is frequently added to the project near the end of the study. The timing is different in qualitative inquiry, but the literature is still essential. Qualitative, subjectivist, inductive work progresses toward an explanatory argument that can be serious only if it reflects a careful review of the existing theory.

The essential questions about previous studies and formal theory are simple. Does a theory help to explain the data? Does it help us to understand what we have encountered? Does it help us to build a stronger argument? While fitting the data, the theory must be helpful for understanding and explaining it. It is comforting to import well accepted theory into a study. It is sometimes tempting to force the data to fit the theory. The investigator must judge whether the fit is adequate and use theory that both fits and explains. As we stated several times, the theory and the data are drawn together through a prolonged, iterative, confirmatory process.

The mechanics of the literature review process are familiar. Guided by the emerging outline of concepts and code words, the investigator searches the literature using familiar language and imagination. Your first choice of vocabulary when selecting code words and search terms may or may not lead to a successful literature search. It is often necessary to adjust the language of the search, perhaps after consultation with thoughtfully chosen colleagues. There are then the familiar tasks of finding, scanning, reading, extracting and taking notes. For qualitative work there is the additional process of adding codes to notes taken from the literature indicating how the noted theory may fit together with the data and the argument the investigator is crafting. The same code words that are gradually inserted into the data (field notes) can be inserted into notes taken in the library. Library time is almost certainly a part of the project, but colleagues and other consultants, often in unfamiliar domains and departments, also play an important role in guiding the investigator toward useful theory. As noted in the introduction to this chapter, adding colleagues to the team can be intellectually complex but substantively rewarding.

Many projects can be strengthened through an effort to go beyond the theories and literature the investigator considers familiar. Without pretending real expertise, she can turn to new concepts and arguments, reaching for new explanatory power. In our Up-To-Date case study, for example, after searching the literature on new initiatives in informatics, she might turn to the literature on the implementation of new treatments and technologies in medicine. Going farther afield, she might look into studies of innovation in business or in the military. There are certainly limits to the general points and differences within each field and situation, but Up-To-Date is not facing a novel circumstance.

Planning

Subjectivist work is complicated. Facts and possibilities offer themselves constantly and unpredictably at different degrees of clarity. Planning is the thinking involved in maintaining control over the process. Much qualitative thinking is intuitive and spontaneous. Much is analytical and deliberate. During the four kinds of thinking described above, potential next steps to take occur to you, and much is lost if the ideas are not captured and organized. In general, planning can be understood as specifying action steps to be taken to extend your work in relation to the other four kinds of qualitative thinking.

Ordinarily, the notes you prepare during any time set aside for a particular kind of thinking include short comments on other ideas as they arise. (See the discussion above about trigger notes and field notes.) The action ideas that represent different areas of planning should be captured in brief notes whenever they occur. In trigger notes they would be brief, and in field notes they are expanded.

In relation to sensing the data, planning might identify specific people, places, or records to be approached tomorrow.

"Ask Bill about the decision they reached."

"Spend some time in the coffee lounge."

"How many people are arriving late for the sessions?"

"Do the minutes include any indication of that disagreement?"

"Look for other times when she makes written notes."

"Look back over my notes from the meeting on annual results."

In relation to finding useful theory, planning might specify steps toward new authors, consultants, or theoretical vocabulary.

"Check this situation with X's dissemination model."

"Include the term 'practice' in the literature search."

"Send Dr. Smithers the page I wrote about the fight yesterday."

"Reread Brown's article on organizational tension."

"Ask Sandy for a name I can call in the psychology department."

In relation to reflection on your own experience, planning might mark questions to be considered in a private time, people to contact, or memories to be clarified.

"This is like the problem using new radio procedures in Vietnam."

"Why am I avoiding that administrator?"

"Where have I seen this before?"

"I need a break this weekend!"

In relation to interpretation and argument building, planning might suggest specific places for focused thought and exploration or alternatives to be considered.

"Write a page about fatigue in the clinic."

"How does the quiet staff meeting fit with the conflict idea?"

"Check these data with the loyalty idea, not just conflict."

Keeping simplified notes about the action ideas, across the four other kinds of thinking, increases the likelihood that we will eventually take some of the next steps and recognize some of the possibilities associated with them. It also keeps these ideas in a familiar place for careful review during periods of review. As the ideas occur—during a period of observation, for example—they are quickly recorded but not judged or developed. Later, more deliberate planning refines some ideas and eliminates others.

Apart from a momentary effort to keep track of action ideas, planning includes more extended times for deliberate effort to organize action in the next stages of the study. There should be blocks of time, perhaps on a routine basis, in which you reverse the priorities. Instead of making quick notes of plans and setting them aside to continue with another kind of thinking, you now set the other kinds of thinking aside to concentrate on planning. These planning sessions, whether 5 minutes at the end of each day, an hour once a week, or sometimes a whole day at the end of a major stage of the project, help you keep track of all the important but inherently complicated elements of good subjectivist work.

As a final point on planning, there is an additional urgency involved when multiple investigators are involved. In one sense there are more planning ideas to be recorded, reviewed, and implemented. In another sense, there is a continuing need to keep all members of a team up to date on the plans so each member can seize appropriate opportunities as they continue with their individual roles.

As we noted at the beginning of this section, the five kinds of thinking inherent in subjectivist work are not neatly sequential or independent but overlapping and interactive. Our discussion here has emphasized the substance and practicalities of sensing the data, reflecting on subjective experience, building an argument, reviewing relevant theory, and planning. Throughout the process of any study, one important skill is the ability to acknowledge and make note of "distracting" thoughts while concentrating primarily on something else.

Safeguards to Protect the Integrity of the Work

The objectivist approach to research and evaluation includes a variety of strategies to safeguard the data, the analysis, and ultimately the conclusions reached. There are safeguards in subjectivist work, too, and they imply a deliberate rigor to achieve a descriptive and explanatory argument that can be used by others with confidence. The literature includes an extensive discussion of the potential dangers and useful safeguards. Lincoln and Guba offered a useful chapter on Establishing Trustworthiness.[13] In general, apart from the continuing effort to find discrepant data in the exploration-confirmation cycle, there are five strategies that should be considered part of every qualitative work.

Triangulation

Triangulation means supporting an argument with data from different sources, different investigators, or both. It is not enough to quote one subject. It is not enough to refer only to interview data, certainly not if only one investigator did the interviews. It is better to include multiple investigators or to support the specifics and the overall argument with different kinds of data. It is best to use both different kinds of data and different investigators. Although this simple sounding principle is true, it is difficult to apply.

With regard to data, it is rarely possible to have different kinds of qualitative data line up exactly to support the same point. Intellectually, this process is much less precise than the radio direction finding (RDF), which triangulation suggests. (In fact, even with RDF the multiple bearings on a transmitter always define an area, not a precise spot.) It is important to work for confirmation from different data sources, but the final declaration of support requires an interpretive step, not just a moment of observation.

Similarly, combining support from multiple investigators almost inevitably means colleagues who know each other, who work together on the project, who discuss the facts repeatedly, and who plan to write together. Achieving agreement on all or part of the argument is a necessary step, and the process strengthens the argument; it requires, however, an interpretive step beyond a simple comparison of the conclusions the people reach "independently." Can the different investigators agree on a common statement? In fact, it is best to cultivate a sense of positive disagreement, expecting that the debates that arise will often lead to a stronger argument in the end.

It is worth noting a variation on the triangulation strategy. As suggested above, the investigator should work repeatedly to find data that conflict with the argument she is building, constantly aware of the natural tendency to ignore data that do not support current thinking. If she is able to show that she searched for but did not find the contradicting data, she has a different kind of multiple data support.

Triangulation is a general strategy to guide the process of analysis and interpretation throughout a study. Illustrations and evidence of the effort to triangulate should be presented with any report on the project. It cannot, however, reach the level of precision objectivist studies employ. Triangulation cannot be as precise as "random sampling" or "blinded independent judgment," as discussed in Chapters 5 and 6.

Member Checking

Member checking is an effort to have subjects in the study confirm that the investigator's findings are reasonable. This strategy can be used in many ways and on numerous occasions. At one extreme, the investigator can mention a hunch to a friendly subject as he walks out of the building and then listen carefully to the response. At the other extreme, he can ask carefully selected subjects to read drafts of his overall argument. He may approach a person whom he does not yet know well. He may recruit selected subjects to take on the advisory role repeatedly, perhaps becoming members of an informal group. In each case he is asking if his argument captures the life of the subject. When they confirm that he does understand, he has another kind of support for his argument.

You should not expect that, when subjects and respondents agree, you are right or that when they disagree you are wrong. When they agree with your idea, it may be that you have correctly identified part of the image they want you to see or that they accept themselves as a part of their organizational culture. Stopping at that point might mean missing some related points that are not as popular among or well understood by the subjects.

Returning to the Up-To-Date Clinic, the consultant might correctly sense that the staff complains about the computerized patient record system because it appears to be changing the individuality they have valued in their medical practice up to this point. When the consultant shares this "insight" with two physicians, they may agree with her because of the popularity of the complaint among the clinical staff. Their support may mask an unspoken sense among the physicians that the business approach to medicine will improve their private lives through a more predictable schedule. Because it is not as "legitimate" as the concern about the character of medicine, this potential consequence of the business perspective is not discussed openly.

This example also suggests that when subjects disagree with an insight it does not always mean the insight is wrong. There are times when the investigator has simply made an uncomfortable but reasonable point or has unwittingly but necessarily taken sides in an organizational conflict. Ideally, a subject who gives feedback on the investigator's ideas (often called a respondent) could come to see the strength of the insight despite the discomfort involved. This possibility suggests the importance of developing a good relationship with selected subjects.

In general, after checking with a subject about any aspect of his emerging argument, the investigator must make a final judgment about the results. Although it is gratifying to be confirmed and discomforting to be challenged, neither response is inherently accurate. Each might be accurate or might mask another important point. After careful attention to a subject's response, and after fitting the response into the overall pattern of data, the investigator makes a decision about how to proceed. It is rarely a black or white decision, and it always requires interpretation and judgment for which the investigator must accept responsibility.

Note also that the process of member checking, like many other elements of the subjectivist approach, has an effect on the subjects and the study. The simple act of offering a new way to understand the situation can alter the subject's personal view of the situation or their reputations if others know that they have been involved this way. The fact that the study will or may have an effect on the situation can be both positive and gratifying, even if it conflicts with the principles of objectivist research, which hold that the investigation should not change the subject of the study.

Qualitative work in general almost always changes the situation under study, no matter how quiet the researcher tries to be. Probing a subject's thoughts in an interview changes the way the subject thinks. Even passive observation can make the subjects conscious of their situation in new ways. It is easy to overestimate the potential to induce change, as complex situations are sustained by a wide array of social and organizational forces. Subjects routinely return to their established ways soon after the subjectivist investigator departs. Even so, the investigator must choose her tactics knowing that the change is possible. This caveat particularly holds true during program evaluation, depending on the nature of the final report and the ways it is used by program managers.

In one relatively radical stream of subjectivist research, known as critical theory, the possibility of change is seen as a positive goal.[6] If a project reveals something morally wrong, it is appropriate for the study to induce change. This point obviously implies that someone must make the moral judgment and raises the question of who has that role.

In the context of organizational development, which overlaps with subjectivist (e.g., action) research and evaluation, it is also appropriate that the investigator is involved in change. In this case, however, the change is understood as appropriate from the beginning, made explicit in the project negotiations and under the control of the program managers.

As a general rule, the subjectivist investigator should acknowledge that change may follow from the details and the outcomes of a study, but the change should not be a deliberate part of the investigator's work. Some would go further and say that the investigator should be deliberate in working to minimize the immediate effects of the study, allowing for change to be undertaken as a deliberate process under the manager's control after the study is complete. This policy implies that the investigator must anticipate the use of the results and consider the possibility of hidden agendas in the negotiations that surround the beginning of the study.

Neutral Partner

One of the principal threats to the integrity of qualitative work is the potential that you become too involved, representing some people and their interests carefully given the warm personal regard the intimate contact of qualitative study can produce. Is the argument or the report distorted by friendship or animosity? A different threat is that you, the investigator, can become stuck on a point, overprotective of an idea even when conflicting data become evident. This danger is often marked with a passionate tone in your argument, a sense of excitement and defense. The standard safeguard is to find a neutral partner, someone with whom you can speak freely while withdrawing from the study from time to time. If you can build a sufficiently trusting relationship with this partner that allows you to listen when he points out your blind spots and mistakes, you can expect that the discussion will lead to a more legitimate argument. Recruiting this partner and then working to find conclusions together can be an awkward process, not least because the two people have different investments in the work. This safeguard can be considered a variation on triangulation if the partner studies the data thoroughly enough to form an interpretation of his own.

The neutral partner can offer a range of other support as well. When the investigator shifts into an extended time for planning, is bored with the data, or is unsure how far to follow a new theoretical possibility, a partner can help her regain a sense of control of the project. At some point, the partner may even begin to suggest that she is getting close to the end. It can be good to hear that the argument is becoming clear, or that it is time to polish a draft report to be submitted for formal review.

Saturation in the Field

It takes time to become familiar with the facts and dynamics of the situation. Certain features can become evident early, even during the initial stage of entering the field, but real understanding takes time. Saturation in the field implies that you spend enough time to see beyond the novelties and the obvious issues to find the underlying factors that deserve your attention. In general, there is a cycle of immersion, saturation (temporary), withdrawal from the field, reflection and interpretation, and re-entry for another cycle. (This process is related to the "iterative loop" and is described in Chapter 8.) Each of the stages of immersion ends with a sense of saturation that routinely dissipates with rest, reflection, interpretation, and contact with other people and other issues. At the end of each cycle, new possibilities, questions, tactics, and theories guide the investigator back into the field and the data.

At some point in the life of the study, however, the next cycle in the field seems flat. Nothing new comes into view. The search for confirmation and contradiction supports the argument that has emerged.[12] Member checking offers a basic support for the findings. The study becomes almost boring. There are other feelings, such as a sense of fear that nothing significant will ever emerge, which can be confused with the boredom that marks the final stages in the field. There is also a stage beyond the boredom during which the study is drawn to a close, and the relationships formed in the process are either ended or changed. At the end, however, there is a confidence which comes from moving through all five kinds of thinking completely enough to take a stand.

There is no way to predict how much time a study will take. Ordinarily, the constraints of the resources available and the investigator's other roles limit the project and compel him to find an end sooner than the end might come through a natural sense of saturation. It is one of his responsibilities to sense the depth of the understanding he has achieved and to temper his argument with recognition of the time he might have spent.

Audit Trail

The audit trail is a record of the project that allows someone else to follow its history to determine if the investigation was an adequate basis for the argument. The record would reveal the course of the project:

Origin of the project and the initial steps

Sequence of contacts in the field

Evolution of the code words and interpretation/argument

Details of the interviews, field notes, and relationships

Nature and basis of the major strategic decisions

Specifics of personal involvement

Such a record would enable someone else, even an outsider, to follow the history of the argument to determine if there are flaws at the level of the research process. Maintaining the records is a major task, but if the investigator has maintained files of her field notes, a chronology of her code words and outlines, notes on her efforts to find contradicting data, and a diary of her personal experience, the audit trail is essentially complete. Although it might be difficult for someone else to read or understand the records, even if they had free access, the basic elements of the audit trail are inherent in the files of the five kinds of thinking we have discussed, and the record can be reviewed by someone else. In that sense, the trail is the result of good thinking and good project management, which should give an investigator confidence. Keeping the records is imperative to building a sound argument, even if no one else ever sees them.

Some proponents of the audit trail suggest a variety of specific formats. Lincoln and Guba offered a useful overview.[13] In general, however, as with objectivist studies, the investigator is not asked for the files. Others might ask to see some parts of the record. At times the investigator requests some level of review. Some parts of the record are almost certainly private documents, in part because of the ethical requirement that the subjects' anonymity must be protected. Having the record and being able to point to it is in fact important; but unless the findings are officially challenged, it is unlikely that the record will be shared with anyone in its entirety. The audit trail is more a concept and a procedural standard than a prospect that the work will be reviewed.

Special Issues of Subjectivist Evaluations

Subjectivist approaches offer the potential to produce important answers to evaluation questions. At the same time, there are a number of special issues that demand more attention for subjectivist than for objectivist approaches. The most significant issue is based on the fact that subjectivist studies place the investigator in much more intimate contact with the activities and the people involved. With the extended time, direct observation, open questions, and careful listening subjectivist work implies, more of the details of the program and the people become apparent. This problem is a delicate one because there are real people involved, not just machines or instruments or tests.

Particularly after the subjects get over the novelty of the study, the data include facts that represent a candid picture with realistic but potentially embarrassing details. It may include people liking and disliking each other, helping and harassing, impressing and disappointing, manipulating and posturing. A study reveals the politics of the organization based on the multiple interests of the various stakeholders. The investigator will encounter unprofessional behavior, familiar enough in other settings (including her own) but never flattering. She will encounter feelings, and people customarily consider their feelings private property not public data. Because she is just as human as the people she is studying, the investigator will react to all of this personally as well as professionally.

The up-close character of subjectivist studies produces problems of trust and utility. Much of what the investigator comes to know helps him build his argument, and the argument potentially changes the program for the better. He is in a position to hurt people in ways that would never be possible for an evaluator who works only with quantitative outcome measures in the isolation objectivist approaches consider essential. Any evaluation can have an impact, positive or negative, on a program and its people. Subjectivist evaluation multiplies the possibilities because the deeper understanding it provides also involves details that are typically extraneous in other approaches. Operationally, even if the investigator works to provide an analysis that protects individuals, it is often difficult to conceal identities.

Because the details recorded throughout the study represent the data on which the argument is built, the problem of intimacy requires careful decisions about which quotes and descriptions to include in the reports at the end of the study. The first step is to decide which points lie outside the boundaries of the study, however interesting these points may appear. There are often details that attract attention but which have no significance within the project.

In the Up-To-Date Clinic project, if the consultant discovered that one of the senior physicians was planning to leave to take another position but had not yet told anyone, would he use the sensitive knowledge? He probably would mention it in a report, after checking with the physician, if the decision was in any way related to the new patient record system (e.g., management's decision to impose the new system was the final straw in the physician's decision to leave). Otherwise, even if the departure would have an important impact on the clinic, there would be no reason to mention it. The investigator must be particularly careful about "leaking" news.

In general, if a point cannot be usefully related to the overall argument, it should simply be omitted. There are obvious limits to this policy: Criminal behavior would not go unreported. The policy affects many less obvious decisions, though, some of which require careful thought. This problem is another example of the potential value of discussions with a neutral partner, as described above under Safeguards.

If a point is legitimately within the argument, it should be included, with careful attention to a basic principle: protect the anonymity of subjects. In general, no data should be reported that would reveal the identity of the subject who provided it. This goal is difficult to achieve, particularly in small organizations, and may imply some adjustment in the way findings are reported. Furthermore, the client of a given evaluation may well apply pressure to learn the identity of certain sources. The pressure must be resisted, making reference to a confidentiality agreement that should be included in the official agreement that provides the basis for the evaluation.

We cannot say "Do no harm" in subjectivist work because the argument may of necessity include points that work to the disadvantage of some participants. It is imperative, however, that potentially damaging points be fully analyzed to be sure the argument does not represent a one-sided version of the situation.

In conclusion, the intimacy of subjectivist evaluation calls extra attention to the need for careful negotiation at the beginning of a project. Subjectivist evaluation involves an ethical dimension on a daily basis. The investigator must accept responsibility for monitoring the ethics of the study and ensuring that the work remains on solid ethical ground. In the agreement formed between investigator and client at the beginning of a study, the details of participants' confidentiality should be made explicit. In the evaluation agreement, it is important to clarify the investigator's promise to treat all of the details confidentially, including the important issue of editorial rights with regard to the final report and publication rights after the study is complete.

Special Problems When Reporting on Subjectivist Work

It would be unreasonable to offer a lengthy statement here on the art of writing, but it is worth some space to point out that subjectivist reports require some adjustments in familiar styles and language. We make five points.

First, the report sequence in objectivist literature is not just a simple formality but a custom with features that add to the image of rational, linear, "scientific" objectivity. The standard format assumes that the investigator did the study by proceeding from question to literature to method to data to conclusions. That image is more or less accurate for an objectivist study, but the traditional format forces a subjectivist study into contortions. With subjectivist writing, the language of the report must fit the reality of the inductive, emergent, nonlinear work.

The introduction should express the issues and questions the investigator is ready to address when the project is complete without pretense that the questions were clear from the beginning. The literature section includes the theory the investigator finds useful at the end to explain the events. The methods section describes the major steps that evolved during the conduct of the study, with some effort to suggest the details and the variations within the design. The findings section inevitably incorporates interpretation, which is traditionally saved for the conclusions section in objectivist studies. The conclusions section resembles the conclusions in objectivist studies, presenting the essence of the argument, the limitations, and the potentials for further study.

It is important to note a significant problem arises when describing the methods of any subjectivist study. Subjectivist methods cannot be presented as precisely as the statistical methods of objectivist work. It is possible to say that a series of interviews were "semistructured," but there are numerous variations within this category. In one interview the investigator might have probed by asking for an illustrative example of an issue the subject mentions. In another, she might have briefly shared a personal memory and asked if it illustrates the subject's point. Furthermore, between the scheduled interviews, she also probably had innumerable conversations, observed in several ways with many differences in the kinds of interaction she had with the subjects. We can outline the major features of the design. We could not provide a description of each event in the same direct way that the objectivist investigator can refer to use of a t-test. The records of the study include much of the description, but we cannot include enough detail in a report to match the clarity of an objectivist report.

In a different sense, there are style changes to be considered that seem like violations of an unspoken law. Specifically, consider using the first person active voice. Say "We interviewed five physicians." In the more familiar genre you would say "Five physicians were interviewed," pretending that no potentially subjective person was involved. This change is not necessary but is becoming the preferred approach among investigators who use qualitative approaches regularly. Again, expect that it will "feel wrong" given the habits and norms learned in years of training.

Third, including the data in a qualitative report is difficult in several ways. The data consist of quotes and descriptions, all of which take significant page space. Furthermore, there is a limit to the accuracy and detail available in the field notes maintained during the study. Writing effectively requires a thoughtful discipline when deciding which quotes to include to make the argument clearly and convincingly. Using the quotes allows the subjects to speak directly, but the investigator must add his own interpretation and take his own stands. Expressing the data in the report inevitably involves interpretation. The task is to make the interpretive steps clear so readers can see the boundary between the investigator and the raw data.

Fourth, include statements in the report that reflect the safeguards built into the study. The investigator should mention enough about herself to allow the reader to anticipate the biases she may have brought to the project. Illustrate the different kinds of interviews and observations employed in the study. Outline the interpretive cycle. Describe briefly the efforts to triangulate and to ask subjects for confirmation. Give the silent partner(s) credit. Even if the investigator cannot describe the process in complete detail, the effort to mention them indicates that she understands the issues and her efforts to safeguard the study throughout. By including these elements in the report, the "methods section" is as complete, in its own way, as the familiar presentation of methods in an objectivist study.

Finally, be sure that the report includes enough detail about the events and their context so a reader can begin to judge whether the findings can be generalized to fit other circumstances. Some authors believe that subjectivist studies are so fundamentally tied to a specific context they should not include any attempt to generalize for application in other settings. Taken to a philosophical extreme, such a position implies that no knowledge gained in one place can confidently be used anywhere else. We believe that although context is an essential dimension of any event, a rigorous study can yield a theoretical, interpretive argument that can be extended to other circumstances. It is also true, however, that the reader should be the final judge of whether the argument fits their circumstances. In order to make that judgment, the reader needs to know enough about the situation in which the argument was developed to estimate the difference in relation to his own situation. Generalization is not an issue when writing an evaluation report for use within the program being studied. However, many evaluation reports are rewritten, with the client's consent, for publication. At that stage of the evaluation the problem of generalization is the same as in objectivist research.

Conclusions

All of the points we have raised here could become the basis of extended discussion. Most involve numerous variations when they are taken into the field and applied. The many tactics an investigator can use in the midst of a basic interview, for example, could fill a useful chapter. Anyone intent on trying subjectivist work needs the initiative to start, the time to reflect on their experience, the imagination to find new ideas, and the courage to build an argument based on studies that seem clumsy and incomplete. With time, practice, and consultation, the many pieces of the subjectivist approach can become familiar and dependable. We offer a list of references as one support in the process.

It may be encouraging to re-emphasize that there is no single right way to proceed in general or with any particular study. There are a number of principles, and there is a continuing requirement that the subjectivist approaches demand rigor, discipline and time. The investigator is free to build the study, to assemble it from a long series of pieces that are both planned and accidental. The end result must describe and explain, offering an argument about how the events that were studied can be understood. Ordinarily, the investigator finishes with a strong personal sense of expanded understanding and new curiosity. Often he or she cares about the study for some time.

At the end, there is a different kind of problem. Having decided to stop, to write the final draft and move on to something else, the investigator must disconnect from the study. Intellectually, it means encapsulating the insights gained through the process while allowing the new questions to suggest another study. Personally, it means stepping back from the people and the events, changing or ending the intimacy the subjectivist study required. Professionally, it often means living through a brief hiatus while the time, energy, and concern that belonged to the study can be reoriented to other people and projects. In general, it gradually becomes apparent that subjectivist approaches bring more of the investigator into the study. At the end, it takes more time to bring the study to a close.

References

1. Geertz C: The Interpretation of Cultures. New York: Basic Books, 1973:7.
2. Patton MQ: Qualitative Evaluation and Research Methods. Newbury Park, CA: Sage, 1990:44,199–369.
3. Van Maanen J(ed): Qualitative Methodology. Newbury Park, CA: Sage, 1983.
4. Lofland J, Lofland L: Analyzing Social Settings. Belmont, CA: Wadsworth, 1995.
5. Shaffir WB, Stebbins R, Turowetz A: Fieldwork Experience. New York: St. Martin's Press, 1980:23.
6. LeCompte M, Millroy W, Preissle J: The Handbook of Qualitative Research in Education. Orlando, FL: Academic Press, 1992:597–632.
7. Guba E: Toward a Methodology of Naturalistic Inquiry in Educational Evaluation. Los Angeles: Center for the Study of Evaluation, University of California, 1978:6.
8. Bogdan R, Biklen S: Qualitative Research for Education. Boston: Allyn & Bacon, 1982.
9. Kleinman S, Copp M: Emotions in Field Work. Newbury Park, CA: Sage, 1993.
10. Miles MB, Huberman AM, Qualitative Data Analysis. Newbury Park, CA: Sage, 1984.
11. Weitzman EA, Miles MB: Computer Programs for Qualitative Data Analysis. London: Sage, 1995.
12. Glaser B, Strauss A: The Discovery of Grounded Theory. Chicago: Aldine. 1967:3, 61.
13. Lincoln YS, Guba E: Naturalistic Inquiry. Beverly Hills, CA: Sage, 1985:289–331.

Appendix A: Interviewing Tips

Note: These comments apply to a semi-structured interview format.

Preparation

- Do not "wing it." Know in advance what key topics or issues you want to be sure to cover before the interview is over.
- Bring what you need with you. If you are taking handwritten notes, bring paper, something to lean on, a good writing implement plus an extra, and a watch. If you are tape-recording, check the recorder in advance to be sure the batteries work (do not count on a conveniently located AC outlet), and bring an extra cassette and set of batteries. Avoid 120-minute cassettes.

Getting Started

- Explain the purpose and format of the interview. Make it clear that although you have a set of issues you wish to address you are interested in hearing everything the interviewee thinks is important on the subject. If the study plan calls for sending a summary back to the interviewee for approval, state that at the beginning. Give appropriate reassurance about anonymity and confidentiality.
- Tell the interviewee that you will make every effort to end the interview on time, where "on time" is whatever interval has been negotiated. That gives the interviewee a chance to say that it is all right to run overtime—or not.
- Begin the interview with an open-ended question. ("In general, how is this project working out for you?") Or you may want to ask the interviewee to describe his or her role in the project. As a rule, it is easier to go from general to specific than in the other direction. Also, specific questions asked early in the interview constrain everyone's thinking. You may never get back to some issues not in the domain of the first few questions you ask.

Topic Flow and Question Format

- In general, let the interviewee dictate the flow of the topics. However, if half the allotted time passes and you still have not touched on any of your predetermined issues, you may need to take some control of the agenda. Do it with an apology.
- Before making a major change in the subject, ask the interviewee if she or he has anything else to add on this issue.
- Always avoid leading questions. ("You don't approve of the way this is being done, do you?)

- If you think you do not fully appreciate what the interviewee is saying, it is acceptable to ask for clarification. Restatement is a good way to do it. ("Let me tell you what I think you are saying. Correct me if I don't have it quite right.")
- It is acceptable to ask the interviewee to reflect on what others have said about the same issue. It is often tempting to do it at later stages of a study when you are looking for corroboration. Be careful, though, it must be done in a way that preserves confidentiality. Do not quote individuals whose views are so well known you are implicitly identifying them when you cite what they said.

Data Recording

- If you are taking handwritten notes, maintain as much eye contact as possible (difficult). Write as quickly as you can and only as neatly as necessary to allow you to understand what you wrote 24 hours later. You should review your notes within 24 hours. Many investigators key them into a computer at this time.
- As you take notes, try to distinguish between direct quotes, reasonably accurate paraphrases, and complete paraphrases. You know when something worth quoting is being said. Try to capture these statements accurately because quotes add a great deal to a report. You can use standard quotation marks (") to denote a direct quote and apostrophes to delimit (') an accurate paraphrase.
- Keep a topic checklist on a separate sheet of paper. On one side of the sheet, list the issues you want to be sure to cover before the interview is over. Check them off as they are addressed and whether at your instigation or raised spontaneously by the interviewee. On the other side of the sheet, list issues and questions that occur to you during the interview and to which you may wish to return later if time allows. Do not plan to take note directly onto an outline of the interview questions.
- Even if you tape-record the interview, take some notes. These notes focus on your thoughts as the interviewee is speaking. Transcribe the tape as soon as possible and review the transcript while the interview is still fresh in your mind.

Ending the Interview

- When time is up, say so and make it clear that the interview can end now. Many interviewees want to keep on talking. Some save their most incisive remarks until the end. For this reason, do not schedule interviews back to back.
- When the interview is over, thank the interviewee and ask, if appropriate, if he or she has any questions about the study methods and what will happen next.

Appendix B: Observation Tips

Preparation

- Negotiate entry into the site. At the beginning, this implies a careful discussion with "gatekeepers" who can grant access. Throughout a study, negotiation means arranging for future visits and new situations. "I'll be back tomorrow afternoon. Is there anything special I should expect?"
- Set aside the time for observation. It is not realistic to start late or to interrupt the observation to respond to other demands. It may be difficult for others to reach you, depending on where you choose to move as observation proceeds. Set time aside for preparing field notes after the observation is complete.
- Try to anticipate how often you will be observing in this site.
- Clarify the initial questions you have in mind as one basis for directing your attention.
- Dress moderately. You want to be both comfortable and somewhat inconspicuous, neither too casual nor too formal.
- Try to have a guide who can take you into the site without marking you as representing any particular people or positions. Clarify how you want to be introduced.
- Rehearse the way you will introduce yourself. The people working in the field will be curious about you, your motives, and the data you are collecting. A first explanation cannot be as objective as the paragraph you may have written about the purpose of the study.
- Take what you will need, knowing how long you will stay: a small notebook and pens, a watch, a snack, business cards.

Getting Started

- Pick a place in the flow of activity and simply watch for a while. Do not move around at the beginning unless you are getting out of someone's way.
- If you get into conversations, keep them brief and simple at the beginning. If you know there will be more observation time with the same people, minimize your impact on them at the beginning.
- Pay particular attention during transitions in the activities.
- Find one person to talk with for 3–5 minutes near the end of the observation period. Choose thoughtfully. You want someone who will be friendly, and through whom you can begin to meet others. For this contact, avoid controversial figures and people with authority roles.

Data Recording

- Take notes briefly and occasionally; don't make a commotion about getting your notebook out. Writing for 15–30 seconds now and then is better than adding smaller notes constantly.

- Be prepared to show some participants your notes. Explain them briefly.
- Step out of the situation occasionally to work on your trigger notes and to take care of yourself. Be sure you know the schedule so you can re-engage with your subjects when you return.
- If you are using a computer, be sure it is a quiet one. If you are using a dicta-phone or minirecorder, avoid talking into it while close to the participants. Make your recordings when you step aside from time to time.
- Be sure to include notes on your own experience as the observation continues.

Ending a Session

- Excuse yourself quietly. Express your thanks to one or two people and let them know what your next steps will be.
- Try to anticipate something you can do to engage the participants more actively next time.
- Allow 5–10 minutes of quiet time immediately after leaving the site. Avoid moving directly from observation on the site into another kind of responsibil-ity. Leaving the site to rush to a committee meeting disrupts your thinking.
- Review your trigger notes soon after leaving the site. Even a quick reading can boost your memory for the time when you can expand them into field notes.

10

Organizational Evaluation of Medical Information Resources

Bonnie Kaplan

Up to this point, the discussion of evaluation has focused on the information technology itself or on the individuals who use or are affected by the technology. Evaluation from a technology perspective considers hardware, software, telecommunications technology, and databases. Evaluation from a people perspective focuses on training, personnel, attitudes of personnel, ergonomics, and regulations affecting employment. It also is important to consider the nature of the work individuals do and the tasks they perform. Designers and evaluators increasingly are recognizing that compatibility of an information resource with work practices is an important concern, and some new methodologies are premised on the assumption that design must be based on work routines.[1-10]

Beyond the individual as the unit of analysis, a variety of issues arise that have to do with the nature of organizations, organizational structure, and the politics of crossing organizational boundaries. For an evaluation at the organizational level, interactions between technology, people, tasks, and organizational structure should be investigated as well. For example, how an organization responds to an information resource may be due to factors inherent in the resource itself; factors inherent in the individuals affected by the resource; factors inherent in the nature of the work or the nature of the organization; or factors pertaining to the interrelationships between the resource, the individuals affected by the resource, and the organization.[11-13] Moreover, according to a sociotechnical theory of organizations, a change in technology, people, task, or structure results in adjustments by the other three to maintain organizational stability.[14] Considering all factors can help the evaluation include important data and insights.

This chapter considers evaluation at an organizational level. First, the nature of the change processes involved when an information resource is introduced is discussed, followed by a discussion of the nature of organizations. The chapter concludes with evaluation questions and criteria for an evaluation plan. The hospital is taken as the primary example of an organization, although similar issues arise in other settings in which clinical information resources may be introduced, such as physicians' offices or health departments. Furthermore, although the discussion is couched in terms of "an organization," it can be applied at different levels of analysis (e.g., to a department, a single hospital, or a multihospital system).

Change Processes

Three well-known models of change provide useful approaches for evaluation.[15] This section briefly describes each model and then draws implications for evaluation from them.

Models of Change

Havelock et al.[16] described three principal groups of models of change based on an extensive review of research literature in several disciplines. They called them (1) problem solving; (2) research, development, and diffusion; and (3) social interaction models.

Problem-Solving Models

According to problem-solving (PS) models, change agents collaborate with clients to bring about change. Change is viewed as occurring in stages. First, needs are identified and then articulated as problems. Next, solutions are sought, one is selected, and this solution is then applied to reduce the needs that were identified. The main focus is on the client's efforts to solve the problems.

Lewin's work[17] formed the basis for these models. According to his theory, change occurs in three stages: unfreezing, moving, refreezing. First an organization must be made ready for change (unfreezing). The change is then put into place (moving). Lastly, the change must become part of the new organizational routine (refreezing). Lewin's analysis of "force fields" that affect these three stages provides the basis for developing strategies for change. Though Lewin's work originally was empirically based, others have expanded on his initial formulation to provide well-known normative models of change,[18] such as those developed by Kolb and Frohman[19] and by Schein.[20, 21]

The PS models seem to have inspired a focus on the political nature of information systems' development and implementation.[13, 22, 23] In this variant of PS models, the focus is on conflicts between different organizational groups.

Research, Development, and Diffusion Models

Models in the research, development, and diffusion (RDD) group start from research and research products and trace a path toward the consumer. A rational, orderly transition of knowledge from research to development to diffusion to adoption is posited by these models. There is little emphasis on *how* knowledge is developed into useful products or problem solutions. The prime actors, according to this set of models, are researchers, developers, and disseminators; the recipients of the new product or problem solution are treated as essentially passive. Unfortunately, the supposed beneficiaries of this solution may not agree that a problem existed or that the solution can help, and consequently they may reject it.

The RDD models may characterize information resource development effort that is being evaluated. These models also underlie policy in many mission-directed agencies of the United States federal government, including agencies that fund medical computing projects and biomedical research. RDD models also characterize academic research enterprises, too, and many researchers share assumptions of these models.[16, 24]

The RDD models also are held implicitly by many in the information systems field. The models resemble the approach to information systems research that Kling[25] characterized as "systems rationalism." In practice, this is frequently the way systems development is undertaken when experts study current information resources, the organization, and the users in order to propose changes to solve a problem. The information resource that may result is assumed to be one that can, or should, support management goals. As in the Kolb-Frohman model[22] users who do not comply are considered "resistant"[26]; and their behavior is seen as "dysfunctional."[27]

This approach has been criticized by researchers working from within a perspective that Kling[25] described as "segmented institutionalist." These researchers recognize that goals may not be shared, so legitimate conflicts might occur.[13] Some of their work indicates the importance of factors identified in the third class of models Havelock[16] discussed: social interaction.

Social Interaction Models

Social interaction (SI) models emphasize diffusion aspects of change and focus on the individual receiver of the innovation. Like PS and RDD models, SI models are stage models, but the concern in SI models is twofold: (1) the stages through which individuals pass as they decide whether to adopt an innovation; and (2) the mechanisms by which an innovation diffuses through an adopting group. Although the adoption process is an individual one, SI models recognize how much that process depends on group interaction. Within the field of information systems, Kling and Scacchi's web model[28] is similar to SI models.

Rogers's classic diffusion model[29-31] generally is accepted as the paradigmatic SI model. In the wide-ranging empirical work studied and analyzed by Rogers to form the basis for this model, the importance of such factors as opinion leadership, personal contact, social integration, and cultural values and beliefs was thoroughly documented. The Rogers model considers diffusion of innovation as consisting of four elements: an innovation (1) is transmitted through channels of communication (2) over time (3) among members of a social system (4).[30] Unlike in the PS or RDD perspectives, Rogers' model indicates that knowledge does not simply filter down, nor is it generated in neat cycles of needs reduction. Instead, it flows back and forth within a complex of networks and relationships. This model has been used to evaluate computer information resources by focusing on such aspects as networks of and changes in communication or on the role of values and professional norms of users.[12, 32-35]

Example

The model an evaluator chooses influences the evaluation by focusing it on different questions and issues. As an example, consider how one might study the adoption and diffusion of a seminal medical information system, the Problem-Oriented Medical Information System (PROMIS).

PROMIS was begun during the 1960s by microbiologist, clinician, and educator Lawrence L. Weed, who soon was invited to develop it at the University of Vermont College of Medicine. Although developed at an academic medical center, it was intended for use in any medical practice. Weed envisioned PROMIS as an active participant in medical management. Objectives included compliance with a new form of medical record that Weed had developed, the Problem-Oriented Medical Record (POMR), and with a vision of medical practice by health care teams. Weed designed PROMIS to address what he considered the three most pressing problems in American medicine: disorganization of medical data, dependence on physicians' memories, and lack of feedback about appropriate care. PROMIS, therefore, went beyond enforcing the POMR format. It was intended both to impose scientific rigor on the complete medical record and also to direct users in the process of clinical care. Clinicians entered data directly into PROMIS and reviewed data directly from it, but PROMIS also volunteered information to instruct and guide clinical decisions and required users to justify deviations from programmed protocols. Although PROMIS was developed and implemented with active involvement of the nursing staff, the medical staff were not involved during the entire term of the project. Despite initial strong support, as evidenced by the University of Vermont's switching to the POMR and desiring to have PROMIS developed and used there, PROMIS ultimately was removed from the ward on which it was tested. PROMIS has not been widely disseminated or used, though the concepts embedded in PROMIS spawned similar endeavors elsewhere, and Weed inspired many projects in medical computing.

The next section briefly describes how an evaluator might explain the development and diffusion of PROMIS according to each of the three groups of change models, based on an excellent comprehensive evaluation of PROMIS by Lundsgaarde et al.[36] (summarized by Fischer et al.[37]).

Using PS Models

An evaluation from a PS orientation, especially in its political variant, might focus on changes in the status of members of the health care team. PROMIS enhanced the professional role of radiologists, pharmacists, and especially nurses at what seemed to be the expense of medical house staff. It was more readily supported and accepted by these groups than by the house staff. However, the medical staff has primary decision-making power in a medical institution, and PROMIS eventually was removed.

An evaluator also might examine the roles of client and change agent. In this case, Weed diagnosed client needs by focusing on needs of nurses rather than on those of his physician colleagues. He also worked with nurses during the change process. It was nurses who were most enthusiastic about PROMIS. Furthermore, the change process was poorly managed. Little was done to unfreeze, move, or refreeze the house staff, who considered PROMIS to have been imposed on them. House staff likely were not involved in decisions pertaining to PROMIS design or implementation. They did not develop a sense of a need for them to use a computer information systen, which, at the time, was a radical ida. PROMIS staff neither focused on house staff needs nor, as unfreezing requires, paid sufficient attention to changing their attitudes so that they would come to see that PROMIS was a solution to a problem they recognized they had. An evaluator studying the PROMIS implementation might examine the forces for change and the forces opposed to it in order to understand what could have been done to unfreeze the house staff so they would be prepared to accept PROMIS, to move them, and later to refreeze them in their new behavior so they would use PROMIS.

Using RDD Models

By taking an RDD approach, Weed could be considered right and the physicians on the medical staff resistant. Weed is a medical practitioner and educator keenly aware of the problems in medicine and sincere in his attempts to remedy them. Surely any physician, from an RDD viewpoint, should share his goals of improving medical practice and medical education. Weed's inspiring vision and evangelical promotion of his ideas did influence many others. Weed followed the process of change that RDD models posit. He is a devoted expert with a visionary solution to a pressing set of problems. His research and development work resulted in a product that should have been beneficial.

Despite Weed's efforts and the potential that PROMIS held, house staff circumvented it. They reported that PROMIS adversely affected their relationships with patients, changed staff communication patterns, and increased the amount of time spent in record keeping activities. In contrast, the study showed that PROMIS did not substantially change the amount of time house staff spent on these activities, thereby raising the question of why house staff thought that it did.

An evaluator using an RDD model would interpret the house staff's behavior and attitudes as resistance. This resistance would most likely be attributed to the house staff's irrationality, perhaps because the medical system itself, from an RDD perspective, is not considered rational or optimal.[26, 35] The problem, then, as in PS models, becomes one of overcoming physician resistance. In RDD models, better education, further technological development, or perhaps requiring that the information resource be used are suggested solutions.[35]

Using SI Models

The SI models would lead an evaluator to focus on any one of four elements of innovation: an innovation, transmitted through channels of communication, over time, among members of a social system. One possibility for an evaluation would be to trace these communication patterns. Anderson and Jay[33] used network analysis to do just that when studying how the adoption of a medical information system spread or did not spread along social networks of physicians associated with a hospital.

PROMIS also could be studied by examining relationships and interactions between the social system where it was introduced, adopter characteristics, and innovation characteristics. Some of these interactions are apparent in the differences in goals and values held by PROMIS's promoters and by potential adopters so that Weed's intentions to revolutionize medicine through the use of PROMIS conflicted with dominant professional values and norms. This conflict contributed to house staff's perceived status change and to their negative perceptions of the changes in communication, record keeping, and relationships with patients.[34] Furthermore, PROMIS's inflexibility deterred adoption and diffusion at its development site because it prevented productive reinvention (explained below) of this information resource by house staff.[38]

Implications of Change Models

Introducing an information resource into an organization necessarily involves change. As these models show, change is a process that takes place over time and involves numerous individuals. Evaluation, then, may document not only what changed but also the processes by which it changed. This area has three important implications for evaluation design.

The first implication concerns a recognition in all these models that change involves communication. Communication may be thought of as one-way, in which change agents disseminate the innovation to potential adopters. The models share an assumption that innovation originates from some expert source and is diffused from a central location out to the periphery. Schön[39] characterized this top–down approach as the "center–periphery model" and criticized it for ignoring decentralized diffusion systems in which innovations may come from multiple sources and evolve as they diffuse along networks of peers. In decentralized systems users modify ("reinvent") the innovation and share decision making. As Rogers pointed out when he modified his classic diffusion model so it was applicable to organizations as well as to individuals, the change process involves participants creating and sharing information with each other. The complex, multidirectional nature of communication involved in the change process means that evaluation must consider these communication activities. Thus, some possible evaluation questions might be the following.[30]

- How are users', organizations', and societies' needs and problems communicated to medical information resource developers? What role do systems analysts, user liaisons, and other agents play in translating these needs and problems into projects?
- What are the key linkages and interrelationships among the various individuals, groups, and organizations involved in the process? They might include, for example, linkages among those developing and disseminating a medical infor-

mation resource, or among those using related resources (e.g., organizations, groups, or individuals linked by computer networks, involved in users' groups, or involved in standards setting).

- How do those who are supposed to use the medical information resource view it? What are the boundaries of the innovation involved (i.e., What do users think is changing, and why do they think so? How do users make sense of the new resource, and how do they explain their behavior with respect to it?)
- In what ways do users and intended users affect the development of the information resource? How have they reinvented the resource? Do "resistance" and reinvention indicate that important aspects of the resource, or assumptions underlying the resource, should be brought to light in the evaluation?

A second implication is the value of making an evaluation longitudinal. More than one time-point is needed to see change. Instead of "snapshot" pictures, research designs providing "moving pictures" of processes through time are needed.[30] Rogers[30] recommended (1) field experiments, (2) longitudinal panel studies, (3) use of archival records, and (4) case studies of the process from multiple respondents.

The third implication of these models of change also is methodological. An evaluator can employ methods that capture why, how, and what changes occurred and the processes that were involved in it. For this reason it is helpful to use a variety of methods, including both qualitative and quantitative ones.

Process theories, too, are especially important for evaluation in order to capture the change processes. Mohr[40] and Markus and Robey[41] described process theories by contrasting them to variance theories. Variance theories are the kind in which various selected factors are measured before and after the introduction of a change. Most commonly it is done through quantitative methods and controlled experimental design. This kind of evaluation is useful for documenting what changes occur. Process theories, however, investigate why changes occurred. To do this, the process of change itself is studied, often by qualitative methods. Qualitative methods are especially useful for understanding the context in which changes occur, how participants experience and conceptualize the changes, and how changes emerge from complex interactions between an information resource, the organizational environment into which it was introduced, and the kinds of individual and technological factors discussed previously in this text.[42]

Thus the same repertoire of methods may be used when evaluating an information resource from the organizational perspective as when evaluating it from the people or technology perspective. Methods are dictated by evaluation questions, however, and some evaluation questions change when taking an organizational perspective. Some of this is implicit in the above discussion. Some becomes more apparent as you understand more about organizations. Therefore the next section discusses organizations per se. Then we return to more specific discussion of evaluation issues.

Nature of Hospital Organizations

Organizational Structure

Formal organizational structure helps an evaluator know how each organizational unit fits with another and what the official role of each individual is within the organization. An evaluator also should be aware that every organization, and organizational unit, has a potent informal structure, too. There are numerous ways in which an organization operates that are not documented on any organizational chart. For example, a renowned surgeon may be influential even if he or she occupies no high-level formal position in the organization. Effective members of an organization know and use this informal structure. They know whom to call to get something done, who the real decision makers are, who has influence over what or whom, and so on. An evaluator can obtain important data by investigating this informal structure as well as the formal structure, though it is more difficult.

The formal structure of an organization generally is conceptualized as dividing an organization along two dimensions. The chain of command and control within an organization—the organization's hierarchy—divides an organization along the vertical dimension, as shown in Figure 10.1. An organization is divided along the horizontal dimension into functional lines. (If an organization has more than one unit, these divisions form the first horizontal level, and they in turn are divided as already described.)

The formal structure generally is readily available by asking about reporting relationships and inspecting an organization chart. An organization chart provides a picture of how an organization is arranged into units (e.g., divisions or departments) and functions—read *across* the page—and which of these units reports to whom—the organizational hierarchy, read *up* the page—as illustrated in Figure 10.2. Each of these two dimensions is described more fully below.

Organizational Hierarchy

In Western societies, organizations typically are thought of as pyramidal in shape, with the point at the top, as depicted in Figure 10.1. The pyramid represents both organizational hierarchy and the relative number of people at each level. Roughly speaking, the pyramidal shape is reflected in an organizational chart (Fig. 10.2). Small or informal organizations may have much flatter pyramids than the description that follows.

At the top of the pyramid, or organization chart, is a chief decision maker who is responsible for running the organization, often the chief executive officer (CEO) or president. A small group of senior executives or senior managers, known as "top management," reports to this individual. For example, Figure 10.2 shows various administrators reporting to the Senior Executive Officer, who reports to the President of the Health Alliance. This president reports to the Senior Vice President/Provost for Health Affairs, who reports to the president of the university of which this hospital is a part. This president, who is not shown in Figure

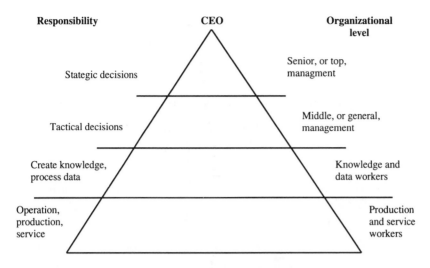

FIGURE 10.1. Organizational hierarchy.

10.2, is the CEO of the university. In some organizations, there also is a governing body or board to whom the CEO reports. Senior management is responsible for strategic decisions concerning the organization. These decisions pertain to long-range planning and the overall purpose of the organization.

At the next level is a group of general managers. Each reports to a senior manager, and each is responsible for a particular area within that major division of the organization. Given their position in the hierarchy, these individuals are called "middle management" (Fig. 10.1). They are responsible for carrying out plans created by senior managers. To do so, they make tactical, or short-range, decisions.

The next, bottom level of the organization is operational (Fig. 10.1). This level consists of the large number of individuals who do the work of producing whatever the organization produces and providing the services needed. Managers and supervisors at the operational level oversee the routine, day-to-day operations of the organization and are responsible for operational level management. The chain of command within an organization goes from top management, through middle management, to the operational level.

Often an additional organizational level is added to the traditional three, as shown in Figure 10.1. This level is for what has come to be called "knowledge workers" and "data workers." Knowledge workers tend to be professionals (e.g., financial analysts or research scientists) who are expert at some specialized area. Their reporting structure is much looser, and they generally are not considered part of the chain of command in a traditional sense. They are far more independent and often function in a consulting role within the organization. Sometimes data workers, including secretarial and clerical staff, also are included in this level,

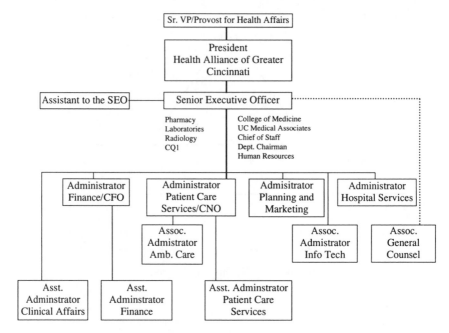

FIGURE 10.2. University of Cincinnati Hospital organization chart. Reprinted with permission from the author.

though in some organizations they are operational/production workers. Knowledge workers are distinguished from data workers by the degree to which knowledge workers create knowledge instead of primarily using or processing data.

The organizational hierarchy applies to hospitals as well as to other organizations. However, hospitals differ from other organizations in important respects. They have at least two lines of authority (chains of command), and they have a large proportion of knowledge workers, who in hospitals consist of the clinical staff. Moreover, clinical departments may have considerable autonomy, especially if they are large revenue producing units. In teaching hospitals the faculty also are knowledge workers.

Hospitals follow the chain of command common in business organizations in that they have a chief executive officer, vice presidents of various areas, department managers, and clerical workers and other production personnel (e.g., cooks, custodians, laundry personnel, police). This line of authority typically is called "administration." Figure 10.2 illustrates the administrative structure of a hospital. Hospitals also have a clinical line of authority, in which there are a senior medical officer, heads of clinical divisions, chairmen of clinical departments, and clinical staff. In some instances the same person occupies two roles; for example, the director of the clinical laboratories may be part of the clinical staff and part of the administrative staff as well. The two lines of authority in a hospital may conflict

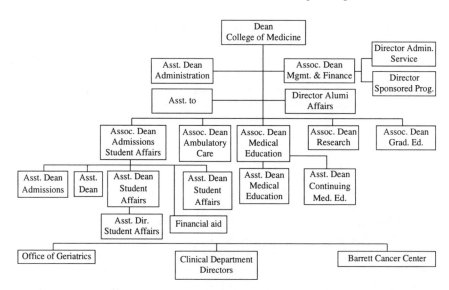

FIGURE 10.3. University of Cincinnati Medical School organization chart. Reprinted with permission from the author.

with each other, as when administration pushes for cost containment measures that clinical staff believe interfere with delivery of patient care. In teaching hospitals, there also is an educational hierarchy that largely coincides with the clinical hierarchy, though it may be part of a different organization, such as a medical school faculty. In such a case, the medical school and the hospital are administratively different, even though they share facilities and personnel. Figure 10.3 is an organization chart of a medical school. Note that the College of Medicine depicted in Figure 10.3 also appears in Figure 10.2; although not shown on this chart, the Senior Vice President/Provost functions as the chief academic officer of the medical school in his role as Provost. Sometimes the dean of the medical school may be one of several deans involved in health care concerns.

Organizational hierarchy also occurs within units and subunits of an organization, so a department may have not only a chair but also vice chairs or division heads and subspecialty heads. In one hospital, for example, the Department of Pathology and Laboratory Medicine was headed by a pathologist who also headed the Pathology Division. Within that division, there were heads of the cytology laboratory, the histology laboratory, and so on. Another division was Laboratory Medicine, headed by a clinical chemist. The heads of clinical chemistry, hematology, and toxicology laboratories reported to him. The larger of these laboratories had assistant heads or chief supervisors. Chief supervisors had supervisors reporting to them, and they in turn had laboratory technologists reporting to them. All the heads of the laboratories were either MDs or PhDs. They served not only on the clinical staff but, because it was a teaching hospital, were on the medical school faculty as well. Thus these directors were part of hospital administration, part of clinical staff, and part of the faculty of the medical school. As shown in Sometimes individuals in a department similar to the one just described could be hospital employees or College of Medicine faculty.

Functional Divisions in Organizations

Typically there are four functional areas within an organization: human resources, accounting and finance, marketing and sales, and production and operations.[43] Just as the size and complexity of an organization determine the number of layers in the organizational hierarchy, they determine the division of labor along functional lines. A small office practice exhibits all these functions, but the functions may be divided among a very few people, some of whom fill more than one function. For example there may be one person in charge of bookkeeping (accounting function) and hiring clerical staff (human resource function). In a hospital setting, administration is represented in all four of these functional areas. Highly educated clinical personnel, who on the whole are considered knowledge workers in the organizational hierarchy, are largely part of the production and operations function since they deliver health care, which is the primary "product" of a hospital.

Organizational Environment

Evaluation requires understanding the organization where an information resource is being installed, at least insofar as it affects both the evaluation and the resource being evaluated. When analyzing an organization, environmental features are important to consider. There are many dimensions along which one can analyze organizations: size, expenditure, number of employees, and so on. Hospitals typically are characterized by number of beds and by their ownership or financing. For example, there are university hospitals, community hospitals, city hospitals, proprietary hospitals, hospitals administered by government agencies, and military hospitals. The different missions, populations served, administrative structure, and financing of these different hospitals makes a difference to how they operate. An evaluator should know the size and type of hospital in which the information resource is being installed because it affects how it is used and perhaps even why it was installed. These aspects often are considered part of the environment of an organization.

Other aspects of organizational environment also are important. Organizational environment can be divided in two ways. First is the distinction between general environment and task environment. Second is the distinction between external and internal environment.

General Environment and Task Environment

An organization's general environment includes the economy, political situation, international situation, and state of technology and science. Task environment includes customers, suppliers, competitors, regulators, and stockholders.[43] For a hospital, they may include patients, pharmaceutical companies, other hospitals, government agents, and contributors, respectively. Environmental factors may affect an information resource significantly. For example, one clinical laboratory planning to purchase a new laboratory information system required a certificate of need to be approved by the appropriate government agency. The hospital waited for more than a year to get this approval. The delay stalled their planned conversion, dampened staff enthusiasm, and resulted in considerable new planning.

External and Internal Environments

An organization also can be thought of as having an external environment and an internal environment. The external environment includes regulations governing hospitals, the type of population being served, epidemics that may occur, government policy concerning financing of health care, and the supply of physicians. These factors can be divided into economic resources, complexity, and turbulence.[43] Economic resources include availability of supplies and labor. Complexity concerns the number of different services a hospital offers, the diversity of the population it serves, the dispersion of hospital units throughout a region, the sources of staffing, and so on. Turbulence has to do with how stable the environment is, for example how quickly prices, demand, reimbursements and government policy change, and, of particular importance, for information resources technology changes.

A hospital's internal environment concerns conditions within the hospital. Internal environment can be divided into four broad areas: management, culture, bureaucracy, and politics.[43] Management issues have to do with the strategic plan of an organization, the style of management, and the degree of management control. Organizational culture has to do with the norms and practices common within an organization. In hospitals the primacy of patient care is an important cultural concern. Professional autonomy is another. These concerns affect if and how clinicians use an information resource.[43, 44] Bureaucracy concerns the organizational structure, hierarchy, and division of labor, as described above, and the procedures used to get work done in an acceptable manner. For example, understanding the bureaucracy aspects of a drug order involve knowing that often in hospitals in the United States a physician gives the order, a nurse writes the order, a ward clerk transmits the order, and the hospital pharmacy receives the order. This set of procedures might well change when a hospital information system is installed. Lastly, politics involves political issues within an organization. They can be, for example, differences in opinion between administration and clinical staff, labor union issues, or decisions concerning allocation of space or work. Often information resources raise political issues and can serve as a focus for carrying out political agendas within an organization.[13, 45–48] Management, culture, bureaucracy, and political issues often are interrelated, as the next section illustrates.

Evaluation Questions

Introducing a technology such as a computer information system can cause both anticipated and unanticipated changes. People tend to use computers as a general-purpose tool to gather and distribute information and to communicate with one another. These social uses of computers influence how people organize their work. Introducing a new computer system thereby changes the organization where it is introduced, because changing the social context changes the organization.[49]

There are three categories of changes that may occur when introducing a new technology or an information resource. First, there are intended technical effects, which are the effects that are planned. Often they are used to justify the introduction of the technology or resource. Second, there are transient effects, which are effects that were not intended. They are short-lived and eventually disappear after an organization has adjusted to the new technology or resource. The third category of effects is unintended effects, which include permanent changes in the organization of social activities and work activities. For example, installation of an elevator had the unanticipated effect of many people who did not know each other suddenly realizing they work in the same building.[49] When evaluating information technology and information resources, it is important to build in ways of considering unanticipated events as well as the anticipated ones, and to distinguish transient from permanent changes.

Anticipated Effects

The organizational background presented so far suggests evaluation questions and areas to investigate concerning anticipated effects. The implementation and use of medical information resources can affect an organization by causing change in (1) decision-making, (2) operations, (3) quality of information, (4) organizational structure, (5) personnel's attitudes, (6) staffing, and (7) costs of operation and information processing.[50] Any of these, or other, changes could be a focus for evaluation.

Evaluation might focus on reasons for initiating projects to implement information resources. Some specific evaluation questions follow, organized according to common reasons for initiating a project. Projects may be initiated to improve capability, control (as in control of data), communication, cost, or competitive advantage.[50] An evaluation can focus on whether any of these areas has, in fact, changed.

1. *Capability:* Increased capability is a measure of a technology's performance, which may affect staffing. Laboratories, for example, were able to increase

their workload substantially without increasing staffing when laboratory information systems were installed.[51] Thus a possible evaluation question might be: Has the information resource changed the way an operation is performed?

2. *Control:* Increased accuracy of data has organizational implications. For example, transmitting drug orders more accurately may improve patient care. Evaluations may include investigating changes in accuracy and completeness of the information users receive.

3. *Communication:* Enhancing communication, such as by increasing access to patient record information for consulting physicians, may improve patient care. An evaluator might investigate changes in the timeliness of information and reports, number of individuals with access to data, interactions among members of an organization, data generation, and data ownership. An evaluator can consider changes in patient care in light of these changes. Enhancing communication for members of an organization also may raise political issues concerning access to patient data or changes in organizational communication and control (discussed below). Evaluation questions might include the following: Has the information resource changed reporting structures or data access privileges? Has it centralized or decentralized control?

4. *Cost:* Hospitals increasingly are monitoring and attempting to control costs, at times by using information technology to monitor organizational resource usage, as in laboratory utilization or the length of stay of patients in various categories. These practices raise concerns about organizational and professional culture and, in particular, about professional autonomy.[34, 47] Issues of conflict and change in professional autonomy make excellent evaluation concerns. An evaluation also might include measuring changes in the cost of an operation, productivity, or amount of effort expended for decision making.

5. *Competitive advantage:* Competitive advantage, though usually not discussed in those words in health care settings, arises as a concern, for example, when attracting patients and personnel. Increased technological capability can provide the wherewithal for other changes. One result can be improved competitive advantage in the form of greater efficiency, a more pleasant place to work, or improved patient care.

Although the original intent of implementing an information resource might serve as a starting point for an evaluation, an evaluation also might ask questions similar to those above, independent of original intent. Additional general evaluation questions of this kind include.[11]

- Does the information resource work as designed?
- Is the information resource used as anticipated?
- How well have individuals been trained to use the information resource?
- Does the information resource produce the desired results?
- Does the information resource work better than the procedures it replaced?
- Is the information resource cost-effective?

Although these questions can be narrowly focused, on technology for example, they also can be investigated by considering how organizational issues shape what happens, or how an information resource affects an organization in these respects.

Unanticipated Effects

The questions listed above take into account the effects of a new information resource on an organization and will help answer whether the changes are for the better. However, no information resource works as anticipated unless individuals use it in appropriate ways. Fifteen years ago, an estimated 45% of computer-based medical information systems failed because of user sabotage[52] (e.g., a user speaking ill of the project or deliberately entering erroneous data). These kinds of reactions are, of course, unintended. Consequently, evaluation also should focus on organizational issues of direct concern to users so as to better understand their behavior. These organizational issues may result from unanticipated effects during and after implementation.

Evaluators also should consider questions concerning unanticipated effects that illuminate organizational processes and issues that can significantly affect users' reactions to a new information resource. For this, broad evaluation questions are needed to raise issues and to obtain data that could not have been included explicitly in the original research design. Four general categories are helpful to keep in mind when considering unanticipated effects of a new medical information resource: communication, care, organizational control (in contrast to control over data, as discussed above), and context. I call these the 4Cs of evaluation.[53] (A fifth C—cost—could be added.) Although these categories can be anticipated, often the consequences of the effects of the change cannot. The 4Cs can be addressed by considering both anticipated and unanticipated effects when seeking to answer the following evaluation questions,[11] which concern issues of communication, context, care, and control, respectively.

- What are the anticipated long-term impacts on how departments interact?
- To what extent do impacts depend on practice setting?
- What are the long-term effects on the delivery of medical care?
- Will the computer information resource have an impact on control in the organization?

Often direct questions concerning the 4Cs cannot be asked. Instead, an evaluator needs to be sensitive to these issues when collecting and analyzing data. Furthermore, answers to each of the above questions likely are related, as the example from the evaluation of a clinical laboratory information system in the next section illustrates.

Example of the 4Cs

A commercial clinical laboratory computer information system replaced a manual system for order entry and results reporting in a 650-bed university hospital. The laboratory information system was used in all nine laboratories within Laboratory Medicine. A study was done to investigate two evaluation research questions.[54-58] One question was to determine the impact of the laboratory information system on work in the clinical laboratories. The other was to identify what happens when a manual order entry and results reporting system is replaced by an automated one. Laboratory directors were interviewed and laboratory technologists surveyed. Observations also were conducted in each laboratory and at laboratory management meetings.

Communication

Prior to implementation, laboratory directors expected the laboratory information system to improve results reporting. They thought results reporting would be faster, more legible, and more complete. Seven months after implementation technologists indicated that the laboratory information system did improve results reporting in these ways and that there was better communication of laboratory results.

Laboratory managers also had expected the laboratory information system to decrease the number of telephone inquiries about laboratory results. In some laboratories technologists said the system reduced the number of calls, which some technologists reported made them "happy." They liked having fewer calls because telephone calls not only interrupt their work but can be unpleasant when the technologists are blamed for slow results or other problems.

Not all technologists focused on these benefits. Some said they still got harassing phone calls, only now they also were being blamed for problems—such as "lost" results—they believed were due to the laboratory information system. Some technologists also focused on how their paperwork and clerical duties had increased. For example, because instruments were not on line, they had to enter test results into the laboratory information system.

The study identified two groups of technologists that differed according to how they responded to the laboratory information system. How technologists saw this system was related to how they conceptualized their jobs. One group of technologists had a product orientation toward their jobs. For them, the job of a laboratory technologist was to produce results and provide a service. The laboratory information system supported the service they were providing. These technologists focused on improved communication and service through better results reporting, and they liked the laboratory information information system more than the other group. The other group had a process orientation toward their jobs. These technologists considered the job of a laboratory technologist to be primarily benchwork, the process of doing laboratory tests. For them, the laboratory information system interfered with this process. They focused on how it had increased work and led to communication problems and other difficulties. Thus how technologists saw the laboratory information system was related to how they saw the role of communication in their jobs and how they saw their jobs altogether. Not all technologists viewed the laboratory information system in the same way, even within the same laboratory. Instead, their job orientation and their views of the laboratory information system were related.

Context

Laboratories as a whole also differed in their response to the laboratory information system. Some laboratories were more process-oriented, and others were more product oriented. Thus the response to the laboratory information system varied with the setting because the job orientation context was different in each laboratory.

Care

Laboratory information systems typically are installed to improve the timeliness and accuracy of laboratory information, which in turn is believed to improve patient care. Altough the laboratory technologists did not report increased accuracy, perhaps because they already thought their performance was good, they did report other ways in which the laboratory information system might improve care. For example, they though that having access to all laboratory data on a patient enabled them to be more connected with patient care because they had what they considered a more complete view of the patient.

Control

Two illustrative control issues arose during the implementation of the laboratory information system. The first concerned the nature of laboratory work and the job of the laboratory technologist. The second concerned whether their department (Laboratory Medicine) would maintain control over all laboratory work in the hospital.

Nature of Laboratory Work

Study results indicated that different laboratory technologists conceptualized their jobs differently, as explained above. This difference raised two issues: What is the technologist's job? Who defines it? There were several ramifications to how these questions were answered.

Laboratory directors did not expect that technologists' jobs would change as a result of the laboratory information system. They reported this assumption during the same interviews as when they said that technologists would have fewer phone calls, fewer repeat tests, and would have to enter data. Even though laboratory directors did not consider these changes in tasks to be changes in the job, some technologists clearly thought that their jobs were changing. They reported increased paper work and more hassles after system implementation. Qualifications for the job of laboratory technologist also were changing. Hiring and retention decisions started to include assessment of a technologist's computer skills.

Another factor indicating job change was that technologists saw experience with the laboratory information system as a way to improve themselves professionally. Some wanted to be appointed as liaison individuals with the systems group so as to improve their job mobility and status. In these ways, technologists thought their jobs were changing, even though directors did not. This made it difficult for directors to plan appropriately for these changes.

Control Over Laboratory Work

A second control issue concerned who controlled laboratory work within the hospital. The intensive care unit, emergency unit, and operating room wanted their own laboratories. At times throughout the study each of these units used the laboratory information system as a reason to argue for having its own laboratory. They claimed that even with the new system they did not get results quickly enough. Hence the laboratory information system served as a focus for political battles.

Implications

This example illustrates that issues of communication, context, care, and control are interrelated in ways that affect what happens when an information resource is introduced. A laboratory information system may improve communication between laboratories and clinical units. However, even technologists who recognize this improvement may find the system incompatible with their work patterns. Laboratory management did not recognize that technologists' jobs were changing and that some technologists would consider these changes to conflict with their understanding of what their job was. Consequently, management could not plan for the ways in which technologists would react to the changes. Changes in communication directly affected changes in work, thereby raising control issues.

These changes can be used as an excuse for playing out existing political agendas. Having other departments claim inadequacies in the laboratory information system and argue that they should have their own laboratory provides an example of how existing organizational control issues may affect, and are affected by, information resources.

Another implication of this study is that it is important to consider different levels of analysis when considering organizational context. The study indicated differences not only between individual technologists but also between laboratories. This finding suggests the importance of distinguishing between settings, instead of, for example, grouping laboratories together into one unit of analysis and treating them all together as the "Department of Laboratory Medicine."

Evaluation Plan: Methodological Guidelines

Five methodological guidelines can be useful when developing a plan for evaluating a complex computer information resource from an organizational perspective. To some extent they are a reiteration of the "evaluator's mindset" first put forward in Chapter 2. The evaluation should:

1. Focus on a variety of technical, economic, and organizational concerns
2. Use multiple methods
3. Be modifiable
4. Be longitudinal
5. Be formative as well as summative

These guidelines serve to integrate into an evaluation plan the organizational considerations discussed in this chapter. Kaplan[5] provided an example of how the plan was used to evaluate a clinical imaging system.

Focus on a Variety of Concerns

An evaluation could include study of a variety of technical, economic, and organizational concerns. These concerns can be examined during the entire process affected by the information resource, with attention to system use, organizational context, and work practices in multiple specialties or functional areas. One way of organizing this evaluation is to use a matrix. One possible matrix, among many possibilities, is shown in Figure 10.4. This sample matrix has, as one dimension, stages of patient treatment[59] and as a second dimension beneficiaries of the information resource.[60] To conduct the evaluation, a variety of questions such as those already presented in this chapter may be asked about each cell in the matrix.

Use Multiple Methods

Evaluations often benefit from multiple research methods. Select the methods that best fit the questions. In the laboratory information system evaluation, a variety of methods was used. Surveys included scaled response and open-ended questions. Laboratory directors were interviewed. Laboratory work and laboratory management meetings were observed. Laboratory documents and memos could have been analyzed. Staff could have been asked to keep logs of critical incidents involving, for example how the laboratory information system changed communication between clinical staff and laboratory staff. The PROMIS study, discussed earlier in the chapter, also used multiple methods. Users were interviewed, observed, and surveyed. Time–motion studies were performed. Two wards, one with PROMIS and one without, were compared.

	Beneficiary		
Stage	*Patient*	*Insurer*	*Physician...*
Examination			
Hospital stay			
Follow-up outpatient care			

FIGURE 10.4. Sample evaluation matrix.

The approaches and methods discussed in other chapters also may be used when evaluating information resources at the organizational level. For example, questionnaires can include scaled response questions as well as open-ended questions, collecting both quantitative and qualitative data. The open-ended questions may be analyzed quantitatively by counting various attributes contained in the data, as in content analysis, or, as is more common for qualitative data analysis, by seeking patterns and themes.

Using a rich variety of evaluation research methods provides several advantages.[32, 42, 56, 61] A combination of methods to evaluate information resources has been advised owing to the diverse and diffuse nature of these resources' effects and to combine results in a way that maximizes understanding of causal links.[62, 63] Combining measurement, experimental techniques, and observational approaches allows collection of a variety of data, each set of which might provide partial information needed for a complete evaluation.[63] Combining qualitative with quantitative methods allows focusing on the complex web of technological, economic, organizational, and behavioral issues.[28, 42] Putting together data collected by a variety of methods from a variety of sources strengthens the robustness of research results through the process of triangulation. Lastly, a multiplicity of methods can help ensure that issues and concerns that were not included in the preliminary design can be integrated into an evaluation later. This can happen in two ways. First, multiple methods increase the chances for such issues and concerns to emerge during the course of an evaluation. Second, the study design then can be modified in light of evaluation findings.

Be Modifiable

Because some important issues and concerns might arise during a study rather than a priori and some effects cannot be anticipated, there are benefits to designing an evaluation that can be modified. Such a plan allows the addition of new phases, methods, or research questions. As discussed in Chapter 9, there are well-established ways of being modifiable without losing rigor or threatening the veracity of a study's findings. A modifiable plan takes account of information resource changes during development and implementation,[64] thereby changing the context from the one when the evaluation originally was planned. Moreover, as individuals become more proficient at using an information resource or more aware of its attributes and effects, they too change the context. Consequently, important new issues and concerns are likely to arise or new knowledge may become available during the course of an evaluation. Periodically reviewing and modifying an evaluation plan in light of this new information can help keep the plan relevant to key evaluation concerns and fit it to the changing nature of the information resource, the organization, and the users.

Be Longitudinal, Formative, and Summative

Advantages of longitudinal evaluation were discussed above, and considerations concerning formative versus summative evaluation are presented in other chapters. Taking a long-term view and attempting to use evaluation to aid implementation processes are of value when studying relationships between an organization and an information resource.

Conclusion

An evaluation at the organizational level is similar in many ways to evaluations discussed in other chapters. What differs most are the focus of evaluation questions and the levels of analysis. An organizational focus includes questions concerning how an information resource, organizational structure, procedures, and general policies[50] mutually affect each other. Also, the political nature of the evaluation is more evident because there are more actors involved with different concerns. This chapter discussed organizational context, evaluation guidelines, and examples to help formulate evaluation questions and approaches that could be useful when considering organizational changes of interest to an evaluation effort.

Acknowledgments. I wish to than Dr. Nancy M. Lorenzi for her invaluable help in providing diagrams for this chapter.

References

1. Fafchamps D, Young CY, Tang PC: Modelling work practices: input to the design of a physician's workstation. Proc Symp Comput Applications Med Care 1991; 15:788–792.
2. Graves W III, Nyce JM: Normative models and situated practice in medicine: towards more adequate system design and development. Inf Decis Technol 1992;18:143–149.

3. Greenbaum J, Kyng M (eds): Design at Work: Cooperative Design of Computer Systems, Hillsdale, NJ: Lawrence Erlbaum, 1991.

4. Holtzblatt K, Bryer HR: Apprenticing with the customer. Commun ACM 1995; 28(1):45–52.

5. Kaplan B: A model comprehensive evaluation plan for complex information systems: clinical imaging systems as an example. In: Brown A, Remenyi D (eds) Proceedings, Second European Conference on Information Technology Investment Evaluation. Birmingham, England: Operational Research Society, 1995:174–181.

6. Kaplan B: Fitting system design to work practice: using observation in evaluating a clinical imaging system. In: Ahuja MK, Galletta DF, Watson HJ (eds) Proceedings, First Americas Conference on Information Systems. Pittsburgh: Association for Information Systems, 1995:86–88.

7. Kaplan B: Information technology and three studies of clinical work. ACM SIGBIO Newslett 1995;15(2):2–5.

8. Nyce JM. Graves W III: The construction of neurology: implications for hypermedia system development. Artif Intell Med 1990;2(2):315–322.

9. Nyce JM, Timpka T: Work, knowledge and argument in specialist consultations: incorporating tacit knowledge into system design and development. Med Biol Eng Comput 1993;31:HTA16–HTA19.

10. Suchman L: Representations of work. Communications of the ACM 1995;38(9): 33–35.

11. Anderson JG, Aydin CE: Overview: theoretical perspectives and methodologies for the evaluation of health care information systems. In: Anderson JG, Aydin CE, Jay SJ (eds) Evaluating Health Care Information Systems: Approaches and Applications. Thousand Oaks, CA: Sage, 1994:5–29.

12. Anderson JG, Aydin CE, Kaplan B: An analytical framework for measuring the effectiveness/impacts of computer-based patient record systems. In: Proceedings of the Twenty-Eighth Hawaii International Conference on Systems Science, HICSS-28, 1995:767–776.

13. Markus ML: Power, politics, and MIS implementation. Commun ACM 1983; 26(6):430–444.

14. Leavitt HJ: Applying organizational change in industry: structral, technological and humanistic approaches. In: March JG (ed) Handbook of Organizations. Chicago: Rand McNally, 1965.

15. Kaplan B: Models of change and information systems research. In: Nissen HE, Klein HK, Hirschheim R (eds) Information Systems Research: Contemporary Approaches and Emergent Traditions. Amsterdam: North Holland, 1991:593–611.

16. Havelock RG, Guskin A, Frohman M. Havelock M, Hill M, Huber J: Planning for Innovation through Dissemination and Utilization of Knowledge. Ann Arbor: Center for Research on Utilization of Scientific Knowledge, Institute for Social Research, University of Michigan, 1971.

17. Lewi, K. Group decision and social change. In: Maccoby E, NewcombTM, Hartley EL (eds) Readings in Social Psychology, 3rd Ed. New York: Henry Holt, 1958:197–211.

18. Ginzberg MJ: Key recurrent issues in the MIS implementation process. MIS Quarterly 1981;5(2):47–59.

19. Kolb DA, Frohman AL: An organization development approach to consulting. Sloan Manag Rev 1970;12(1):51–65.

20. Schein EH: Management development as a process of influence. Indust Manag Rev 1961;2(2):59–77.

21. Schein EH: Professional Education: Some New Directions. New York: McGraw-Hill, 1972.
22. Keen PGW: Information systems and organizational change. Commun ACM 1981; 24(1):24–33.
23. Kling R, Iacono S: The control of information systems developments after implementation. Commun ACM 1984;27(12):1218–1226.
24. Etzioni A, Remp R: Technological Shortcuts to Social Change. New York: Russell Sage Foundation, 1973.
25. Kling R: Social analyses of computing: theoretical perspectives in recent empirical research. Comput Surv 1980;12(1):61–110.
26. Kaplan B: Barriers to medical computing: history, diagnosis, and therapy for the medical computing "lag." Proc Symp Comput Applications Med Care 1985;9:400–404.
27. Wetherbe JC: Systems Analysis and Design, 3rd Ed. St. Paul, MN: West Publishing, 1988.
28. Kling R, Scacchi W: The web of computing: computer technology as social organization. Adv Comput 1982;21:2–90.
29. Rogers EM: Diffusion of Innovations. New York: Free Press, 1962.
30. Rogers EM: Diffusion of Innovations, 3rd Ed. New York: Free Press, 1983.
31. Rogers EM, Shoemaker FF: Communication of Innovations: A Cross-Cultural Approach. New York: Free Press, 1971.
32. Anderson JG, Aydin CE, Jay SJ (eds): Evaluating Health Care Information Systems: Approaches and Applications, Thousand Oaks, CA: Sage, 1994.
33. Anderson JG, Jay SJ: Computers and clinical judgment: the role of physician networks. In: Anderson JG, Jay SJ (eds) Use and Impact of Computers in Clinical Medicine. New York: Springer-Verlag, 1987:161–184.
34. Kaplan B: The influence of medical values and practices on medical computer applications. In: Anderson JG, Jay SJ (eds) Use and Impact of Computers in Clinical Medicine. New York: Springer-Verlag, 1987:39–50.
35. Kaplan B: The medical computing "lag": perceptions of barriers to the application of computers to medicine. Int J Technol Assess Health Care 1987;31:123–136.
36. Lundsgaarde HP, Fischer PJ, Steele DJ: Human Problems in Computerized Medicine, University of Kansas Publications in Anthropology, No. 13. Lawrence: University of Kansas, 1981.
37. Fischer PJ, Stratmann WC, Lundesgaarde HP, Steele DJ: User reaction to PROMIS: issues related to acceptability of medical innovations. Proc Symp Comput Applications Med Care1980;4:1722–1730. Reprinted in: Anderson JG, Jay SJ (eds) Use and Impact of Computers in Clinical Medicine. New York: Springer Verlag, 1987:284–301.
38. Kaplan B: Development and acceptance of medical information systems: an historical overview. J Health Hum Resources Admin 1988;11(1):9–29.
39. Schön DA: Beyond the Stable State. New York: Random House, 1971.
40. Mohr LB: Explaining Organizational Behavior. San Francisco: Jossey-Bass, 1982.
41. Markus ML, Robey D: Information technology and organizational change: causal structure in theory and research. Manag Science 1988;34(5):583–598.
42. Kaplan B, Maxwell JA: Qualitative research methods for evaluating computer information systems. In: Anderson JG, Aydin CE, Jay SJ (eds) Evaluating Health Care Information Systems: Approaches and Applications. Thousand Oaks, CA: Sage, 1994: 45-68.

43. Laudon KC, Laudon JP: Business Information Systems: A Problem Solving Approach. Chicago: Dryden Press, 1991.
44. Kaplan B: Reducing barriers to physician data entry for computer-based patient records. Top Health Inf Manag 1994;15(1):24–34.
45. Aydin CE: Occupational adaptation to computerized medical information systems. J Health Soc Behav 1989;30:163–179.
46. Aydin CE. Computerized order entry in a large medical center. In: Anderson JG, Aydin CE, Jay SJ (eds) Evaluating Health Care Information Systems: Approaches and Applications. Thousand Oaks, CA: Sage, 1994:260–275.
47. Kaplan B: National Health Service reforms: opportunities for medical informatics research. In: Lun KC, et al. (eds) Medinfo 92: Seventh Conference on Medical Informatics. Amsterdam: Elsevier, 1992:1166–1171.
48. Williams LS: Microchips versus stethoscopes: Calgary Hospital MDs face off over controversial computer system. Can Med Assoc J 1992;147(10):1534–1597.
49. Keisler S: The hidden messages in computer networks. Harvard Bus Rev 1986; 64(1):46–60.
50. Senn JA: Information Systems in Management, 4th Ed. Belmont, CA: Wadsworth, 1990.
51. Flagle CD: Operations research with hospital computer systems. In: Collen MF (ed) Hospital Computer Systems. New York: Wiley, 1974:418–430.
52. Dowling AF Jr: Do hospital staff interfere with computer system implementation? Health Care Manag Rev 1980;5(4)23–32.
53. Kaplan B: Implementing and Evaluating Computer-Based Patient Records: The 4Cs of Success, Technical Report 94-001. Hamden, CT: Department of Computer Science, Quinnipiac College, 1994.
54. Kaplan B: Impact of a clinical laboratory computer system: users' perceptions. In: Salamon R, Blum BI, Jørgensen JJ: Medinfo 86: Fifth Congress on Medical Informatics. Amsterdam: North-Holland, 1986.
55. Kaplan B: Initial impact of a clinical laboratory computer system: themes common to expectations and actualities. J Med Syst 1987;11(43):137–147.
56. Kaplan B, Duchon D: Combining qualitative and quantitative methods in information systems research: a case study. MIS Quarterly 1988;124:571–586.
57. Kaplan B, Duchon D: A job orientation model of impact on work seven months post implementation. In: Barber B, Cao D, Quin D, Wagner G (eds) Medinfo 89: Sixth Conference on Medical Informatics. Amsterdam: North-Holland, 1989.
58. Kaplan B, Duchon D: Combining methods in evaluating information systems: case study of a clinical laboratory information system. Symp Comput Applications Med Care 1989;13.
59. Dwyer SJ, Templeton AW, Martin NL, et al: The cost of managing digital diagnostic images. Radiology 1982;144:313–318.
60. Crowe BI: Overview of some methodological problems in assessment of PACS. Int J Biomed Comput 1992;30:181–186.
61. Brewer J, Hunter A: Multimethod Research: A Synthesis of Styles. Sage Library of Social Research no. 175. Newbury Park, CA: Sage, 1989.
62. Bryan S, Keen J, Buxton M, Weatherburn G: Evaluation of a hospital-wide PACS: costs and benefits of the Hammersmith PACS installation. In: SPIE Medical Imaging VI: PACS Design and Evaluation, 1654. 1992:573–576.
63. Keen J, Bryan S, Muris N, Weatherburn G, Buxton M: A model for the evaluation of PACS. In: Boehme JM, Rowberg AH, Wolfman NT (eds) Computer Applications to Assist Radiology, SCAR 94. Carlsbad, CA: Symposia Foundation, 1994:22–29.

64. Berg M: Formal tools and medical practices, getting computer-based decision techniques to work. In: Bowker GL, Gasser L, Star L, Turner B (eds) Bridging the Great Divide. Proceedings of an International Conference on Computer Supported Cooperative Work. Paris: CNRS, 1992:47-64.

11

Proposing, Reporting, and Refereeing Evaluation Studies; Study Ethics

This final chapter addresses a set of issues focusing on communication. These are the often "hidden" but important considerations that can determine if a study receives the resources that make its conduct possible, if a study in progress encounters procedural difficulties, and if a completed study leads to improvement or adoption of an information resource. Whether a study is funded depends on how well the plan for the study is represented in a proposal; whether a study encounters procedural difficulties depends on the investigator's adherence to general ethical standards as well as more specific stipulations built into an evaluation contract; whether a study leads to improvement or adoption of a resource depends on how well the study findings are represented in various reports.

We see that studies can succeed or fail for reasons other than the technical soundness of the evaluation design, considerations that have occupied so much of this volume. Conducting an evaluation study is a complex and time-consuming effort, requiring negotiation skills and the ability to compromise between conflicting interests. The investigator conducting an evaluation must be a communicator, manager, and politician, in addition to a technician.

This chapter provides a glimpse into this set of issues. We focus on proposals that express study plans, reports that express study results, the process of refereeing other people's proposals and reports, and a set of ethical and legal considerations. We are aware that the treatment each of these issues includes just the rudiments of what a fully accomplished investigator must know and be able to do. We encourage the reader to make use of the references and additional readings listed at the end of the chapter.

Writing Evaluation Proposals

Why Proposals Are Necessary and Difficult

A proposal is a plan for a study that has not yet been performed. A proposal usually also makes a case that a study should be performed and often that the recipient of the proposal should grant resources to make the study possible. In most situations, evaluation studies are represented in formal proposals before a study is undertaken. This occurs for several reasons. First, if the investigator requires resources to conduct the study, granting agencies almost always require a proposal. Second, students conducting evaluation studies as part of their thesis or dissertation research must propose this research to their committees, with formal approval required before the work can begin. Third, human subjects committees (institutional review boards, or IRBs) require written advance plans of studies to ensure that these plans comply with ethical standards for the conduct of research. Field studies of medical information resources usually involve patient data, which requires that they carry IRB approval; laboratory studies may also require approval if data that reflect on the clinical competence of practitioners, who may be the subjects of these studies, are collected.

When evaluations are nestled within information resource development projects that are internally funded, a formal proposal of the study may not be technically required. Nonetheless, a proposal is still a good idea. Sound evaluation practice, as first discussed in Chapters 1 and 2, includes a process of negotiation with important members of the client group for whom the study is conducted. These negotiations cannot occur without some written representation of the study plan. An evaluation contract based on an unwritten understanding of how a study is conducted, absent a written proposal, is bad practice. A written evaluation plan, even when not required, is also an important resource to study planning and execution. Conducting a study without a written plan is like building a house without a blueprint. The investigator is always feeling her way along. Changes in a plan are always possible, but it is helpful for the study team to be keenly aware from what originally conceived plan they are changing. Although they are described differently, subjectivist studies can be reflected in proposals just as readily as objectivist studies. There is nothing ineffable about the subjectivist approaches that defies clear description.

It turns out that evaluation studies in informatics are difficult to propose.[1] Writing a study proposal is difficult largely because it requires the author to describe events and activities that have not yet occurred. For most investigators, writing a plan is intrinsically more difficult than describing in retrospect events that have occurred and have been experienced by the people who would describe them. Writers of proposals must portray their plans in ways that are logical and comprehensible. Uncertainty about what ultimately will happen when the study is undertaken must be acknowledged but constrained. In addition to having a clear idea of what they want to do, proposal writers must know what constitutes the complete description of a plan (what readers of the plan expect will be included), the format these descriptions are expected to take, and the style of expression considered appropriate.

Writing a persuasive proposal is part art, part science. Although this assertion is impossible to confirm, it is likely that much potentially excellent research never is performed because the investigator is not able to describe it satisfactorily in a proposal. Finally, evaluation as a relatively young field has fewer models for good proposals, leaving authors somewhat more in the dark than they would be in mature fields where it would be relatively easy to locate a successful model proposal for a project addressing virtually any topic.

Format of a Study Proposal

To describe evaluation studies, we recommend use of the proposal format embodied in the U.S. Public Health Service Form 398 (PHS 398) even if the investigator is not planning to apply to the Public Health Service for funds.[2] This recommendation has several bases. Most important, this format provides a sound, proved generic structure for articulating a study plan. (Writing a proposal is difficult enough; having to invent a format is yet one more challenging thing for the investigator to do.) Even though was developed by a U.S. research agency, the format is universally applicable. Another reason to use the format of PHS 398 is that many, perhaps most, readers have grown accustomed to reading study plans in this format and write their own proposals using it. They then tacitly or overtly expect the plan to unfold in a particular sequence. When the plan in fact does develop in the expected sequence, it is easier for readers to understand. Copies of PHS 398 can be obtained from any university research or grants office, or by writing directly to the National Institutes of Health.[*]

A complete proposal using PHS 398 has 13 parts, proper completion of which is important if one is applying for research funding. We focus here on the one part of the form that expresses the research plan, which itself consists of nine sections, as shown in Table 11.1. The discussion here focuses primarily on sections a–d, where the investigator expresses what she plans to do. In proposals submitted for U.S. federal funding, the total page length of sections a–d is strictly limited, with recommended lengths of each. Investigators preparing evaluation proposals for other purposes may not need 25 pages to express their ideas. Nonetheless, it is wise to maintain the lengths of sections a–d roughly in the recommended proportion.

For proposals that are submitted for funding, investigators usually find themselves challenged to make their proposals terse enough to comply with the page length restriction. Writing proposals is thus usually an exercise in editing and selective omission. Rarely are investigators groping for things to say about their proposed studies. We recognize that in many cases a single proposal is written to describe a large development project of which evaluation is one component. We explore how the situation is managed.

Suggestions for Expressing Study Designs

Here we provide specific guidance for writing proposals using PHS 398. A checklist for assessing compliance with this guidelines is found in Appendix A.

---

[*] Grants Information Office, Division of Research Grants, NIH, 6701 Rockledge Drive, MSC 7762, Bethesda, MD 20892-7762; e-mail girg@drgpo.drg.nih.gov

TABLE 11.1. PHS form 398 research plan format

---

a. Specific aims (recommended 1 page)
b. Background and significance (recommended 2–3 pages)
c. Preliminary studies/progress report (recommended 6–8 pages)
d. Research design and methods

   (Length of sections a–d not to exceed 25 pages)

e. Human subjects
f. Vertebrate animals
g. Literature cited
h. Consortium/contractual arrangements
i. Consultants

---

1. *Specific aims:* In this section of the proposal the investigator describes what she hopes to achieve in the proposed work. The format of this section consists of a preamble, which provides a general rationale for the study, followed by an expression of the specific aims as discrete entities. It is best to number the discrete aims (e.g., Aim 1, Aim 2) so that later in the proposal the aims can be referenced by number. As a general rule of thumb, a study should have three to five specific aims. If the investigator finds herself expressing the study with one or two aims, the aims may be too general; if so, they can be subdivided. Correspondingly, if a study is expressed with six or more aims, the study itself may be too broad or the aims may be stated too specifically. Even though specific research questions might change in an emergent, subjectivist study, the "orienting" questions used to guide the study from the outset can be stated here.

2. *Background and significance:* This section should establish the need for this study/project, not a general need for studies of this type. After finishing this section, the reader should be able to answer the question, "How will we be better off if the aims of this study are accomplished?" Although it is not solely a literature review, this section makes its points with appropriate citations to the literature. For evaluation studies, the need to cite the literature may be less than for more traditional research studies. However, the investigator must think creatively about what is included in the literature. For evaluations, the pertinent literature might include unpublished documents or technical reports about the information resource under study. In general, it is not a good idea for the investigator to cite too much of her own work in this section.

3. *Progress report/preliminary studies:* This section describes previous relevant work undertaken by the investigators and her collaborators. When the proposal describes a new line of research, this section is called "preliminary studies." When the proposal describes a continuation of a line of work already begun, the section is called "progress report." This section emphasizes results of this work and how the proposed study builds on these results. If measurement studies have been performed by the investigator, for example, this section describes the methods and results of these studies. Any pilot data and their implications are included

here. Although it is tempting to do so in this section, it is not the place for the investigators to paraphrase their curricula vitae or describe their awards and accomplishments. In PHS 398, this is accomplished in a separate part of the proposal where the investigators include their biographical sketches.

4. *Design and methods:* This section contains a description of the study being proposed. It includes the following:

- *Restatement of the study aims:* Because the study aims were expressed in section a, this repetition helps the reader bring the study back into focus.

- *Overview of the study design:* Again, to give the reader the "big picture," this part include the evaluation approach being employed as described in Chapter 2 of this book and the type of study as discussed in Chapter 3. If a field study is proposed, it is important to explain how the study will fit into its patient care or educational environment. If the study is objectivist, explain whether the design is descriptive, comparative, or correlational— and why this choice was made. Give an overview of the study groups and the timing of the intervention. If the study is subjectivist, give a sense of what data collection procedures will be employed.

- *Study details:* For *objectivist studies,* this part must include specific information about subjects and their sampling/selection/recruitment; experimental procedures with a clear description of the intervention (the information resource and who will use it, in what forms); description of the independent and dependent variables; how each of the variables will be measured (the instrumentation, with reliability/validity data if not previously reported); a data analysis plan (what statistical tests in what sequence); and a discussion of sample size, which in many cases includes a formal power analysis. Samples of any data collection forms, or other instruments, should be provided in an appendix to the proposal. For *subjectivist studies,* the study details include the kinds of data that will be collected (who is anticipated to be interviewed, the types of documents that will be examined, the types of activities that will be observed); how will study documents be maintained and by whom; the plan for consolidating and extracting patterns and themes from the data. Some readers may find the "Five Kinds of Thinking," described in Chapter 9 a useful structure for describing in advance how a study will be conducted. The reader of the proposal, if conversant with subjectivist methods, will understand that many of the ideas expressed in this section may change as the study unfolds.

- *Project management plan:* For evaluations, it is important to describe the study team and its relation to the resource development team and how decisions about the course of the study will be made.

- *Reporting plan:* For evaluations, it is important to explain the report(s) to be developed, by whom, and with whom they will be shared in draft and final form.

- *Timeline:* The proposal should include, preferably in chart form, a timeline for the study. The timeline should be as detailed as possible.

General Strategies

Evaluations Nested in Larger Projects

Many evaluations are proposed not in a free-standing manner but, rather, as part of a larger development project. In this case the evaluation is best expressed as one specific aim of the larger study. The background and significance of the evaluation is then discussed as part of the "Background and Significance" section of the proposal; the same would be true for the "Preliminary Studies" section of the proposal. The evaluation methods would be described in detail as a major part of the "Design and Methods" section. It inevitably requires the evaluation to be described in condensed form. Depending on the scope of the evaluation, this may not be a problem. If insufficient space is available in the main body of the proposal, the investigator might consider including one or more technical appendices to provide further detail about the evaluation.[*]

Unresolvable Design Issues

At the time they write a proposal, investigators often find themselves with a design issue that is so complex it is not clear how to resolve it. In this case, the best strategy is not to try to hide the problem. An expert, careful reader will probably see that the problem is there. Hence, the investigator should admit she has an unsolved problem, show she is aware of the issues involved, and, above all, how others in comparable situations have addressed issues of this type. This strategy often succeeds in convincing the reader/reviewer of the proposal that although the investigator does not know what to do now she will make a good decision when the time comes during the execution of the study.

Cascade Problem

A related issue is the so-called cascade problem which occurs when the plan for stage N of a study depends critically on the outcome of stage N-1. There is no simple solution to this problem. The best approach is to describe the dependencies, how the decision will be made, and possibly describe in some detail the plan for stage N under what the investigator considers the most likely outcome of stage N-1. Some proposal writers consider the existence of a cascade problem to indicate the boundaries of what they will define as one study. If the outcome of stage

---

[*] Some caution is required here if the proposal is to be submitted for federal funding. The guidelines for Form 398 specifically state that the appendix should not be used "to circumvent the page limitations of the research plan."[2] If one includes specimen data collections forms in the appendix and provides more technical information about the forms also in the appendix, that is probably all right. However, if the main body of the proposal says that "the evaluation design is described in Appendix A" and the appendix in fact contains the entire description, the proposal will likely be returned by the funding agency for modification.

N depends on stage N-1, stage N is considered to be a different study and is described in a separate proposal.

Writing Reports of Completed Studies

Generic Issues of Report Writing

Once a study is nearing completion, much data will have been collected and many possible interpretations discussed. These alternative interpretations of the data usually have been fueled by reports of other studies in the literature. As a result, those responsible for writing up the study usually have access to a mass of raw and interpreted data and comparisons between their results and those of others. Deciding what to include in any written report is often difficult. The key question, as when deciding what to study,[3] is what is necessary, in contrast to what might be interesting, to include for the audience or audiences who are the "targets" of the report.

Because evaluations are carried out for specific groups with specific interests, the task of report writing can be clarified through attention to what these groups need to know. If the report is for a single reader with a specific decision to make, that individual's interests guide the contents of the report. More typically, however, the investigator is writing for a range of audiences, perhaps including clinicians, medical informaticians, methodologists and computer scientists. Each of these audiences expect more detail in the areas of most interest to them, potentially making for a lengthy report. There is a conflict between making a report brief enough to reach a wide audience, often by publication in a widely read journal, and describing the information resource, clinical problem and setting, the subjects studied, origin of cases, and study methods in enough detail to allow others to reproduce them.

One strategy in any sizable evaluation study is to publish details of the information resource, clinical problem, and setting in one paper and then refer to this publication in subsequent evaluation reports. Rightly, however, clinical journals are reluctant to accept publications that merely describe an information resource and its potential application without evidence of effectiveness - or at least accuracy. However, some medical informatics journals thrive on descriptions of novel information resources, making it easier to publish some of this technical detail separately. Once measurement studies are complete, these too can be separately published, especially if they describe methods and instruments that measure attributes of general interest, such as the dilemmas faced by primary care physicians,[4] the quality of medication prescribing, or user attitudes to information resources. The paper describing the demonstration study can then focus on the details of the study methods, the results, and the conclusions drawn in the context of the literature.

As time goes on and the field of informatics becomes more mature, public resources such as libraries of test cases and published, validated measurement instruments accumulate. Once they are established, reference to these published or otherwise documented resources and methods are enough, as is seen in the biological sciences literature for standard assays and preparation methods. Such references make evaluation study reports briefer, as some detail is published elsewhere.

A useful strategy is to view reporting as a process rather than a single event. It is most useful when a study is conducted for a specific audience which needs to make decisions that previously have been identified, but it also can assist the investigator when the intended foci of the evaluation are less clear. Subjectivist approaches offer an extreme manifestation of this via the process of "member checking" where the investigator continuously reflects her findings and interpretations against the individuals in the environment under study (see Chapter 9). Less extreme applications of this approach include sharing of report drafts with selected audience members. Their reactions to drafts can make a modified report more informative to a wider distribution. Sometimes a study divides itself naturally into sections, each of which must be completed before the next is undertaken. In such cases the investigator could produce and disseminate a report of each section before undertaking the next phase of the study.

In all evaluations, but particularly when reporting is to be a multistaged process as suggested here, the evaluation contract assumes a central role in shaping what will happen. A possible dilemma arises if an audience member, perhaps the director of the resource development project under study, disagrees with the methods or conclusions of a draft evaluation report. The contract, if properly written, protects the investigator and the integrity of the study by giving the investigator the final word on the content of the report. A contract typically stipulates that reactions to draft evaluation reports have the status of advice. The investigator is under no obligation to modify the report in accord with these reactions. More often than not, however, the reactions to draft evaluation reports do not raise ethical/legal dilemmas but, rather, provide crucial information to the investigator that improves the report.

Another dilemma facing authors is whether they should "pass judgment" on the information resource or leave judgment to the reader. Referees and journal editors increasingly expect every statement in an article's conclusions to be justified by reference to the data presented; vague or exaggerated statements such as "this technique has a great potential for wider application" are likely to antagonize readers and lead referees to reject the paper. Thus if conclusions are drawn, they should be specific, justified by reference to study results, and not unduly generalised beyond the settings and information resource studied. The readers are left to satisfy themselves about whether the resource is likely to benefit them. In general, the investigator should remain available to the various audiences of the evaluation to clarify issues and provide information beyond that included in the formal report, should it be requested.

Finally, written, textual communication is not the sole medium for communicating evaluation results. Although they are difficult to make part of journal publications, alternative methods and "multimedia" approaches can be helpful as ways to enhance communication with specific audiences. A useful strategy is to hold a "town meeting" to discuss a written report after it has been released. Another strategy is to take photographs or videotapes of the clinical setting for a study, the people in the setting, and the people using the resource. These images—whether included as part of a written report, shown at a town meeting, or even placed on the World Wide Web—can be worth many thousands of words. The same may be true for recorded statements of resource users. If made available, with permission, as part of a multimedia report, the voices of the participants can convey a feeling behind the words that can enhance the credibility of the investigator's conclusions.

Objectivist Study Reports

The format of scientific papers has evolved over the last century into the well-known "IMRAD" structure.

1. *Introduction* to the problem, review of relevant literature and statement of study goals.
2. *Methods* adopted, including details of statistical tests used, described in enough detail (or by reference to published papers) to allow another investigator to replicate the study.
3. *Results,* often summarized in tables or graphs. Some journals now ask for full data to be sent with the article for the purposes of refereeing. With the authors' agreement, these data can be made available to other interested parties on request.
4. *Analysis* or interpretation of the data.
5. *Discussion* of the results and potential limitations of the study, and conclusions drawn in the context of other studies.

This formula emphasizes clear separation between the study aims, methods, results, and conclusions, in keeping with the objectivist approach to evaluation. This distinction is also seen in the recommended format for study proposals (see above). Writing up an evaluation study using this model encourages authors to be clear about the scientific questions that were tackled, the data that will answer the questions, and if the inferences drawn from the data are justified.

Authors of papers describing studies of information resources should be guided by the above structure but may wish to add further sections or detail within sections where necessary. For example, where novel statistical or computational methods have been used, it is useful to include a paragraph describing them in the methods section; in the case of measurement studies, it is wise to include copies of the relevant instruments for publication as figures or an appendix.

The above structure applies equally to randomized clinical trials, but because of the importance of trials as the most reliable form of evidence about the efficacy of clinical interventions[5] additional guidelines about reporting trials have been published, including the work of the Standards of Reporting Trials group.[6] Some journals are now requiring that all clinical trials be reported according to these standards. This practice will aid groups such as the Cochrane Collaboration, who are writing systematic reviews or meta-analyses of the literature.[7] Equally, because bibliographic systems increasingly store the abstract along with the citation, many journals are now requesting that authors structure the abstract of an article into sections resembling the IMRAD structure of the article and keep the length of abstracts to a strict word limit.

Subjectivist Study Reports

The goals of reporting a subjectivist study may include describing the resource; how it is used; how it is "seen" by various groups; and its effects on people, their relationships, and organizations. This means that the subjectivist researcher needs to include direct quotations, interesting anecdotes, revealing statements, lessons learned, and examples of the insights, prejudices, fears, and aspirations that study subjects expressed— all with due regard to the contract or memorandum of understanding negotiated at the study outset.

Reports of qualitative studies raise a number of special issues, which are discussed briefly below:

- In comparison with an objectivist study, writing a subjectivist report is less formulaic and more challenging to the written communication skills of the investigator. Conveying the feelings and beliefs, and often the hopes and dreams, of members of a work environment in relatively few words can require the talents of a poet. Reports typically require numerous drafts before they communicate as intended.

- Respecting the confidentiality of study subjects. The main concerns about potential breakdown in confidentiality are clear from the way effective field work is conducted, and the measures to be taken to protect subjects should be laid out in the memorandum of understanding. This memorandum may need to be altered to address difficult problems or conflicts as they emerge. Before distributing the report, the evaluator must show each subject any relevant passages that might allow them to be identified and allow the subject to delete or modify the passage, within limits, if there are major potential implications or if they are in any doubt about the subject's concerns.

- The study report is typically an evolving document, written in consultation with the client group. Version control is important, and it is often unclear when the report is "finished." Here again, the evaluation contract may be helpful for determining when "enough" work has been done.

- The report can itself change the environment being studied by formalizing and disseminating insights about the information resource. Thus evaluators must adopt a responsible, professional approach to its writing and distribution.

- It can be difficult to summarize a subjectivist study in 10 to 20 manuscript pages without losing the richness of the personal experiences subjectivist studies strive to convey. There is a danger that journal articles describing such studies can be unpersuasive or come across as more equivocal than the underlying data really are. To counteract this problem authors can use extracts from typical statements by subjects or brief accounts of revealing moments to illustrate and justify their conclusions in the same way objectivist researchers summarize a mass of patient data in a set of tables or statistical metrics. If there exists a more lengthy report, they can attach it when submitting their paper to aid editors or referees in assessing the shorter report; journals could make such longer reports available to interested third parties in the same way they make detailed data from objectivist studies available.

- Few articles describing subjectivist studies are published in clinical journals, but this may be gradually changing, with a recent *British Medical Journal* series describing subjectivist methods.[8] Also, a variety of subjectivist studies relevant to medical informatics have been reported.[9–11] We believe there is no intrinsic or insurmountable reason why subjectivist studies should be unpublishable in the traditional archival literature. The key points if one is writing for a journal are to be brief but describe comprehensively the data collection and interpretation methods used, give illustrative examples of results (data collected and analyzed) to support the conclusions, and avoid any implication that the subjectivist methods are ineffable, intuitive, or irreproducible. Such implications would play into the biases of many reviewers against subjectivist methods. All investigators, objectivist and subjectivist, are guided significantly by intuition, and the entire scientific community tacitly acknowledges that fact.

Refereeing Evaluation Studies

We discuss here briefly how one goes about reviewing a proposed study submitted for funding or a completed study that has been submitted for publication. Many funding organizations or journals provide referees with a checklist of questions they would like addressed, which obviously take precedence over the generic advice that follows. In general, the questions that referees can ask themselves include the following.

- Is there a study question, and is it clearly formulated? Often there is more than one question per study
- Is the study question worth answering, or is the answer already well established from other studies?
- What methods would you have adopted to answer the study questions?
- Are the methods described in sufficient detail to be sure what was done or is being proposed?
- Are these methods appropriate to answer the study question, given the potential biases and confounding factors, that is, is the study internally valid?

- Is the study setting sufficiently typical to allow useful conclusions to be drawn for those working elsewhere, that is, is the study externally valid? This point may not always be crucial for an evaluation done to satisfy a "local" need.
- In the case of requests for funding, is it feasible for the investigators to carry out the methods described within the resources requested? Does the proposal meet the standards given in Appendix A?
- In the case of completed studies, are the data reported in sufficient detail? In objectivist studies, do all summary statistics, tables, or graphs faithfully reflect the raw data; or is there, for example, a suspicion of non-normality in the data that may make parametric statistical tests inappropriate? In subjectivist studies, is the writing sufficiently crisp and evocative to lend both credence and impact to the portrayal of the results?
- Does the interpretation of the data reflect the source of the data, the data itself, and the methods of analysis used?
- Are the conclusions valid given the data, the study design and setting, and other relevant literature?

Ethical and Legal Considerations During Evaluation

Ethical Issues

Evaluation raises a number of ethical issues. One of the most common ethical concerns raised at the outset of an evaluation project is the need to maintain the confidentiality of the clinicians and patients studied. It is of special concern when data must be processed off-site or includes items likely to be sensitive to patients (e.g., their HIV status or psychiatric history) or clinicians (e.g., their performance or workload). One approach is to "anonymize" the data by removing of obvious identifiers, altough, especially in the case of rare diseases or clinicians practicing in unusual specialties, people with certain skills and access to a number of related databases may still be able to identify the individuals concerned by a process of triangulation.[12] Physical security measures and shredding of discarded paper are underutilized but effective methods of restricting access to confidential data.[13] Software access controls on databases and encryption of data sent by insecure methods such as the Internet are also useful. The need to respect the anonymity of informants in subjectivist studies has been discussed above and in Chapter 9.

Another ethical concern is whether it is right to make an information resource available to care providers during a demonstration study without requesting the approval of the patients whose management it may indirectly influence or, conversely, to withhold advice of an information resource from the physicians caring for a control group. In anything other than a straightforward case, such as providing doctors with the CD-ROM equivalent of a standard textbook, it is essential to request the approval of an IRB before starting a health care impact study and to follow the advice of the IRB regarding whether, for example, to obtain informed consent from patients whose care providers are participating.

The final ethical problem discussed here concerns the evaluator's integrity and professionalism.[14] Evaluators are in a strong position to bias the collection, interpretation, and reporting of study data in such a way as to favor—or disfavor—the information resource and its developers. To prevent it, they should typically be independent agents, commissioned by an independent organization with no strong predispositions toward or profit to be made from specific outcomes of the evaluation. In the extreme case, the developers of an information resource should avoid the temptation to be the sole evaluators of their own work unless there is an external audit of decisions taken and data collected. Otherwise, no matter how careful the methods and clear the results, there may remain a suspicion that 19 negative studies were conducted and their results suppressed before the twentiethth study, which revealed a favorable result statistically significant at the 5% level. When the evaluation group for a project includes the same people as the development group, it is advisable to create an "advisory committee" for the evaluation that can perform an auditing, validation, and consultative function for the evaluation.

Legal Issues

The developers and users of medical information resources may be concerned about the possible legal implications should a patient take legal action against a clinician who had access to an information resource during a demonstration study and who might have based the patient's care in part or whole on the advice of the resource. This topic is complex,[15] but in summary both developers and clinician-users would probably be immune from negligence claims if they could show that:

1. The information resource had been carefully evaluated in laboratory studies
2. The information resource provided its user with explanations, well-calibrated probabilities, or the opportunity to participate in the decision-making process
3. No misleading claims had been made for the information resource
4. Any error was in the design or specification of the information resource rather than in its coding or hardware
5. Users had been adequately trained and had not modified the information resource

The intent of these measures is to persuade a court that system developers had acted responsibly and were providing clinicians with a service to enhance their professional skills, not a black-box product. This diminishes a developer's risk exposure because those who provide services are judged by whether they acted responsibly (the Bolem test)[15]; those who provide products are deemed negligent once a fault is proved, no matter how much care they have taken to avoid faults: "strict" product liability.[15]

Conclusions

Planning and running an evaluation study is a complex, time-consuming effort that requires both technical skills and the ability to compromise between often conflicting constraints. Once the study is complete, it must be reported in such a way that the context, results and implications are clear. Evaluation does raise a number of ethical and legal issues that must be carefully considered; the separation of the information resource developer from the evaluators is now becoming an accepted part of medical informatics.

References

1. Miller RA, Patil R, Mitchell JA, Friedman CP, Stead WW: Preparing a medical informatics research grant proposal: general principles. Comput Biomed Res 1989; 22:92–101.
2. US Department of Health and Human Services, Public Health Service. Grant Application (PHS 398). Form approved through September 30, 1997, OMB No. 0925-0001.
3. Miller PL, Sittig DF: The evaluation of clinical decision support systems: what is necessary versus what is interesting. Med Inf (Lond) 1990;15:185–190.
4. Timpka T, Arborelius E:. A method for study of dilemmas during health care consultations. Med Inf (Lond) 1991;16:55–64.
5. Sackett D, Haynes R, Guyatt G, Tugwell P: Clinical Epidemiology: A Basic Science for Clinical Medicine, 2nd Ed. Boston: Little Brown 1991
6. SORT: Standards of Reporting Trials Group. A proposal for structured reporting of randomised controlled trials. JAMA 1994;272:1926–1931.
7. Chalmers I, Altman DG: Systematic Reviews. London: BMJ Publishing, 1995
8. Jones R. Why do qualitative research? BMJ 1995;311;2 [editorial].
9. Lindberg DA, Siegel ER, Rapp BA, Wallingford KT, Wilson SR. Use of MEDLINE by physicians for clinical problem solving. JAMA 1993;269:3124–3129.
10. Forsythe DE. Using ethnography in the design of an explanation system. Expert Syst Applications 1995;8:403–417.
11. Osheroff JA, Forsythe DE, Buchanan BG, et al: Physicians' information needs: an analysis of questions posed during clinical teaching in internal medicine. Ann Intern Med 1991;114:576–581.
12. Anderson R: NHS-wide networking and patient confidentiality. BMJ 1995;311:5–6.
13. Wyatt JC: Clinical data systems. II. Components and techniques. Lancet 1994;344:1609–1614.
14. Heathfield H, Wyatt JC: The road to professionalism in medical informatics: a proposal for debate. Methods Inf Med 1995;34:426–433.
15. Brahams D, Wyatt J: Decision-aids and the law. Lancet 1989;2:632–634.

Suggested Reading

Smith NL (ed): Communication Strategies in Evaluation. Beverly Hills, CA: Sage,1982. [A somewhat old but very interesting book that outlines many nontraditional modes of communicating evaluation results is.]

Popham WJ: Educational Evaluation. Englewood Cliffs, NJ: Prentice-Hall, 1988. [An amusing, widely applicable chapter on reporting evaluations.]

Appendix A: Proposal Quality Checklist

A. Specific aims
  1. Establishes a numbering system (Aim 1, Aim 2...)
  2. Includes preamble followed by a list of numbered aims
B. Background and significance
  1. Establishes the need for this study/project (not a general need for studies of this type)
  2. States how we will be better off if we know the answers to these questions
  3. Uses the literature extensively (30+ references)
  4. Does not cite too much of the investigator's own work
C. Progress report/preliminary studies
  1. Describes relevant previous work of principal investigator or collaborators
  2. Emphasizes results of this work and how proposed study builds on these results
  3. Does not paraphrase investigator's curriculum vita
  4. Reports pilot data
D. Design and methods
  1. Does the proposal use the structure of the aims to organize the research plan? Are the following included?
     a. (Re)statement of aims and specific hypotheses or questions
     b. Overview of design
     c. Management plan
     d. Reporting plan
     e. Timeline in as much detail as possible
  2. For objectivist studies
     a. Subjects and their selection/recruitment
     b. Experimental procedures/intervention
     c. Independent and dependent variables
     d. How variables will be measured (instruments and any reliability/validity data not previously reported)
     e. Data analysis plan (what statistical tests in what sequence)
     f. Power analysis and discussion of sample size
  3. For subjectivist studies
     a. Kinds of data that will be collected
     b. From whom data will be collected

    c. How study documents will be maintained

    d. Plan for consolidating and generating themes from data

E. In general

  1. Does the format/layout help the reader understand the project?

  2. If there is an unsolved problem, does principal investigator show awareness of the issues involved and how others have addressed them?

  3. Is the cascade problem (if any) adequately addressed?

  4. Are specimen data collection forms included in the Appendix?

Glossary*

Accuracy: (1) Extent to which the measured value of some attribute of an information resource, or other object, agrees with the accepted value for that attribute or "gold standard" (q.v.[†]); (2) extent to which a measurement in fact assesses what it is designed to measure (roughly equivalent to "validity").

Alerting system: System that monitors a continuous signal or stream of data and generates a message (an alert) in response to patterns or items that may require action on the part of the care provider.

Analysis of variance (ANOVA): General statistical method for determining the statistical significance of effects in experimental studies. The F test is the basic inferential test statistic for analysis of variance (see Chapter 7).

Attribute: Specific property of an object that is measured, similar to "construct."

Baseline study: Study undertaken to establish the value of a variable of interest prior to an intervention such as the deployment of an information resource.

Bias: (1) *Measurement bias:* Any systematic deviation of a set of measurements from the truth. (2) *Cognitive bias:* A set of consistent tendencies of all humans to make judgments or decisions in ways that are less than optimal.

Bug report: User's report of an error in a program. The rate of bug reports over time may provide a measure of improvement in a system.

Calibration: Extent to which estimates of the probability of an outcome of interest are accurate, in comparison to the percentage of subjects actually developing that outcome.

---

* This glossary was adapted from an earlier version produced by the authors for a conference on evaluation of knowledge-based systems, sponsored by the National Library of Medicine and held December 6–8, 1995. Some terms defined here are not explicitly used in this book but may be encountered elsewhere by readers as they read evaluation reports or the methodological literature. We thank Bruce Buchanan, Gregory Cooper, Brian Haynes, Henry Schoolman, Edward Shortliffe, and Bonnie Webber for their suggestions for terms and definitions.

† q.v. = see also

Clinical trial: Prospective experimental study where a clinical intervention (e.g., an information resource) is put to use in the care of a selected sample of patients. Clinical trials almost always involve a second group, formed by random allocation, which receives either no intervention or a contrasting intervention.

Cohort study: Prospective study where two or more groups (not randomly selected) are selected for the presence or absence of a specific attribute, and are then followed forward over time, to explore associations between factors present at the outset and those developing later.

Comparative study: Experimental study where the values of one or more dependent variables are compared across discrete groups corresponding to values of one or more independent variables. The independent variables are typically manipulated by the investigator but may also reflect naturally occurring groups in a study setting.

Confounding: Problem in experimental studies where the statistical effects attributable to two or more independent variables cannot be disaggregated. Also, the "hidden" effects of a bias or a variable not explicitly included in an analysis.

Consultation system: Decision support system that offers patient- and situation-specific advice when a decision-maker requests it.

Content analysis: Technique widely used with narrative data to assign elements of verbal data to specific categories (see Chapter 9). Usually, the categories are defined by examining all or a specific subset of the data.

Context of use: Setting in which a system is situated. It is generally considered important to study a system in the context of use as well as in the laboratory. Synonym: "field."

Contingency table: Cross-classification of two or more nominal or ordinal variables. The relation between variables in a contingency table can be tested using the chi-square or many other statistics. When only two variables, each with two levels, are classified: often called a "two by two table (2×2)."

Control (control group): In experimental studies, the intervention(s) specifically engineered to contrast with the intervention of interest. It can be no treatment other than the normal treatment, an accepted alternative treatment, or no treatment disguised as a treatment (placebo).

Correlational study: Nonexperimental study, conducted in a setting where manipulation is not possible, that establishes correlations or statistical associations among independent and dependent variables.

Cost–benefit: Measuring the effectiveness of an intervention and its costs in monetary terms. The result is a statement of the type "running the reminder system cost $20,000 per annum but saves $15 per patient in laboratory tests."

Cost-effectiveness: Measuring the value of a system by taking into account both the effect/impact of the system and its marginal cost in comparison with care provided without the system. Similar to cost–benefit, but cost-effectiveness analysis does not require expression of system performance in monetary terms. The result is a statement of the type "running the reminder system costs $20,000 per annum but saves one laboratory test per patient."

Critiquing system: Decision support system in which the decision maker describes the patient to the system then specifies his or her own plans to the system. The system then generates advice—a critique—which explores the logical implication of those plans in the context of patient data and medical knowledge.

Decision support system (decision-aid, decision-assistance system, decision-making system): System that compares patient characteristics with a knowledge base and then guides a health provider by offering patient-specific and situation-specific advice. Such systems, by definition, offer more than a summary of the patient data.

Demonstration study: Study that establishes a relation—which may be associational or causal—between a set of measured variables.

Dependent variable: In a correlational or experimental study, the main variable of interest or outcome variable, which is thought to be affected by or associated with the independent variables (q.v.).

Descriptive study: One-group study that seeks to measure the value of a variable in a sample of subjects. Study with no independent variable.

Double-blind study: Clinical trial in which neither patients nor care providers are aware of the treatment groups to which patients have been assigned.

Emergent design: Study where the design or plan of research can and does change as the study progresses. Characteristic of subjectivist studies .

Errors of commission (type I error, false-positive error): Generically, when an action that is taken turns out to be unwarranted or an observed positive result is in fact incorrect. In statistical inference, a type I error occurs when an investigator incorrectly rejects the null hypothesis.

Errors of omission (type II error, false-negative error): Generically, when an action that should have been taken is not taken or a negative test result is incorrect. In statistical inference, a type II error occurs when an investigator incorrectly fails to reject the null hypothesis.

Ethnography: Set of research methodologies derived primarily from social anthropology. The basis of much of the subjectivist, qualitative evaluation approaches.

Evaluation (of an information resource): There are many definitions of evaluation, including (1) The process of determining the extent of merit or worth of an information resource; (2) a process leading to a deeper understanding of the structure, function, or impact of an information resource.

Experimental design: Plan for a study that includes the specification of the independent and dependent variables, the process through which subjects will be assigned to groups corresponding to specific combinations of the independent variables, and how and when measurements of the dependent variables will be taken.

Experimental study: Study purposefully designed by an investigator to explore cause-and-effect relations through use of control, randomization, and analytic methods of statistical inference.

Facet: A source of error that is purposefully explored in measurement studies, analogous to independent variables in demonstration studies.

Feasibility study: Preliminary "proof-of-concept" evaluation demonstrating that a system's design can be implemented and will provide reasonable output for the input it is given.

Field study: Study of an information resource where the system is used in the context of ongoing health care. Study of a deployed system (cf. Laboratory study).

Formative study: Study with the primary intent of improving the information resource under study by providing the developers with feedback or user comments (cf. Summative study).

Gold standard: Expression of the state of the art in health care or the "truth" about a patient's condition, against which performance of an information resource can be compared. In practice, gold standards are usually not knowable, so studies often employ the best approximation to the "truth" that is available to the investigator.

Human factors: Those aspects of the design of an information resource that relate to the way users interact with the system, primarily addressing the issues involved in a user interface design (related to ergonomics).

Impact: Effect of an information resource on health care, usually expressed as changes in the actions or procedures undertaken by health care workers or as outcomes such as patient morbidity and mortality.

Independent variable: In a correlational or experimental study, a variable thought to determine or be associated with the value of the dependent variable (q.v.).

Information resource: Generic term for a computer-based system that seeks to enhance health care by providing patient-specific information directly to care providers (often used equivalently with "system").

Instrument: Technology employed to make a measurement, such as a paper questionnaire. The instrument encodes and embodies the procedures used to determine the presence, absence, or extent of an attribute in an object.

Interval variable: A variable in which meaning can be assigned to the differences between values.

Intervention: In an experimental study (q.v.), the activity or treatment that distinguishes the the study groups.

Judge: Human who, through a process of observation, makes an estimate of the value of an attribute for an object or set of objects.

Knowledge-based system: Class of information resource that provides advice by applying an encoded representation of knowledge within a biomedical domain to the state of a specific patient.

Laboratory study: Study that explores important properties of an information resource in isolation from the clinical setting.

Level: In measurement situations, one of the discrete values a facet can take on. In demonstration studies, one of the discrete values a nominal or ordinal variable can take on.

Measurement study: Study to determine the extent and nature of the errors with which a measurement is made using a specific instrument (cf. Demonstration study) (see Chapters 5 and 6).

Member checking: In subjectivist research, the process of reflecting preliminary findings back to individuals in the setting under study, one way of confirming that the findings are truthful.

Meta-analysis: Method to combine the results of completed studies of the same phenomenon to draw conclusions more powerful than those obtainable from any single study of that phenomenon. (Also refers to a set of statistical techniques for combining quantitative study results across a set of comparable studies.) Basis for systematic reviews or overviews.

Nominal variable: Variable that can take a number of discrete values with natural ordering.

Nonparametric tests: Class of statistical tests that requires few assumptions about the distributions of values of variables in a study (e.g., the data follow a normal distribution).

Null hypothesis: In inferential statistics, the hypothesis that an intervention will have no effect: that there will be no differences between groups and no associations or correlations among variables.

Object (of measurement): Entity on which a measurement is made and to which a measured value of a variable is assigned.

Objective: (1) Noun: state of practice envisioned by the designers of an information resource, usually stated at the outset of the design process. Specific aims of an information resource. (2) Adjective: a property of an observation or measurement such that the outcome is independent of the observer (cf. Subjective).

Objectivist approaches: Class of evaluation approaches that make use of experimental designs and statistical analyses of quantitative data.

Observational study (naturalistic study): Approach to a study design that entails no experimental manipulation. Investigators draw conclusions by carefully observing users of an information resource.

Ordinal variable: Variable that can take a number of discrete values having a natural order.

Outcome variable: Similar to "dependent variable," a variable that captures the end result of a health care or educational process; for example, long-term operative complication rate or mastery of a subject area.

Outcomes: See Impact.

Panel study: Study design in which a fixed sample of respondents provides information about variable at different time periods.

Pilot study: Trial version of a study (often conducted with a small sample) to ensure that all study methods will work as intended or to explore if there is an effect worthy of further study.

Power: Statistical term describing the ability of a study to provide a reliable negative result; if a study design has low power, usually because of small sample size, little credence can be placed in a "negative" result. Power equals one minus the probability of making a type II error.

Practical significance: Difference or effect due to an intervention that is large enough to affect clinical practice. With large sample sizes, small differences can be statistically significant but may not be practically significant, usually because the costs or danger of the intervention do not justify such a small benefit. Similar to "clinical significance."

Precision: In measurement studies, the extent of unsystematic error in the results. High precision implies low error. Similar to Reliability.

Process variable: Variable that measures what is done by health care workers, such as accuracy or diagnosis of number of tests ordered.

Product liability: When a developer or distributor of an information resource is held legally responsible for its effects on patient care decisions, regardless of whether they have taken due care when developing and testing the information resource.

Prospective studies: Studies designed before any data are collected. A cohort study is a kind of prospective study.

Randomized studies: Experimental studies in which all factors that cannot be directly manipulated by the investigator are controlled through random assignment of subjects to groups.

Ratio variable: Continuous variable in which meaning can be assigned to both the differences between values and the ratio of values.

Regression, linear: Statistical technique, fundamentally akin to analysis of variance, in which a continuous dependent variable is modeled as a linear combination of continuous independent variables.

Regression, logistic: Statistical technique in which a dichotomous dependent variable is modeled as an exponential function of a linear combination of continuous or categorical independent variables.

Reliability: Extent to which the results of measurement are consistent (i.e., are free from unsystematic error).

Retrospective studies: Studies in which existing data, often generated for a different purpose, are reanalyzed to explore a question of interest to an investigator. A case–control study is a kind of retrospective study.

ROC analysis: Receiver operating characteristic curve analysis. First used in studies of signal detection, it is typically used with a test that yields a continuous value but is interpreted dichotomously. ROC analysis documents the trade-off between false-positive and false-negative errors across a range of threshold values for the test result.

Sampling strategy: Method for selecting a sample of subjects used in a study. The sampling strategy determines to which population the results of a study can be generalized.

Sensitivity: (1) Performance measure equal to the true positive rate. In an alerting system, for example, the sensitivity is the fraction of cases requiring an alert for which the system actually generated an alert. (2) In system design: the extent to which the output of the system varies in response to changes in the input variables.

Single-blind study: Study in which the subjects are unaware of the treatment groups to which they have been assigned.

Specificity: Performance measure equal to the true negative rate. In a diagnostic system, for example, specificity is the fraction of cases in which a disease is absent and in which the system did not diagnose the disease. Specificity is not defined for an alerting system, as the true negative rate is undefined.

Statistical significance: A difference or statistical effect that, using methods of statistical inference, is unlikely to be due to chance alone.

Subject: In an experimental study, the entities on which independent observations are made. Although persons are often the subjects in informatics studies, systems, groups, or organizations can also be the subjects of studies.

Subjective: Property of observation or measurement such that the outcome depends on the observer (cf. Objective).

Subjective probability: Individual's personal assessment of the probability of the occurrence of an event of interest.

Subjectivist approaches: Class of approaches to evaluation that rely primarily on qualitative data derived from observation, interview, and analysis of documents and other artifacts. Studies under this rubric focus on description and explanation; they tend to evolve rather than be prescribed in advance.

Summative study: Study designed primarily to demonstrate the value of a mature information resource (cf. Formative study).

Tasks: Test cases against which the performance of human subjects or an information resource is studied.

Triangulation: Drawing a conclusion from multiple sources of data that address the same issue. A method used widely in subjectivist research.

Two by two (2 × 2) table: Contingency table (q.v.) in which only two variables, each with two levels, are classified

Validation: (1) In software engineering: the process of determining whether software is having the intended effects (similar to evaluation). (2) In measurement: the process of determining whether an instrument is measuring what it is designed to measure. (See Validity.)

Validity: (1) In experimental designs: internal validity is the extent to which a study is free from design biases that threaten the interpretation of the results; external validity is the extent to which the results of the experiment generalize beyond the setting in which the study was conducted. (2) In measurement: the extent to which a instrument measures what it is intended to measure. Validity is of three basic kinds: content, criterion-related, and construct (see Chapter 4).

Variable: Quantity measured in a study. Variables can be measured at the nominal, ordinal, interval, or ratio levels.

Verification: Process of determining whether software is performing as it was designed to perform (i.e., according to the specification).

Index